LAMINITIS

UNDERSTANDING, CURE, PREVENTION

For all of whom that have led me (back) onto the path of the horse.
For Rajette and Amaghon: "I didn't know better back then".
And, with mixed emotions, for all horses that have been euthanised for scientific research.

Laminitis

understanding, cure, prevention

Remco Sikkel

ISBN 978-94-93034-09-9 (softcover)
ISBN 978-94-93034-08-2 (hardcover)

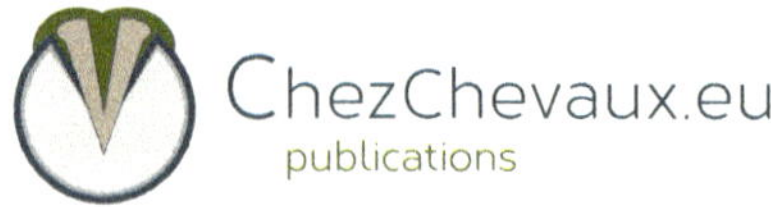

© first Dutch edition 2011, Remco Sikkel, published by Rozhanitsa, Kampen (The Netherlands), ISBN 978-90-79249-26-8
© first English edition 2016, Remco Sikkel, published by ChezChevaux.eu, Clermond-Ferrand (France), ISBN 978-90-825191-1-2

Translation: Heleen Davies
Original title: Hoefbevangenheid : begrijpen, genezen, voorkomen
Photo credits: see page 221

By the same author:
- The Laminitis answer book : over 200 questions answered (ISBN 978-94-93034-10-5)
- The PPID book (ISBN 978-94-93034-20-4)

understandinglaminitis.com
fb.me/understandinglaminitis

This book is not intended as a substitute for the medical advice of veterinarians, hoof care providers or other horse health care specialists. It just provides an overview of the current theories, diagnostic and treatment methods with regard to laminitis. The reader should always consult a veterinarian in matters relating to their horse's health and particularly with respect to any clinical signs that may require diagnosis or medical attention. Neither the author, the publisher, the photographers nor the translator can be held accountable for any resulting damage caused by the application of the information in this book.

TABLE OF CONTENTS

CHAPTERS

INTRODUCTION

HOOF ANATOMY AND HISTOLOGY

DEFINITION

THEORIES AND CAUSES

DIAGNOSIS AND PROGNOSIS

TREATMENT AND PREVENTION

LIVING CONDITIONS

DONKEYS

RESOURCES

APPENDICES

SIDEBARS

PHOTOS

INTRODUCTION

HOOF ANATOMY AND HISTOLOGY

DEFINITION

THEORIES AND CAUSES

DIAGNOSIS AND PROGNOSIS

TREATMENT AND PREVENTION

LIVING CONDITIONS

DONKEYS

FOREWORD

Laminitis. If you own a horse chances are you will be confronted with this disease one day. When it happens (again) and your horse, pony or donkey is unable to move you will feel completely desperate. You will want nothing more but to help.

There is an obvious relationship between laminitis and the unnatural living conditions of the domestic horse. Unfortunately, this relation is often overlooked by many horse owners, veterinarians and hoof care providers. Too often the main focus is on the pathology of the disease. Therapeutic shoeing, box rest, painkillers and anticoagulants are widely used treatments.

The purpose of this book is to convey a broad perspective on what happens in and around the horse's body before and during laminitis. The first chapter places the horse in the context of its long evolutionary history. Hoof anatomy is discussed in the following chapter. The third and fourth chapters describe the disease and the current theories about its causes. Chapter five and six cover diagnosis, treatment and prevention. The seventh chapter fills in more details by focussing on the horse's living conditions. Because donkeys sometimes require a slightly different approach, the eighth and final chapter is devoted to donkeys and laminitis.

This book offers practical solutions and simple preventive measures. The emphasis is on the very important role you have as the horse's owner. In short, after reading this book you will know how to help your beloved horse to recover and remain healthy.

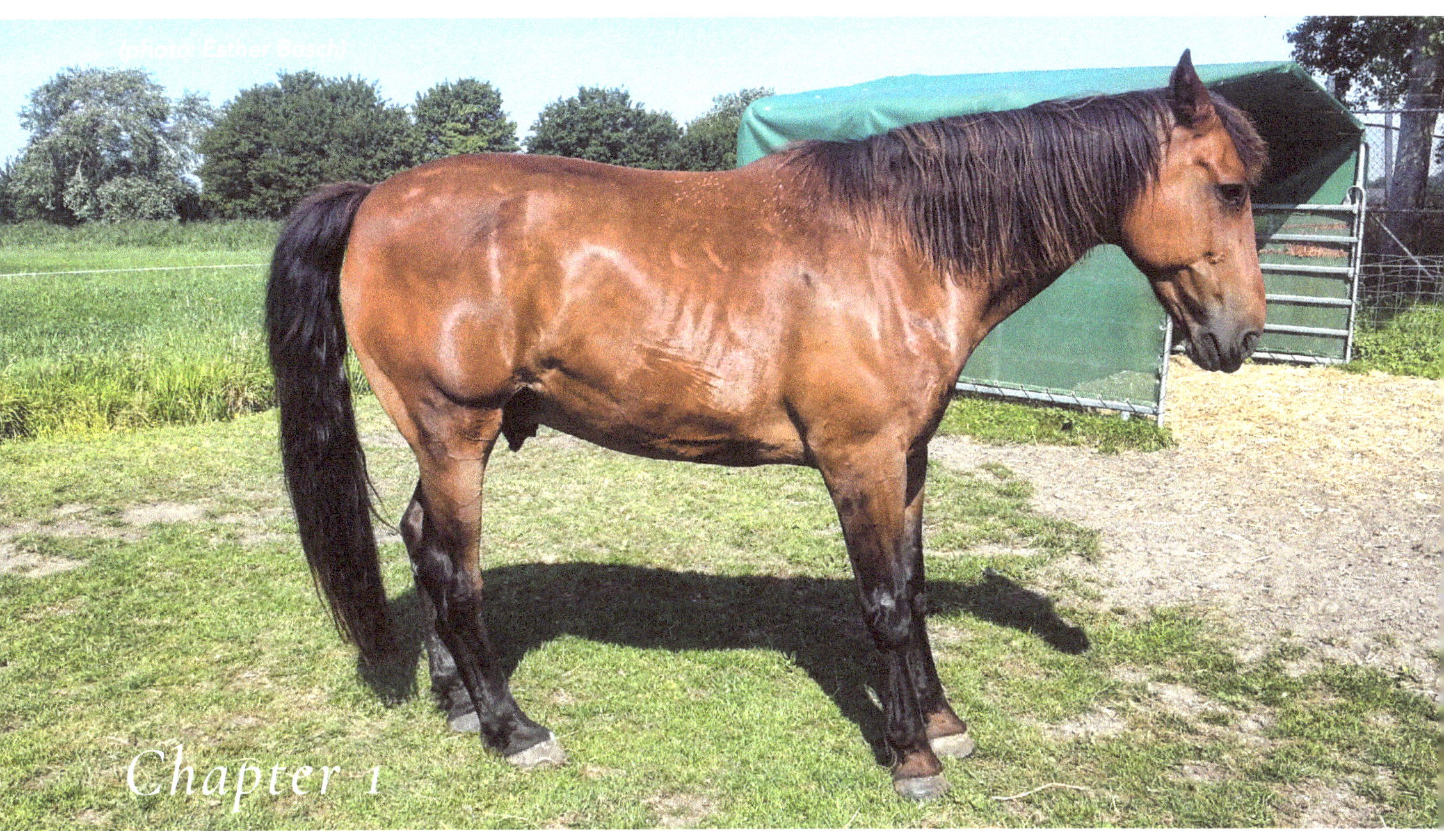
(photo: Esther Boschi)

Chapter 1

INTRODUCTION

In this chapter, we will first determine what laminitis actually is, before delving into all other aspects of laminitis. To do this, we will not only go back in history, but also look at some statistical data in the present time. Finally, we pay attention to the indisputable link between domestication and laminitis.

THE HOOF

About 54 million years ago there lived an animal as big as a fox. This animal, called Eohippus, originally had five toes on all feet, but only used four toes on its front feet and three on its hind feet for walking. In the evolution of the horse the Eohippus was followed by the Mesohippus, that had only three toes on its front feet. The middle toe became longer than the outer two in the Merychippus, that walked the earth between 20 to 10 million years ago. All that remained of the outer toes of its successor the Pliohippus, were two splint bones. A million years ago, the Equus Caballus, our current horse, emerged from the Pliohippus. The full weight of the horse is thus carried by a single toe on each leg: the hoof.

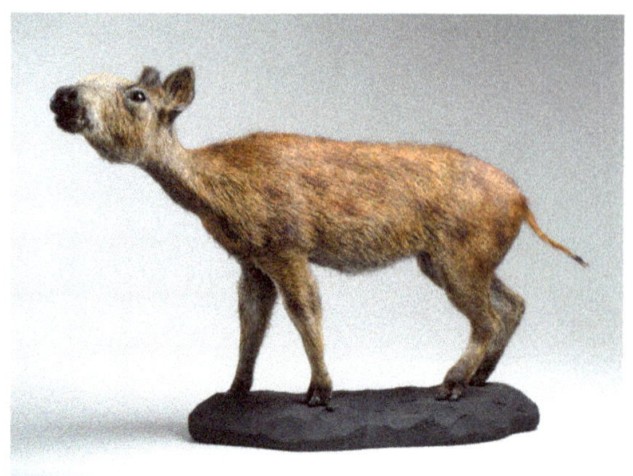

The dawn horse Eohippus
(reconstruction and photo: Museum für Naturkunde, Berlin)

LAMINITIS

Each hoof contains a coffin bone. This bone is equivalent to the last phalanx in our own toes. The coffin bone is attached to the hoof wall by means of an ingenious structure of horn plates and sensitive plates (also called 'lamellae' or 'laminae') that can be compared with extremely strong Velcro. Damage to this structure is called laminitis.

SYMPTOM CONTROL

Laminitis is a complicated condition, many aspects of which are still unknown or misunderstood. Scientific studies are often contradictory. Veterinarians, hoof care providers and nutritionists often strongly disagree about the cause or preferred treatment.

A real understanding of the disease is difficult, which unfortunately creates the large risk that the main focus is on symptom control instead of effective treatment and prevention. Many horses are still bombarded with therapeutic shoeing, anticoagulant and analgesic drugs.

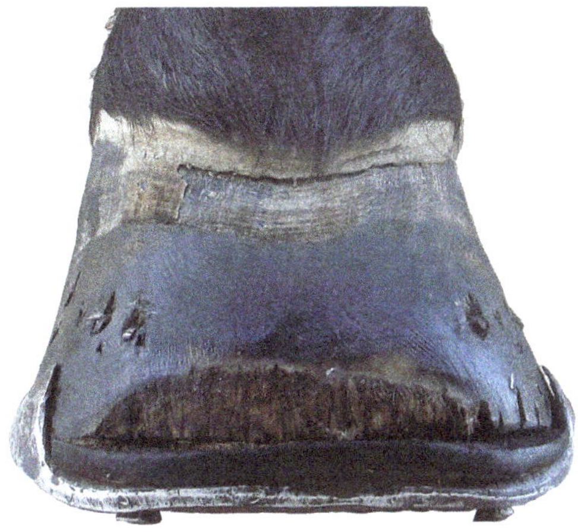

A clear case of symptom control
Shoes with rubber pads

SYSTEMIC DISEASE

Laminitis is not a hoof disease, although laminitis literally means 'infection of the laminae (lamellae)' and the most obvious and severe clinical signs can be found in the hooves. It is a manifestation of problems in one or more parts elsewhere in the horse's body. The intestines, blood vessels and hormonal glands are often involved in the onset of laminitis. Diseases that affect the entire body are called systemic diseases. They are not the result of one single cause, but the effect of multiple factors that influence each other. Often there is an underlying disease, disorder, deficit or surplus that will cause the disease to occur earlier, more frequently or be more severe. It is a misunderstanding of the nature of the ailment that labels laminitis as a hoof disease.

UNNATURAL LIVING CONDITIONS

In the bigger picture, the unnatural living conditions of horses contribute to the onset of laminitis. They cause problems that create the foundation for this disease. Unnatural feeding practices, housing and exercise are especially important factors.

Natural selection

The lack of natural selection as a result of breeding programs and the absence of natural enemies also play a role (see sidebar 'White line separation and evolution' on page 18). The latter is perhaps the only condition we should not change. All other circumstances usually have room for improvement.

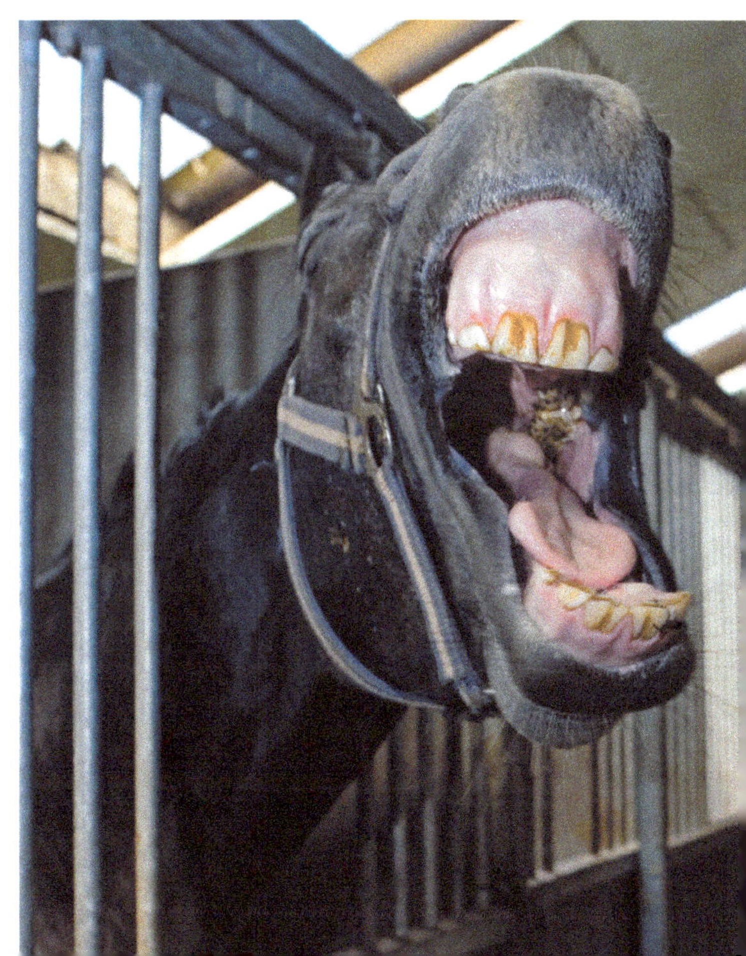

Unnatural living conditions
(photo: Justyna Furmanczyk)

WHITE LINE SEPARATION AND EVOLUTION

The breaking of the lamellar connection is called white line separation. The total rupture of the connection is called a sinker. As soon as there is white line separation or a sinker, movement becomes painful, difficult or even impossible. This is an undesirable situation for a prey animal. From an evolutionary perspective, it is arguable that horses with a low predisposition to developing laminitis have a greater chance of survival and are therefore more likely to reproduce.

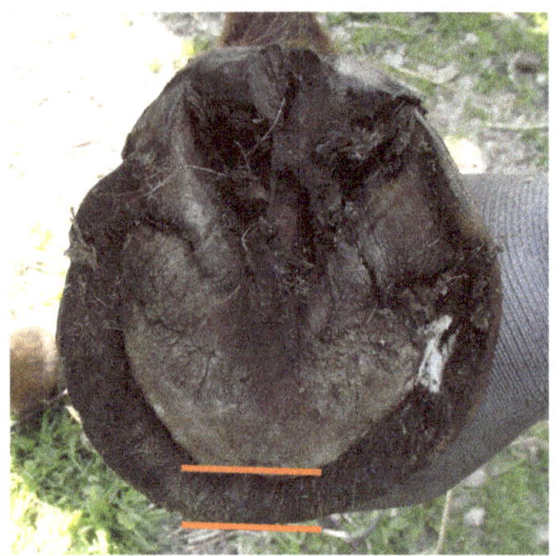

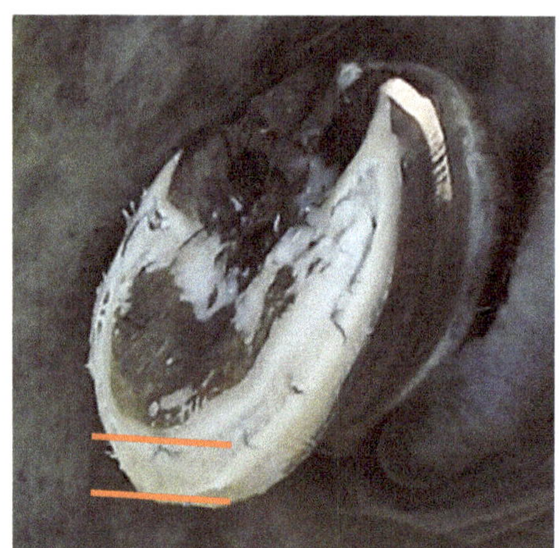

White line seperation

SOME FACTS

HISTORY

References to laminitis dating back to 445 BC can be found in the writings of the Spartan army officer and horseman Xenophon. Even earlier, in 1350 BC the horse trainer Kikkuli describes how the Hittites took care of food and water for their horses in a way that suggests even these ancient people were dealing with laminitic horses. The first unmistakable description of laminitis dates from the early fourth century AD. Acute laminitis is then described by the Greek horse physician Apsyrtus as barley disease. The treatment consisted of diet changes, exercise and bloodletting. Today the first two remedies are still as relevant as 1700 years ago. Up to 1940 bloodletting was still used but since then no longer considered acceptable. Today however, renewed interest in this treatment is on the rise. In the fifth century AD the Roman historian and horse breeder Vegetius Renatus suggested in his veterinary guide castration of stallions when all other treatments were ineffective.

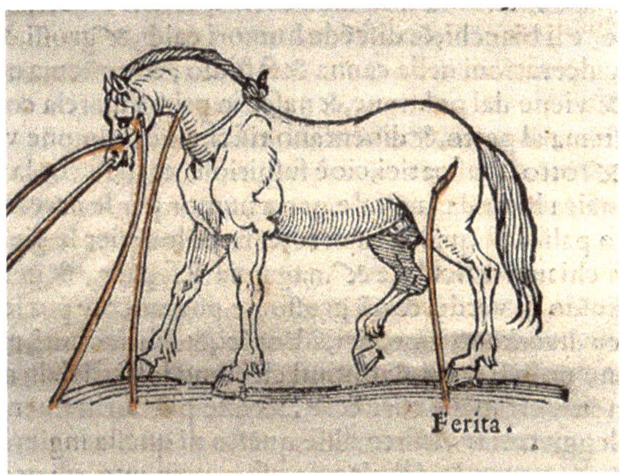

Bloodletting in ancient times

Grass

Only since the 1940s the link between diet and laminitis has been established. However, it is quite possible that around that time changes in the living conditions of the domestic horse contributed to a significant rise of this type of laminitis. For example, grass varieties containing more sugar were being sown in the meadows. In addition, the horse became more of a luxury animal rather than a working animal. He was eating more sugars than before, but his energy requirement was actually lower. Another twenty years later, grass is cited as the culprit in virtually all literature.

FIGURES

- After colic laminitis is the condition that causes most horses to be euthanised.
- Insurance data show that 1 in 20 claims are related to laminitis.
- Approximately 15% of all lameness issues can be traced back to laminitis.
- A 2004 survey showed that according to veterinarians laminitis should be the first ailment to be taken into account for more research.
- In 2010 a large-scale study showed that mares are more susceptible than stallions and geldings.
- Laminitis is relatively common in brood mares. This can be attributed to hormonal changes during pregnancy and lactation as well as to complications such as infection of the udder (mastitis) or lining of the uterus (endometritis) or a bacterial infection after placenta retention.
- Stallions are usually older when they get the disease. On average they are between seven and ten years old as opposed to mares and geldings that are between four and seven years old when they get laminitis for the first time.
- Breeding stallions seem to be more susceptible to developing laminitis. This could be due to their owners' tendency to want to take extremely good care of them. Overfeeding is not uncommon. This increases the risk of hormonal problems, such as EMS/insulin resistance (both disorders will be discussed in detail later in this book). In addition, stallions seem to have a higher tolerance to pain,

especially during the breeding season. This makes it possible that they are already in an advanced stage of laminitis before they show any signs of lameness.

- Ponies have a four times higher risk of developing laminitis than horses, but the effects are usually more severe in horses.
- The number of sunshine hours per month and the occurrence of laminitis are directly related.
- The month of May appears to be the most dangerous month of the year in terms of laminitis.

DOMESTICATION AND LAMINITIS

Wild horses and other wild equids suffer significantly less from laminitis. This seems to indicate a direct relationship between the domestication of horses and laminitis.

The circumstances of most wild horses in relation to nutrition, exercise, environment, social interaction and natural selection are so much better than those of domesticated horses that it is not surprising that laminitis is a typical ailment for our horses or even a lifestyle disease. In the sidebar on the next page you can read about the Kaimanawa horses or how the exception tests the rule.

Wild horses have hardly been subject to evolutionary pressure in regard to laminitis. As a result, recovery from hoof tissue damage in laminitis is relatively slow compared to other types of tissue damage.

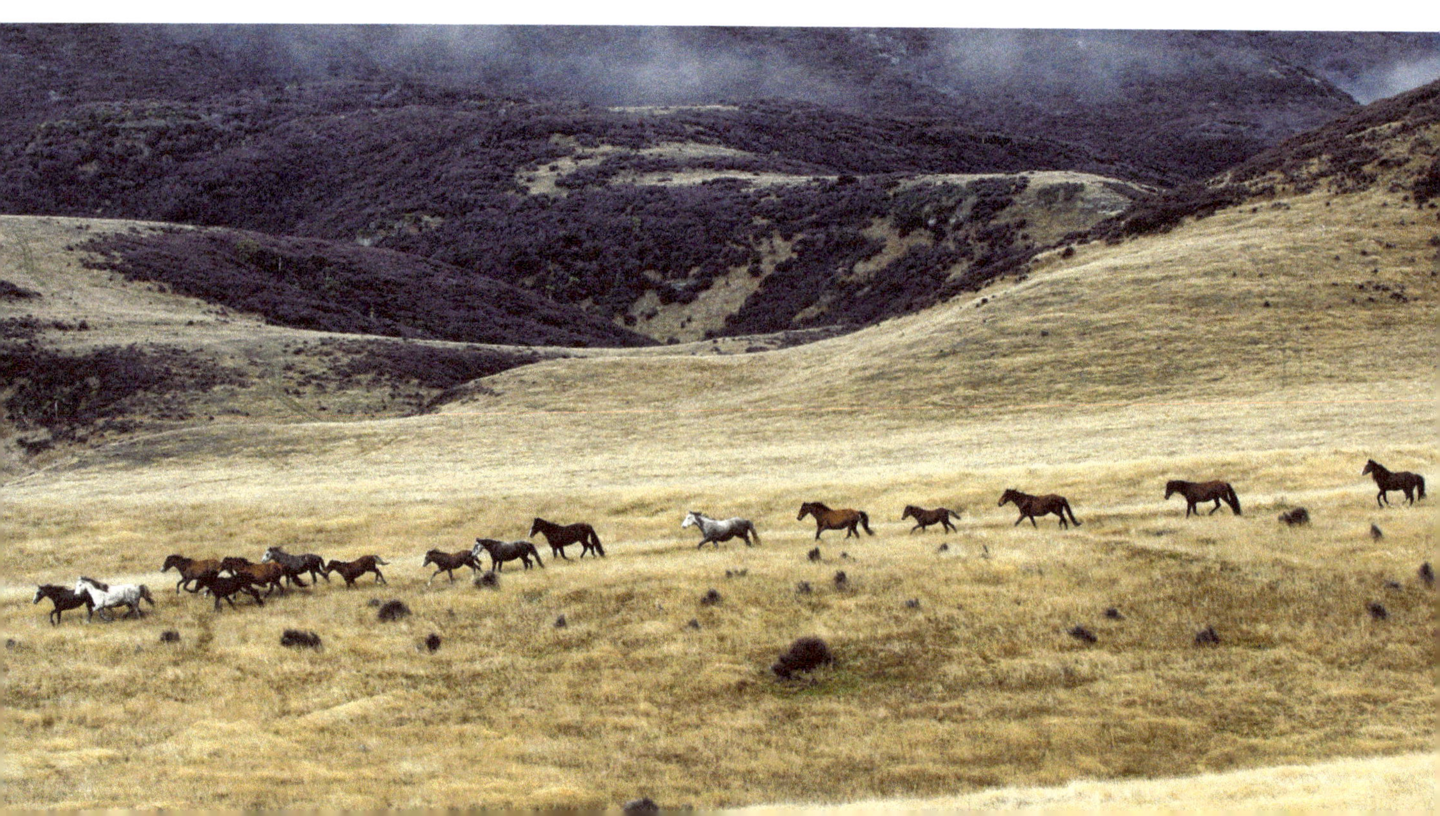

Kaimanawa horses
(photo: Kelly Wilson)

KAIMANAWA HORSES

A study of 56 wild Kaimanawa horses in New Zealand showed many signs of laminitis. Eighteen horses showed the typical laminitic rings in the hoof wall, six horses had bone deformity of at least one coffin bone (ski-tip), two horses had a coffin bone rotation of more than two degrees. White line separation was observed in half of all the horses in this group.

Possible explanations:

- The very soft ground the horses live on.
- Climatic conditions that cause high carbohydrate concentrations in grass and abundant clover growth. Clover provides enhanced nitrogen release and retention. This acts as a natural fertiliser. In addition, clover contains a lot of fructan. More about carbohydrates, nitrogen and fructans later.
- Lack of natural selection because the herds are rounded up for sale and slaughter annually. The horses intended for sale, are usually the better horses with the better feet. They no longer reproduce within the herd. Their good hooves or low predisposition to the development of laminitis are therefore not passed on to any offspring.
- The breed is based on the Welsh and Exmoor ponies brought by immigrants, which both, genetically, have a higher risk of laminitis.

From these explanations you could conclude that domestication is not the major cause in itself. However, disturbance of the natural selection and the narrow base of the breed are also factors of domestication.

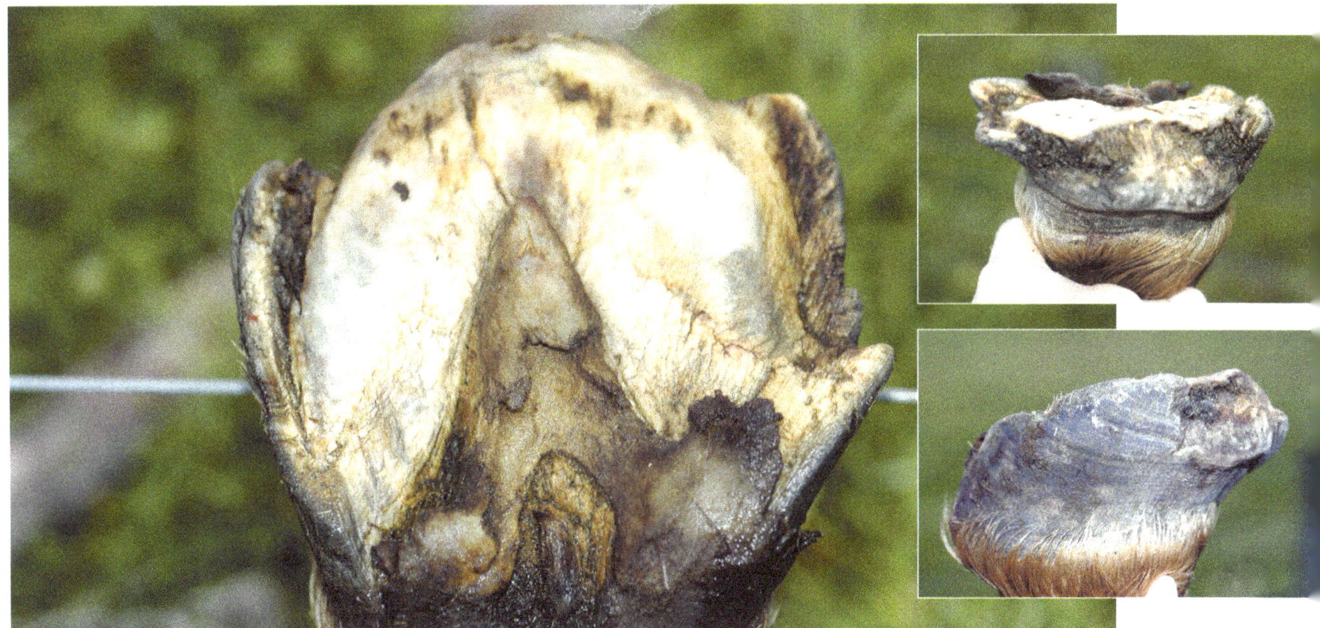

Hooves of a Kaimanawa horse
(photo: Brian Hampson)

(plastinate: Christoph von Horst)

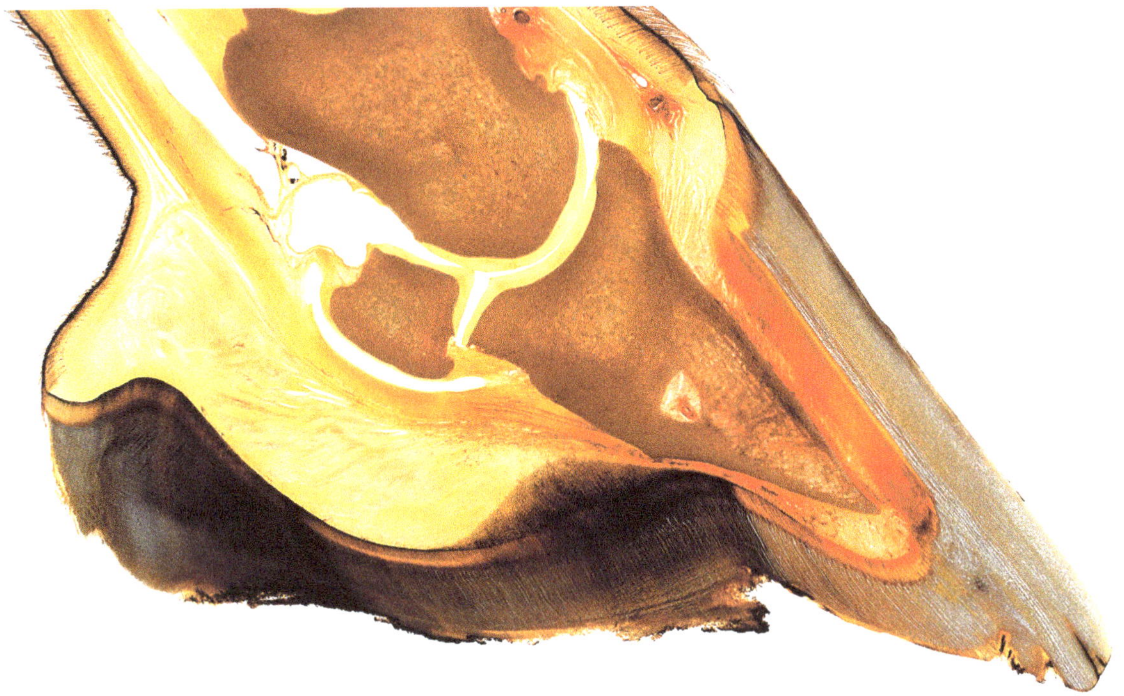

Chapter 2

HOOF ANATOMY AND HISTOLOGY

BEING A PREY ANIMAL THE HORSE IS HIGHLY DEPENDENT ON THE QUALITY OF ITS HOOVES. A HORSE WITH BAD HOOVES CANNOT MOVE WELL AND THEREFORE WILL BE SHORT-LIVED IN THE WILD. HORSE HOOVES HAVE PROVEN TO BE TRUE BIOMECHANICAL MIRACLES OF EVOLUTION.

TO BE ABLE TO UNDERSTAND LAMINITIS IT IS NECESSARY TO KNOW SOME PROPERTIES OF THE HOOF'S STRUCTURE (ANATOMY) AND ITS TISSUES (HISTOLOGY).

Many beautiful books and great DVD's about hoof anatomy and histology are available in which the hoof is described into the smallest details. In this chapter we restrict ourselves to the definitions and properties of the parts of the hoof that are associated with laminitis. Later in this book their function and role in the development of the disease will be discussed in greater depth.

If this chapter contains too much information to take in at once, then use it as reference when you encounter the described parts later in this book. Also study the pictures on the next page carefully.

DEFINITIONS AND PROPERTIES

Looking from the inside of the hoof towards the outside we see:

- Coffin bone and its tendons
- Dermis
- Hoof cartilage
- Digital cushion
- Hoof capsule

Within the hoof capsule we also find a dense network of nerves, blood vessels and capillaries.

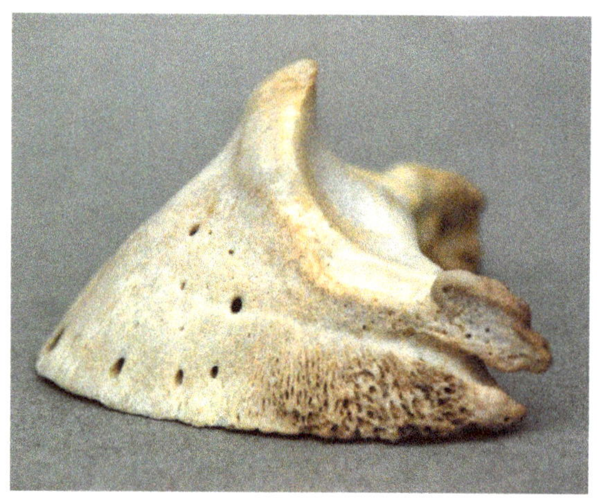

Coffin bone
(photo: Heleen Davies)

COFFIN BONE AND ITS TENDONS

The coffin bone (P3, pedal bone) is the lower bone in the hoof. This bone is similar to the last phalanx in our fingers and toes. Like any other bone it consists of living, active tissue.

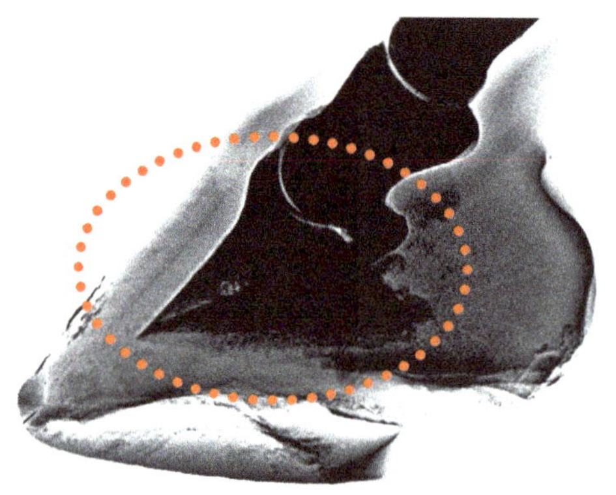

Radiograph of a normal hoof
The coffin bone is encircled
(photo: Alfons Geerts)

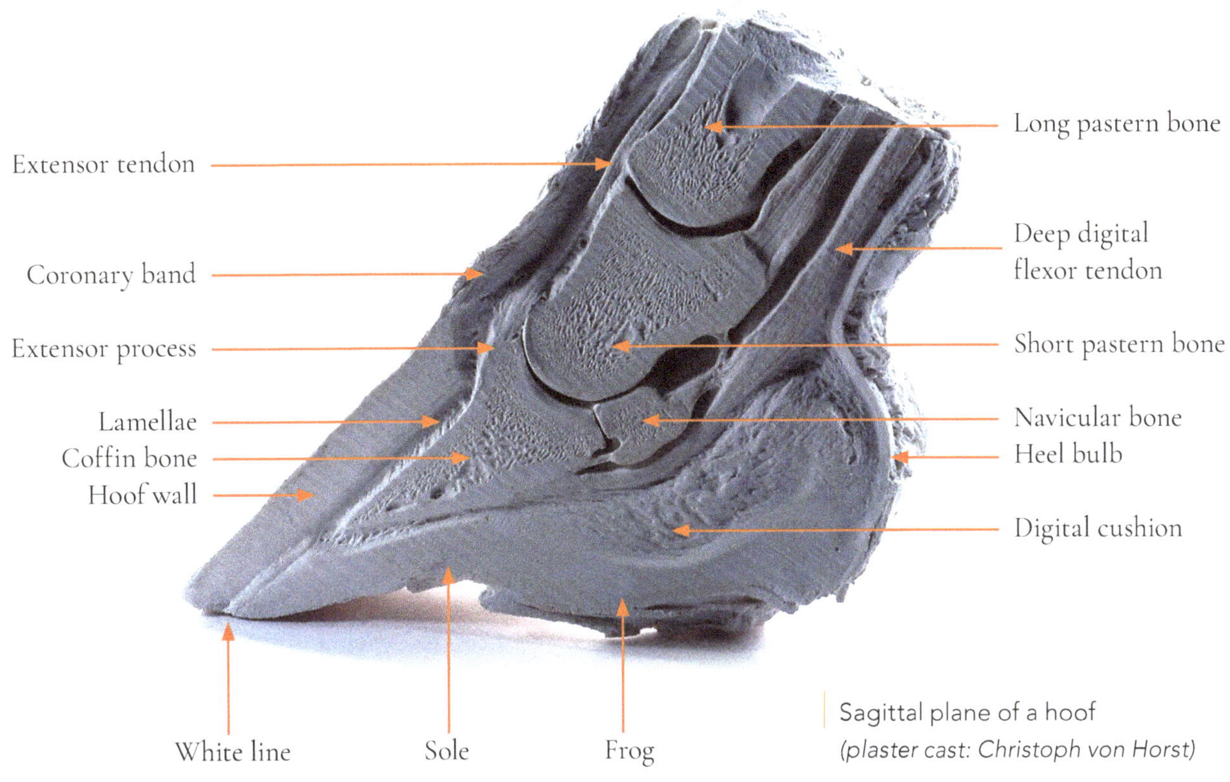

Sagittal plane of a hoof
(plaster cast: Christoph von Horst)

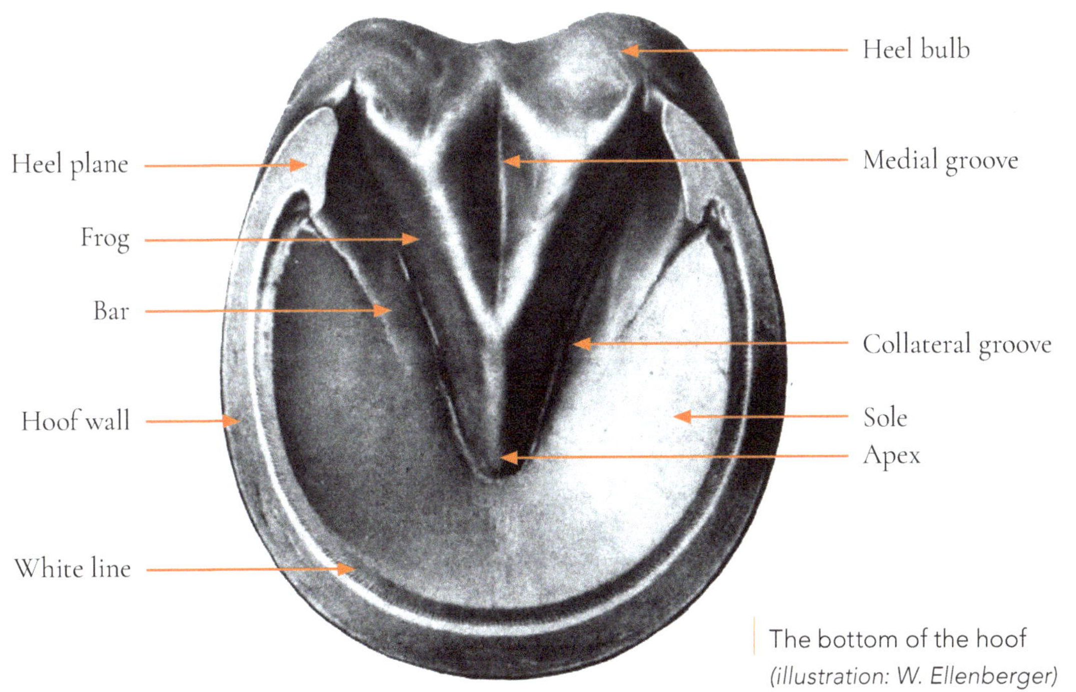

The bottom of the hoof
(illustration: W. Ellenberger)

Deep digital flexor tendon

Tendons connect muscles to bones. The deep digital flexor tendon runs at the back of the leg and is attached underneath the coffin bone. The muscle it is attached to is the deep digital flexor muscle. Together, the muscle and tendon enable the horse to flex the foot backwards. Besides that they generate a basic strength to counterbalance the downward pressure of the body. The white line (that will be discussed later in this chapter) and the extensor tendon provide a strong counterforce to the deep digital flexor tendon.

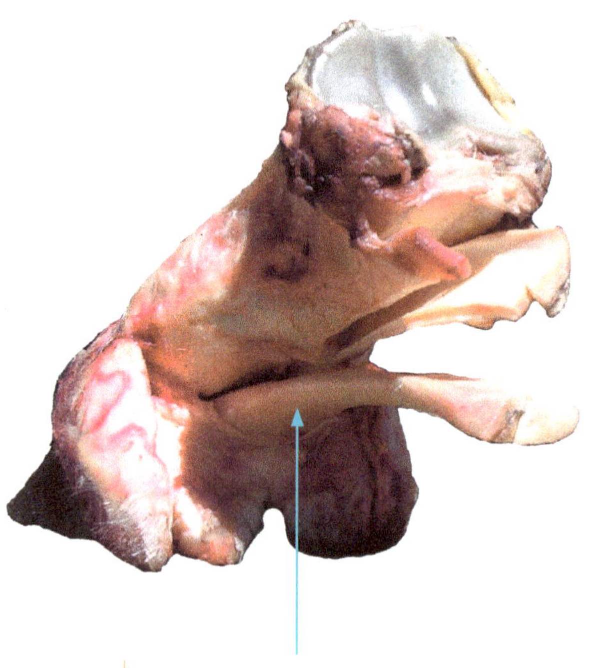

Deep digital flexor tendon
(photo: Cheryl Henderson)

Extensor tendon

The extensor tendon, located at the front of the leg, connects the extensor muscle to the front of the coffin bone. This muscle and tendon enable the horse to stretch the foot forward.

DERMIS

Inside the hoof capsule the whole internal foot is covered with dermis. This is a tendon-like tissue full of arteries, veins, capillaries and nerves. Depending on its location the dermis is called solar, perioplic, wall, coronary, frog, bulbar or bar dermis. These various types of dermis produce different types of horn. For example the frog dermis (sensitive frog) produces frog horn (live frog) and the solar dermis produces sole horn (live sole).

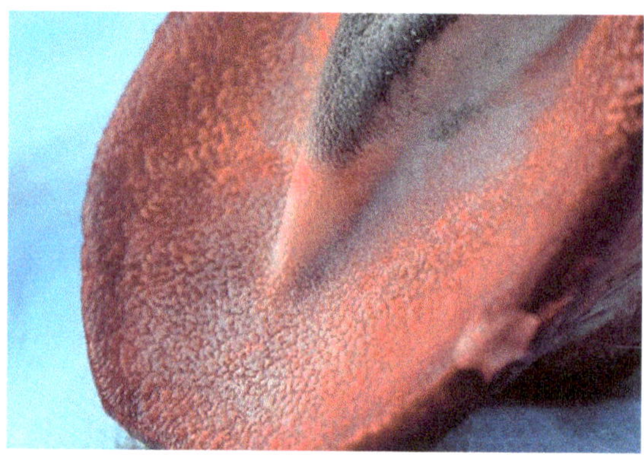

Solar dermis
(photo: Tanja Boeve)

Wall dermis

The wall dermis is (partly) located in between the coffin bone and the hoof wall.

Dermal lamellae

The wall dermis produces primary dermal lamellae (also called sensitive lamellae). The primary dermal lamellae are covered with secondary dermal lamellae.

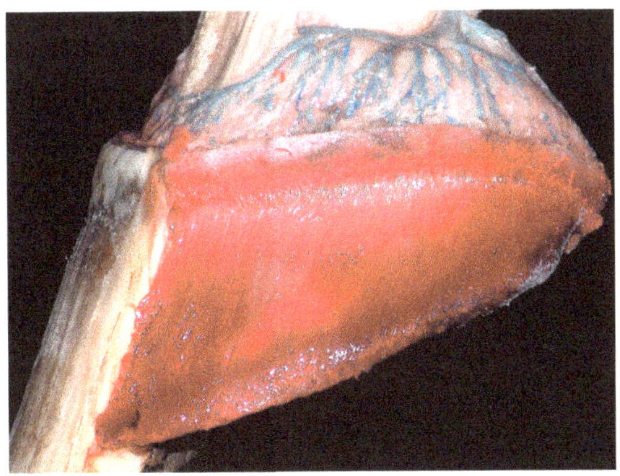

Dermal lamellae
(photo: Hasan Jerbi)

Dermal papillae

Apart from the wall dermis, all other types of hoof dermis are covered with finger-like dermal papillae. They produce new horn cells and provide nutrition to the hoof tissue.

HOOF CARTILAGES

The hoof contains two hoof cartilages, located behind the coffin bone. The coffin bone forms the base of the front half of the hoof, the hoof cartilages give structure to the back half. Because of their resilience the hoof cartilages provide cushioning and flexibility to the foot. The ability to flex is important for the hoof mechanism (see sidebar 'Hoof mechanism' on page 30). Both coffin bone and hoof cartilages are covered with wall dermis and its primary and secondary dermal lamellae.

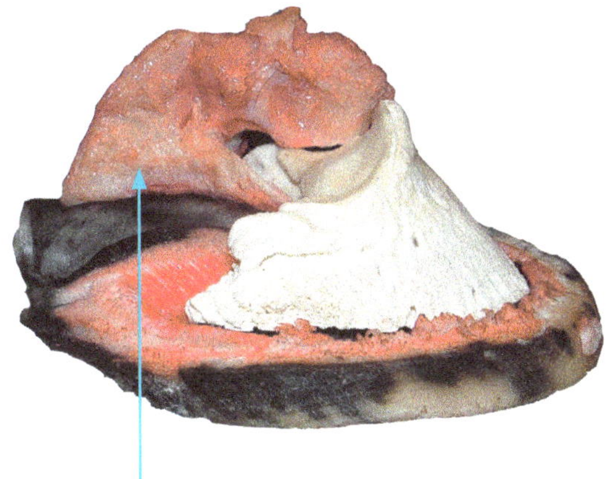

Hoof cartilage
(photo: Cheryl Henderson)

DIGITAL CUSHION

The digital cushion is a wedge-shaped, bulbous, flexible tissue that forms a shock absorber between the sole and the frog below and the tendons, bones and joints above. It consists of collagen, fibrocartilage, fat and glands. A big part of the proprioceptors of the hoof are located in the digital cushion. Proprioceptors are sensory organs that determine where the parts of the body are located. They are very important for locomotion, balance and body awareness.

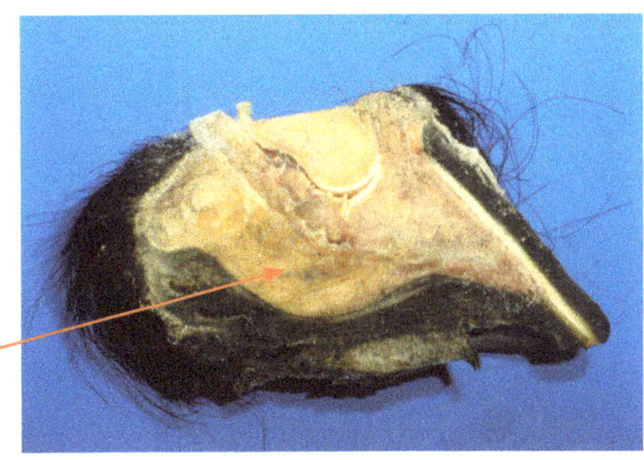

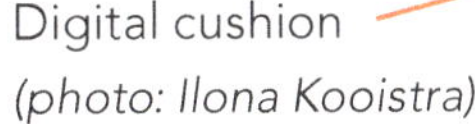

Digital cushion
(photo: Ilona Kooistra)

HOOF CAPSULE

The hoof capsule consists of hoof wall, bars, sole, frog, heel bulbs, white line and perioplic skin.

HOOF WALL

The hoof wall is produced by cell division that takes place in the coronary band and in one part of the lamellae. On the outside the wall consists of tubules and intertubular horn.

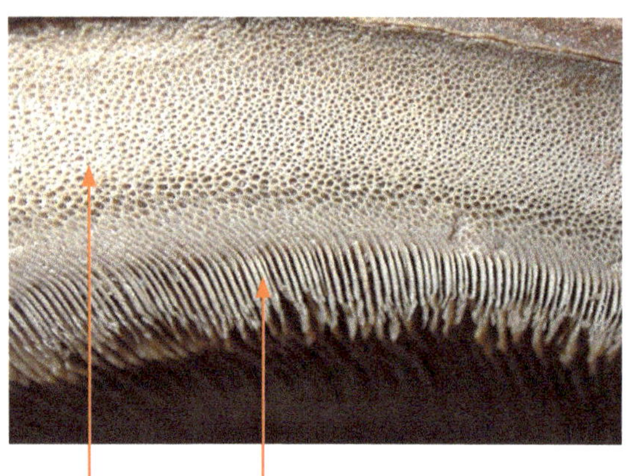

Tubules and epidermal lamellae
(photo: Marion Ryan)

The intertubular keratin mainly gives the hoof wall its strength. Growth rings in the hoof wall can be caused by seasonal changes, food changes, medication, fever, infections or laminitis. In the latter case, they are called laminitic rings.

EPIDERMAL LAMELLAE

On the inside of the hoof wall 550 to 600 primary epidermal lamellae are formed (also referred to as insensitive lamellae). Just like the dermal lamellae each primary epidermal lamella is covered with 150 to 200 secondary epidermal lamellae. The primary and secondary epidermal lamellae hold on to the primary and secondary dermal lamellae. The existence of the secondary lamellae - not present for instance in cattle hooves - enlarges the total surface area. That way a much larger binding surface is created between the epidermal and dermal lamellae. The total surface area of the primary and secondary lamellae of a hoof wall of a standardbred horse is estimated to be approximately 0,8 square meter (8,6 sq ft).

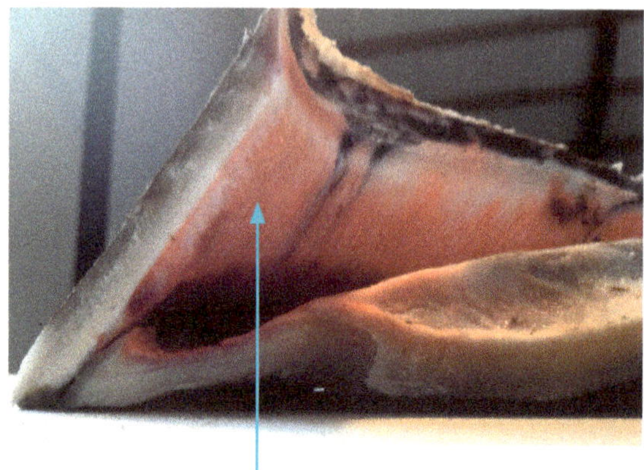

Epidermal lamellae
(photo: Klaas Feuth)

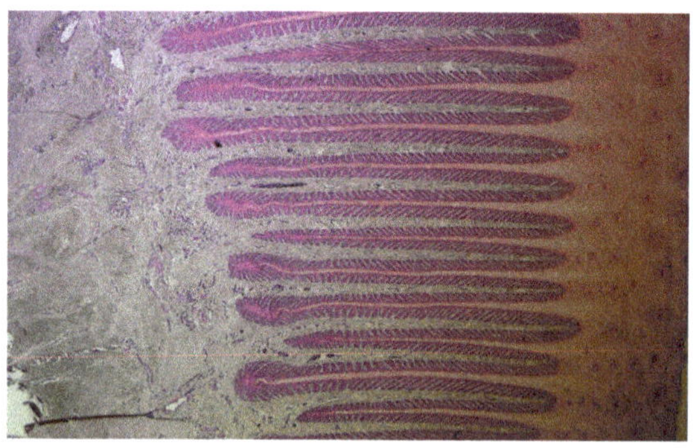

Primary en secondary lamellae
(photo: Brian Hampson)

THE 'SLIDING' HOOF WALL

Hoof wall growth is an amazing process. The hoof wall continues to grow throughout the horse's life without the close connection with the coffin bone suffering from it. The hoof wall slides down over the coffin bone. There are two complementary theories on how this process works:

- The theory of Dr. Chris Pollitt focuses on the connection between hoof wall and coffin bone. Influenced by pro-enzymes the available hemidesmosomes and protein fibres are broken down. This controlled destruction (and the reconstruction that follows) ensures that the connection remains strong while the hoof wall grows down at a cellular level.
- The main focus of Dr. Robert Bowker's theory is on keratinocytes. The secondary epidermal lamellae are made of these horn cells. While they grow out they produce the fibrous protein keratin. A keratinocyte becomes increasingly saturated with keratin. Eventually the cell dies and forms, with many other dead keratinocytes the hoof wall. Because of the death of the cells in the secondary epidermal lamellae their connection with the primary epidermal lamellae is lost. This continuous detachment and the production of keratinocytes enables the hoof wall to grow down.

Renewal of the entire hoof wall takes between eight and fifteen months. The heel is replaced much faster because the hoof is shorter at the back.

BASEMENT MEMBRANE

The basement membrane is located between the secondary dermal lamellae and the secondary epidermal lamellae. This membrane is a connective tissue that attaches the dermal and epidermal lamellae to each other, in the same way as dermis and epidermis are held together in human skin. It is regarded as the most important connection in the structure of the hoof. Besides enabling a firm connection between the lamellae, the basement membrane also has a temperature regulating function and plays a role in the exchange of oxygen and nutrients.

LAMELLAR CONNECTION

The connection between dermal and epidermal lamellae, including the basement membrane, is called the lamellar connection.

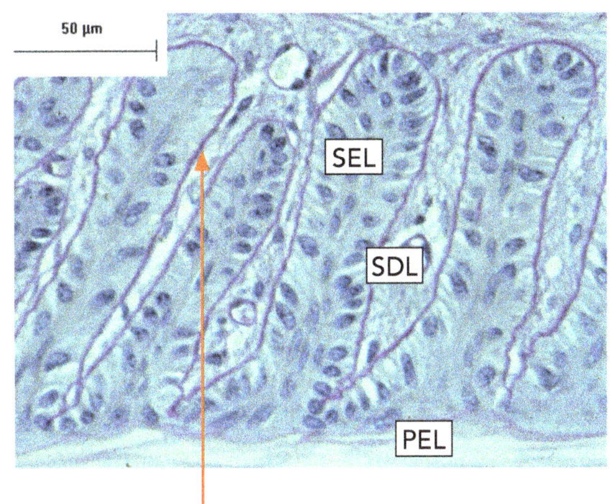

Basement membrane
SEL= secondary epidermal lamella
PEL= primary epidermal lamella
SDL= secondary dermal lamella
(photo: Chris Pollitt)

(continue reading on page 32)

HOOF MECHANISM

Hoof mechanism is the alternate expansion and contraction of the hoof. The expansion occurs when the hoof hits the ground, the contraction as the hoof is lifted of the ground. In the context of laminitis circulation and shock absorption are the key features of the hoof mechanism.

- Circulation
  The expansion and contraction of the hoof creates a pumping action that assists the heart in circulating blood. A well functioning hoof mechanism enables good circulation in the hoof. This ensures the supply of oxygenated blood full of nutrients and hormones and the removal of carbonated blood and waste.

  This cycle is divided into four phases:

  1. The hoof expands when it hits the ground and is loaded by the downward pressure of the horse's weight.
  2. This expansion creates a vacuum that draws oxygenated blood from the arteries of the leg, downwards into the hoof. The vascular system inside the hoof, in the hoof dermis and the cavities of the porous coffin bone, gets filled with blood.
  3. The hoof capsule contracts again once the hoof is gradually unloaded and eventually lifted off the ground.
  4. When the hoof shrinks back to its unloaded shape, carbonated blood is pressed out of the hoof capsule, upwards, via the veins of the leg.

- Shock absorption
  The inertia of blood contributes to the shock absorption. The shock of the landing of the hoof is partially absorbed by the volume of blood inside the hoof. The valves in the superficial coronary, subcoronary, and heel veins also contribute to the shock absorbing function of the blood. This can be compared to the operating principle of hydraulic shock absorbers. As the coffin bone is porous it is capable of containing a large volume of blood. This adds to the total blood mass and increases the shock absorbing ability of the hoof. By simply expanding, the hoof already dissipates energy of the landing of the hoof on the ground. Enabling optimal hoof mechanism will help the laminitic horse to move around as well as possible under its circumstances.

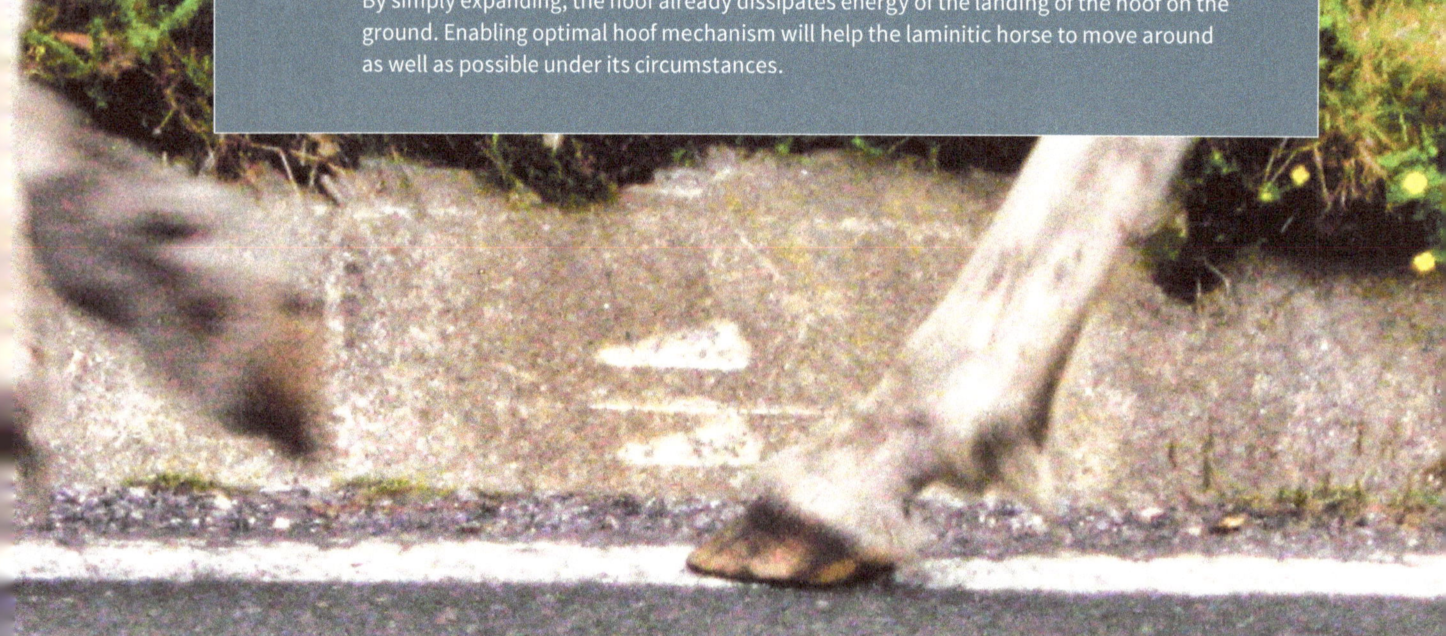

Diagrammatic representation of the hoof mechanism

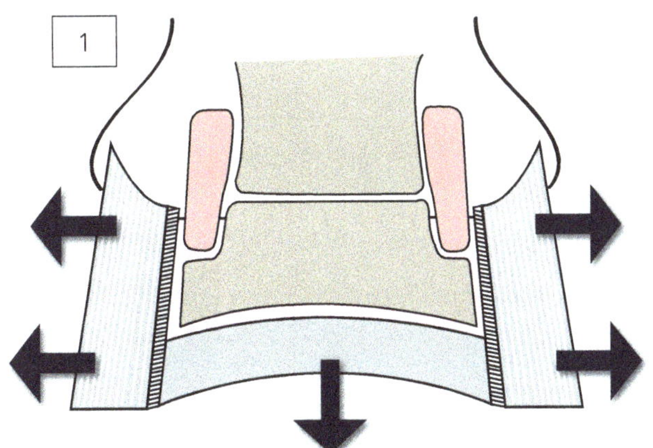

The hoof expands when it hits the ground and is loaded by the downward pressure of the horse's weight.

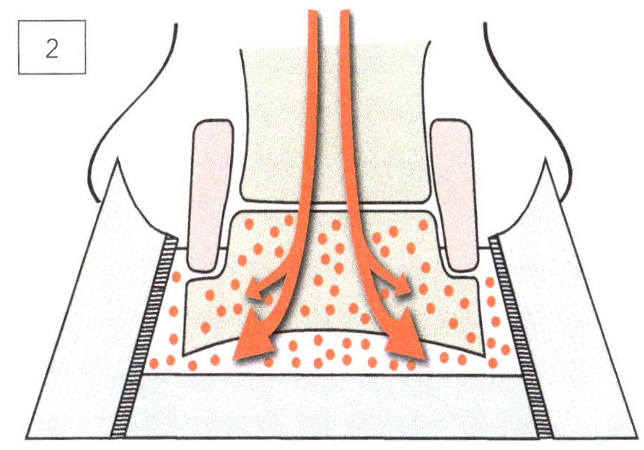

This expansion creates a vacuum that draws oxygenated blood from the arteries of the leg, downwards into the hoof. The vascular system inside the hoof, in the hoof dermis and the cavities of the porous coffin bone, gets filled with blood.

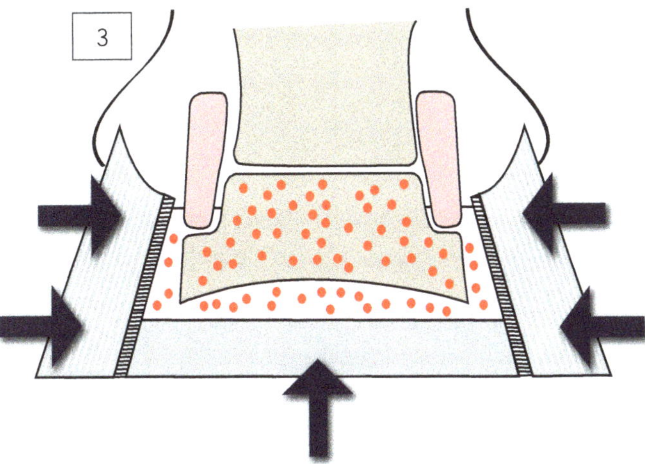

The hoof capsule contracts again once the hoof is gradually unloaded and eventually lifted off the ground.

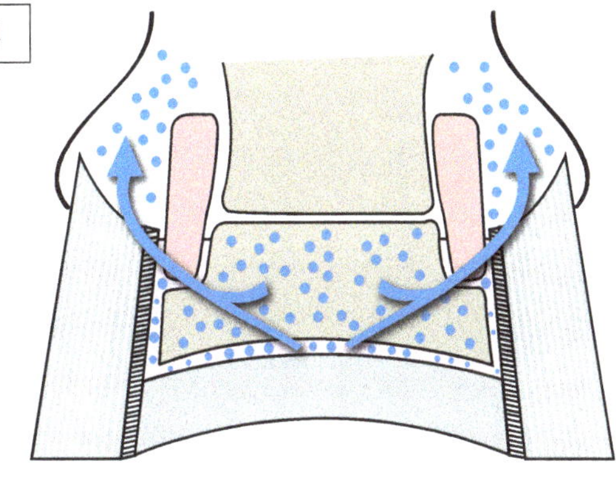

When the hoof shrinks back to its unloaded shape, carbonated blood is pressed out of the hoof capsule, upwards, via the veins of the leg.

FROG CONTACT AND HOOF GROWTH

Ground contact of the frog affects the growth of the hoof. Ground pressure to the frog (and indirectly the underlying digital cushion) contributes significantly to hoof mechanism. Optimum hoof mechanism ensures good circulation in the hoof, providing a constant supply of oxygenated blood and the removal of carbonated blood and waste products. This results in a healthier hoof and improved growth. On the contrary to what many people assume, there is no evidence for the existence of 'growth sensors' in the hoof.

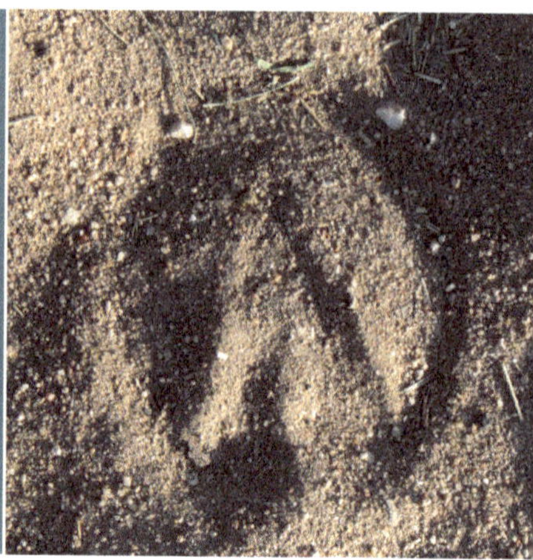

Hemidesmosomes
Hemidesmosomes are protein structures in the cell membrane that enable horn cells to adhere to the basement membrane.

Bars
Bars form the rear part of the hoof capsule. They turn back from the heels into the hoof and run parallel to the collateral grooves.

Sole
Solar horn is produced by the solar dermis. It is quite flexible and provides protection to the coffin bone.

Frog
The frog provides grip to the surface, contributes to shock absorption and plays an essential role in the function of the hoof as a circulatory pump (see sidebar 'Hoof mechanism' on page 30). On either side the frog is bordered by the collateral grooves.

Heel bulbs
The heel bulbs are located where the heels merge into the bulb groove. They also contribute to the shock absorption.

White line
As the growing hoof wall arrives at the level of the sole there are no longer dermal lamellae for the epidermal lamellae to attach to. The connection between the epidermal lamellae of the hoof wall and the sole is formed by a soft type of horn (terminal horn) produced by the terminal papillae that extend from the end of the dermal lamellae. This connection is called white line. At the bottom of the hoof the white line is visible as a yellowish line between the hoof wall and the sole perimeter. This vulnerable part of the hoof is five times weaker than the hoof wall itself. The white line acts as a hinge between hoof wall and sole to facilitate the hoof mechanism.

Perioplic skin
This is an unpigmented, soft epidermis that prevents dehydration of the hoof. The perioplic band, as it is also called, is located just above the coronary band.

NERVES

The hoof contains both sympathetic and sensory nerves. Sensory nerves play an important role in the perception of pain, the sense of touch and the detection of the position of the body parts (the proprioceptors mentioned previously).

HOOF VASCULATURE

The hoof is equipped with a massive vascular system that consists of arteries, arterioles, capillaries, veins, venules and shunts. It runs around and through the coffin bone. It permits the circulation of oxygenated blood, the transport of nutrients, natural chemicals such as hormones and the removal of carbon dioxide and other waste products.

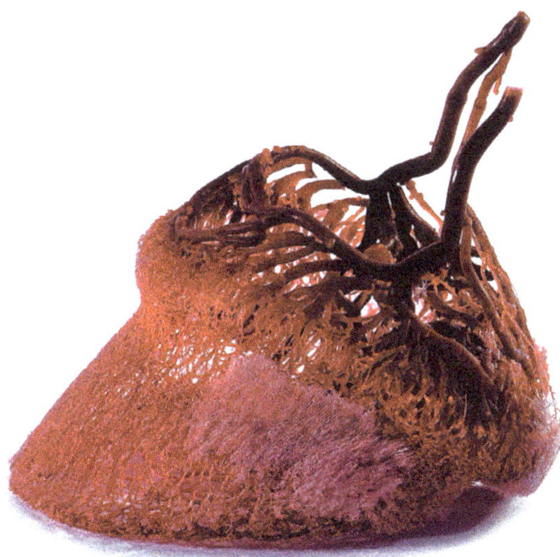

Preparation of the blood vessels of a hoof
Capillaries have been removed, except on the side (preparation: Christoph von Horst)

ANASTOMOSES

Branches of the arteries are interconnected to form 'rings' around the bones. These vascular connections are called anastomoses. Thanks to the aforementioned arterioles, capillaries and these anastomoses, all vascularised parts of the hoof are supplied with blood from different sides. Anastomoses are not to be confused with arteriovenous anastomoses.

ARTERIOVENOUS ANASTOMOSES

Arteriovenous anastomoses (AVA or shunts) are direct connections between arteries and veins. Along these shunts the blood supply to the hoof can be cut short. Shunts are usually closed but open up when the need for temperature regulation occurs. To a certain extent the blood supply to the hoof can be shut down. That way shunts are able to influence the blood pressure inside the hoof. This mechanism is called shunting. It is brought about by smooth muscles which are controlled by the autonomic nervous system.

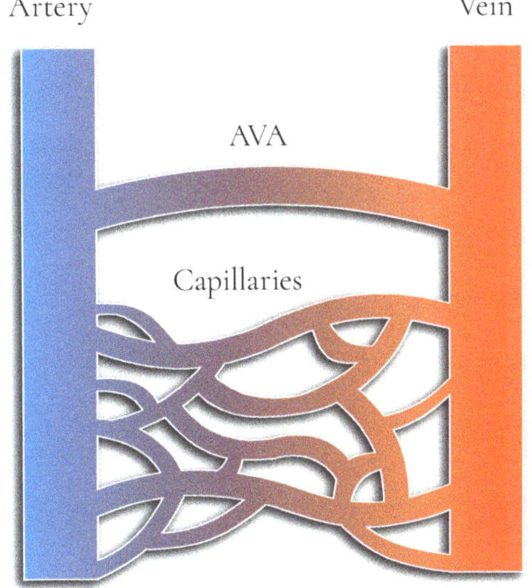

Diagrammatic representation of an arteriovenous anastomosis

SHOCK DISSIPATION AND VIBRATION DAMPING

It is impressive how many different structures of the hoof contribute to shock dissipation and attenuation and vibration damping when the horse's hoof strikes the ground:

- The sole and the soft tissues in the heel region (frog, digital cushion, hoof cartilages and heel bulbs) dissipate a substantial part of the initial forces generated during ground impact.
- Inertia of the blood in the hoof also contributes to shock dissipation and attenuation and vibration damping. The fluid pressure of blood inside the hoof partially reduces the effect of the impact of initial ground contact.
- As the coffin bone is porous it is capable of containing a large volume of blood. This adds to the total blood volume and increases the shock absorbing and vibration damping ability of the hoof. When blood is forced into these blood vessels, the valves in the superficial coronary, subcoronary and heel veins also add to shock absorption. This can be compared to the operating principle of a hydraulic shock absorber.
- The hoof wall acts as a leaf spring. Opening that spring at the back of the hoof takes a lot of energy – energy that will be extracted from the impact with the ground. The hoof wall reduces concussive vertical forces as well by the compression of horn material at ground impact. The more that the hoof wall is compressed, the greater the counteractive compressive stress, and so the greater is the shock absorption. The high moisture content and optimal elasticity of the hoof wall are crucial factors in this.
- Damping takes place at a micro level as well. The wafer-thin layer of articular cartilage in the coffin joint reduces the vibrations. In addition, it ensures an even distribution of pressure on the underlying bone tissue.
- The flexibility and elasticity of the dermis, its dermal lamellae and the subcutaneous connective tissue play a small but important role in vibration damping too.

In a healthy hoof all these structures are in good shape and condition. They work together to minimise any possible damage done to the hoof in the first instance, and therefore to the rest of the horse's body as well.

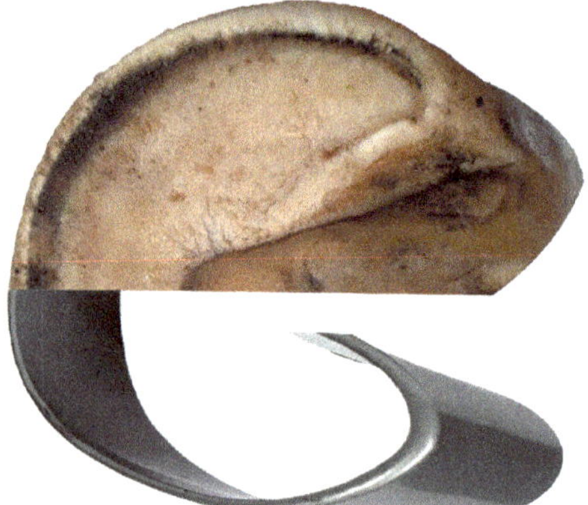

The hoof wall acts as a leaf spring

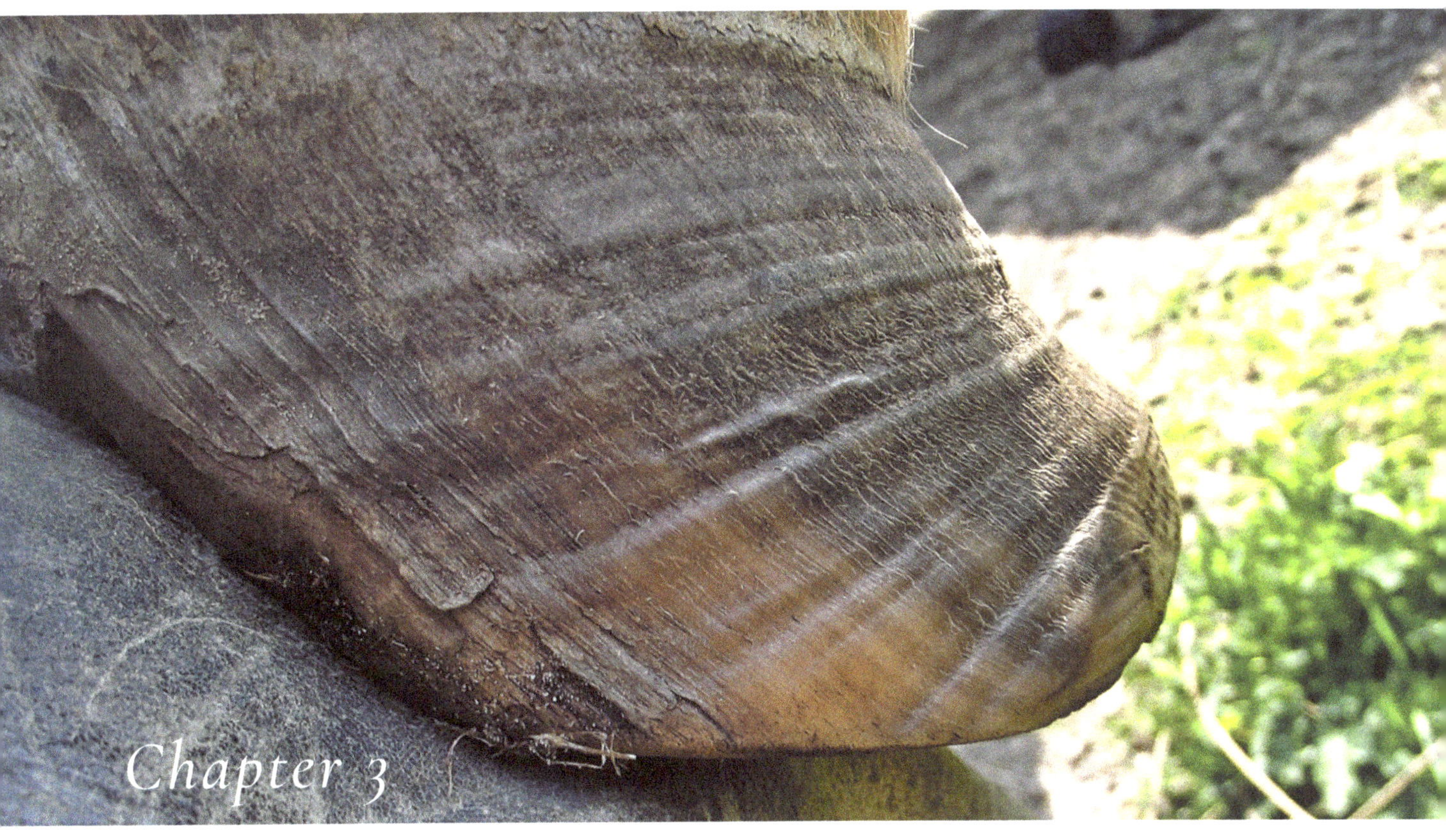

Chapter 3

DEFINITION

Laminitis can be roughly divided into three phases. Each phase has its own clinical signs, which may or may not be immediately visible. The sooner the nature and severity of the disease and its underlying causes are identified, the better the horse's chances of recovery.

This chapter describes the different phases of laminitis. The clinical signs of acute and chronic laminitis are covered extensively. Ahead of what is described in Chapter 5 (diagnosis and prognosis), you will read about the diagnostic options you, your veterinarian and hoof care provider have to establish whether your horse has laminitis and what phase the disease is in.

THE THREE PHASES OF LAMINITIS

Simply said, laminitis is the damage of the connection between hoof wall and coffin bone. This damage does not occur suddenly. It is a development that can be divided into three different phases:

- Developmental phase
- Acute phase
- Chronic phase

In addition to this classification, we find the terms 'subclinical' and 'low-grade' laminitis in veterinary literature.

DEVELOPMENTAL PHASE

The developmental phase starts once the horse has to deal with one of the possible underlying causes. Horses have usually experienced several health issues for a long period of time before the developmental phase sets in. For example, intestines, respiratory, reproductive or digestive systems may have been compromised. But also sudden problems can trigger the onset of laminitis. A classic example is the horse that manages to break into the storage and open the feed bins.

The underlying causes can vary greatly, it can be a single cause or several combined. The sooner and more effectively they are controlled, the greater the chance of cure and the smaller the probability of transitioning into the next phase.

In fact, the word 'underlying' does not do justice to the impact that these causes have on the development of laminitis and the chances of recovery from it. From here onwards we will call them primary causes.

The developmental phase can take between 12 and 48 hours. The lamellae start to detach during this period. This may already have happened after 12 hours. The histological phenomena, such as cell death in the basement membrane, (more about this subject later) already occur after 6 hours.

The difficulty is that by definition horses show no clinical signs of laminitis in this phase so it remains unnoticed. When the first signs of the disease appear, the next phase has already begun.

> Instead of instead of 'symptom', we will use the term 'clinical sign' in this book. The difference lies in the fact that a clinical sign can be determined objectively, while a symptom is a subjective experience of the person suffering from the ailment.

ACUTE PHASE

The acute phase may appear as early as after 12 hours and begins with the first visible or measurable clinical signs. Usually these can be noticed in the front hooves, which does not mean that the hind hooves are not affected.

The primary causes have been present for quite some time. They are now more difficult to identify and control. Basically it is already too late if treatment starts now. This shows how important prevention is. Unfortunately, the first time horse owners are faced with laminitis the disease usually appears completely unexpected.

The acute phase can last between 24 and 72 hours. It ends abruptly when the connection of the lamellae breaks and the coffin bone starts to let go of the hoof wall. The chronic phase has begun.

SUB-ACUTE PHASE

Some horses never enter the chronic phase. Instead they remain in the sub-acute phase. The clinical signs become less severe and the connection of the lamellae remains for the greater part intact. The sub-acute phase, can last for the rest of the horse's life.

CHRONIC PHASE

Once the connection between hoof wall and coffin bone fails and the lamellae let go, the horse enters the chronic phase of the disease. This phase is also called founder. The clinical signs occurring in the hooves can be easily noticed with the naked eye.

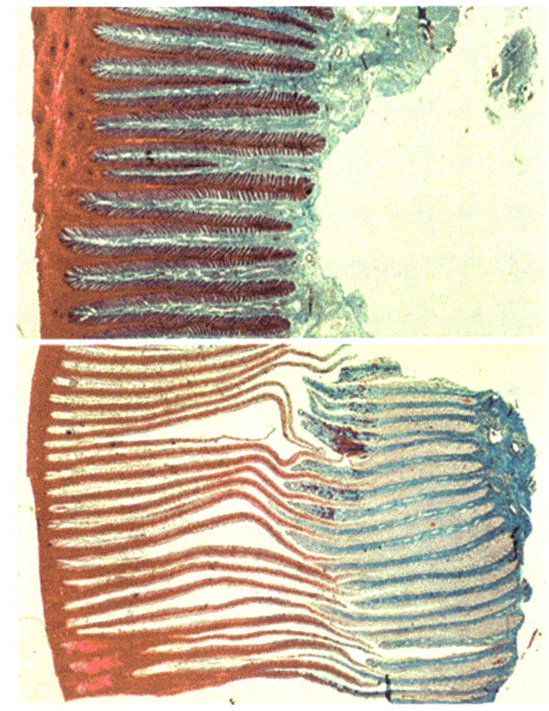

Lamellar disintegration
red=epidermal lamellae
blue=dermal lamellae
(photo: Chris Pollitt)

The horse has to deal with constant pain and lameness. This pain and lameness vary from mild to excruciating. The degree of lameness is indicated by the Obel grading system (see sidebar on the next page).

Later in this phase structural and conformational changes occur in the coffin bone. In extreme cases, the coffin bone penetrates the sole. This is called sole perforation. When the whole connection between dermis and epidermis of the hoof fails, the horse may even lose the entire hoof capsule. This is called hoof sloughing.

THE OBEL GRADING SYSTEM

In 1948 Niles Obel created a classification system for lameness caused by laminitis:

- Obel 0: All movement is without problems.
- Obel 1: Weight shifting from one foot to the other or incessantly lifting of the feet. At the trot a stabbing or shortened stride.
- Obel 2: Stiff movement at a walk. A foot can be lifted off the ground without difficulty.
- Obel 3: Horse moves reluctantly and resists attempts to lift the feet.
- Obel 4: Horse refuses to move.

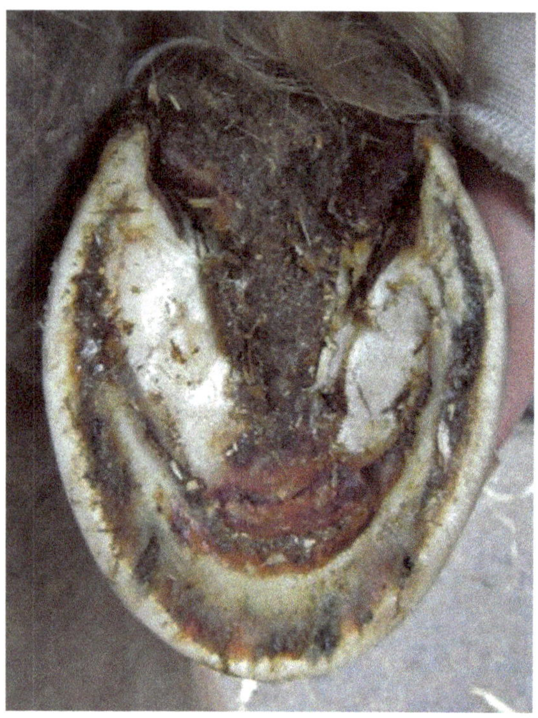

Sole perforation
(photo: Caroline Wang-Andresen)

The primary causes in this phase are also often chronic. Many years of overweight (obesity), PPID (see page 85) or chronic kidney inflammation (nephritis) are good examples of possible primary causes.

The chronic phase is subdivided in a sub-chronic, an active chronic and stable chronic phase:

- Sub-chronic phase: the horse heals completely in a relatively short time (1 to 2 months)
- Active chronic phase: relapse occurs after periods in which improvement is visible
- Stable chronic phase: the coffin bone stabilises, albeit in the rotated position. Hoof wall and sole start to grow again.

The active chronic and stable chronic phase can continue indefinitely. To keep things clear, we combine the three chronic phases usually into one chronic phase.

SUBCLINICAL AND LOW-GRADE LAMINITIS

Subclinical laminitis

A subclinical condition has no recognizable or measurable clinical manifestations. Oddly enough, the term subclinical laminitis is being used here and there to describe clearly visible, diagnosable signs of laminitis, such as a stretched white line, a flaring hoof wall land laminitic rings. These are simply common clinical signs that indicate damage to the lamellar connection.

Actual subclinical laminitis is the situation in which histological changes are taking place, such as cell death in the connective tissue that attaches the dermal and epidermal lamellae to each other (the basement membrane), whilst they are not yet clinically determinable. By definition we are talking here about the developmental phase of laminitis. The subsequent acute phase starts, after all, when the first clinical signs become visible or measurable.

Seasonal condition

Horses with equine metabolic syndrome (EMS, see page 80) are sometimes subject to subclinical laminitis as a seasonal condition. In months when sugar levels of grass are elevated, insulin resistance related to EMS can flare up for them. As a result, histological changes occur in the hoof. The lamellae partly start to detach, without breaking the lamellar connection entirely. The latter even remains for the greater part intact. The transition from the developmental into the acute phase doesn't take place. As soon as sugar levels in the grass decrease or the owner takes the appropriate measures to make sure the horse will eat safely again, the horse recovers.

Living conditions

A non-seasonal change in living conditions can have a negative effect too. An insulin-resistant horse that normally gets a lot of natural movement could stay on the safe side of the line, because of the beneficial effects that this movement has on both blood circulation in the hoof and sugar metabolism. Unfortunately, his laminitis might enter the acute phase if, for example, he is being moved into a place that allows for less natural movement.

Low-grade laminitis

In literature, we come across the term low-grade laminitis. Its definition includes the occurrence of inflammation of the dermal lamellae and/or the solar dermis. These are clinical signs, which define that the disease is in its acute phase. This makes low-grade laminitis a slightly broader definition than subclinical laminitis.

Lameness

To distinguish subclinical from clinical laminitis, the level of lameness is sometimes used as a discriminating factor. The line is drawn between Obel 0, when all movement is without problems and Obel 1, when the first signs of lameness show. This is a disputable distinction. There are plenty of horses whose hooves show a substantially stretched white line, that trot on, seemingly unaffected by their damaged hooves. Even more unsystematic is the distinction between 'sensitive', 'sore' and 'lame'. Numerous horses that are always tender-footed on hard surfaces can thus get the predicate 'low-grade laminitic'. However, their hooves often have a damaged lamellar connection, flares, maybe inflamed dermal lamellae and solar dermis. Nothing low-grade here, as these horses are laminitic. Period.

Red flag

Both terms 'subclinical laminitis' and 'low-grade laminitis' describe the initial stage of laminitis, whilst adequate terminology already exists (developmental and acute phase). However, we should not reject these terms. Their usefulness lies in the cautionary character they have. Hearing the words 'subclinical' and 'low-grade' should raise a red flag right away. No one would want the disease to develop into 'clinical' or 'high-grade'.

Whichever name you wield, there is room for improvement if you recognise the hooves of your horse in what you have just read here. Search for improvement in regards to nutrition, housing, movement and/or hoof care. Don't accept almost-perfect hooves. Go for hooves that are fit as a fiddle. In the chapters 'Treatment and prevention' and 'Living conditions' you can read how to do this.

LAMINITIS OR FOUNDER OR ... ?

The terms laminitis and founder are often used as synonyms, however there is a difference between the two. The suffix -itis always refers to inflammation or infection. In this (etymological) case, an inflammation of the dermal lamellae during the acute phase of the disease. In the chronic phase, once the connection of the lamellae becomes so damaged that the coffin bone starts to rotate or sink into the hoof capsule, the disease is called founder. Founder is an old shipping term used to describe a sinking ship.

Some comments about this nomenclature:

- In relation to the word laminitis it should be noted too much attention is drawn to the aspect of the inflammation. Nowadays the inflammation is regarded rather as a clinical sign or complication than as a cause.
- In addition, it is easy to lose sight of the rest of the hoof when we focus too much on the lamellar connection. In the case of hoof sloughing for example, the sole detaches from the coffin bone as well, while it is not connected by means of a lamellar structure.
- The word founder focuses entirely on the position of the coffin bone and places the other characteristics of the chronic phase to the background.
- By using two different terms it is easy to forget they indicate subsequent phases of the same systemic disease.
- Both words emphasise entirely on the hoof, which is highly debatable in case of a systemic disease. Who knows, the aforementioned Apsyrtus might have been closer to the reality calling it barley disease.

CLINICAL SIGNS

Clinical signs are manifestations of the disease that can be observed by a horse owner, veterinarian or hoof care provider. This means signs can be seen (e.g. black spots on the sole), felt (pulsations at the back of the pastern), counted (increased respiratory rate) or measured (hoof temperature). Sometimes aids are used like radiographs or hoof testers.

The nature and severity of the clinical signs are indications of how badly the horse is affected. Improvement or deterioration of these signs should therefore be monitored carefully. For many of the clinical signs described below it is important to know that what you are observing is different from what it should be when your horse is healthy. Only then it is possible to compare. For example, to feel whether the pulse is higher than usual, it is important to know what the normal pulse feels like. Therefore observe your horse when it is in good health to become familiar with normal values. If you are reading this while your horse already has laminitis you can compare your observations with healthy horses around you.

ACUTE PHASE

Clinical signs of acute laminitis can be divided into:

- Physiological characteristics
- State of the hooves
- Abnormal stance of the horse
- Abnormal movement of the horse
- Abnormal behaviour of the horse
- Characteristics only visible on radiographs

Physiological characteristics

- Strong pulse with an increased frequency (80-120 beats per minute)
  - The pulse is felt in the two digital arteries that are present on each side of the canon bone, on the side of the hoof and near the fetlock.

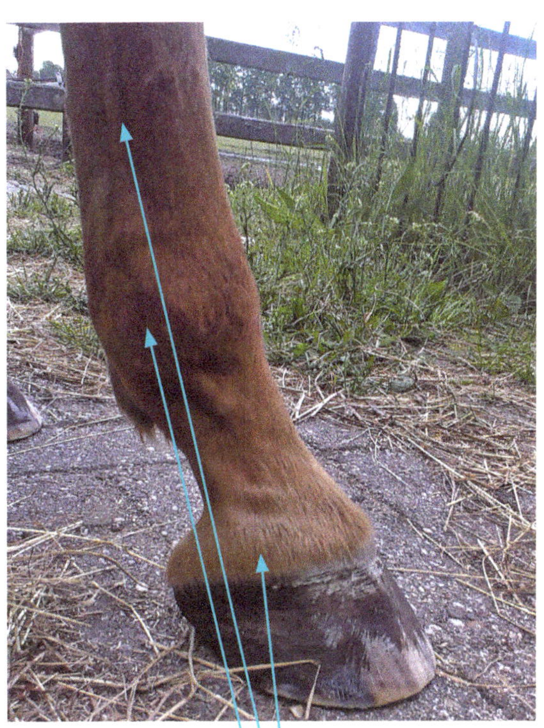

Location of the arteries where the pulse can easily be felt

  - Check the pulse in all four legs.
  - Just an increased pulse is no reason to panic. A horse can have this, among other things, due to work on a hard surface, excitement or a hoof abscess.

Any fluid retention in the leg (oedema) can make it more difficult to detect the pulse.
    - The occurrence of a strong pulse coincides more or less with the beginning of the damage to the lamellar connection.
- Muscle tremors and increased muscle tension
- Sweating
- Signs of dehydration. Pinching a fold of the skin gives an indication of the degree of dehydration. Upon release, the skin should pop back flat within two seconds. This test is certainly not exact. Your veterinarian can determine dehydration accurately with a blood test.

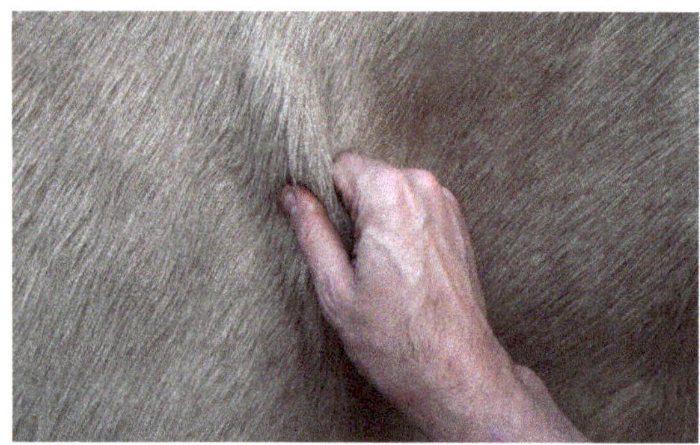

Checking for dehydration

- Dilated pupils
- Excessive blood flow to the eye mucosa
- Widened nostrils
- Ears stiffly turned backwards
- Increased respiratory rate (80-100 breaths per minute)
    - Breathing can be irregular and erratic.
    - Age, high ambient temperature, stress and pregnancy can increase the respiratory rate. Keep this in mind.
- Increase in body temperature to 40-41 °C (104-106 °F).

State of the hooves

- Increased hoof temperature
    - This may be a result of an inflammation of the dermal lamellae or an increased blood flow to the hooves.
    - The hoof temperature can be measured with a laser thermometer. A high ambient temperature makes readings less accurate.
    - Infrared thermography can show the presence of a hoof abscess or laminitis. To establish the difference, the skill and insight of an experienced thermographic photographer are required.
    - Throughout the day the temperature of a laminitic hoof rises and falls. A thermographic image can therefore show a distortion of reality when it is taken at a moment the hoof had a relatively low temperature.
    - A hoof temperature that remains over 30 °C (86 °F) for 24 hours is a clear indication of laminitis.

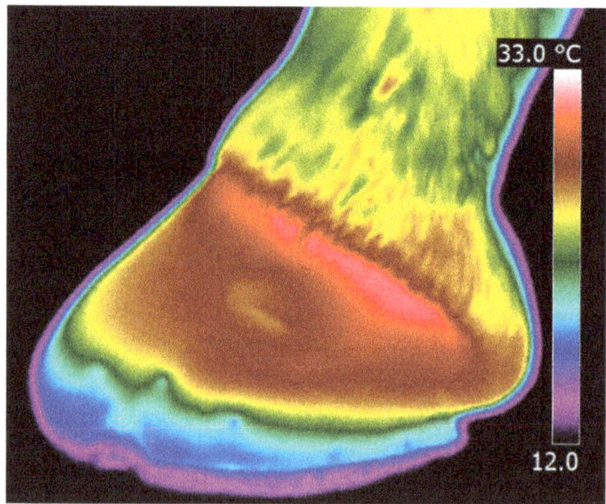

A 30 °C (86 °F) hoof temperature in acute laminitis
(photo: Helen Morrell)

- Sometimes a slightly stretched white line can already be seen. The lamellar connection has deteriorated, but has not yet been torn.

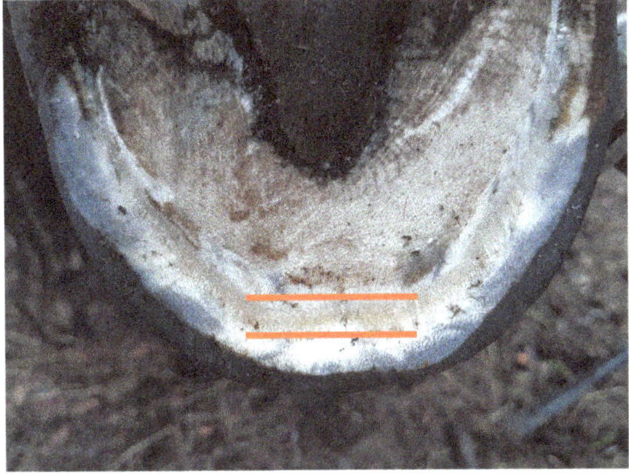

Stretched white line

- One or more abscesses. Necrotic tissue cannot be excreted from the body in the usual way, because of the reduced circulation. It accumulates and causes these abscesses.

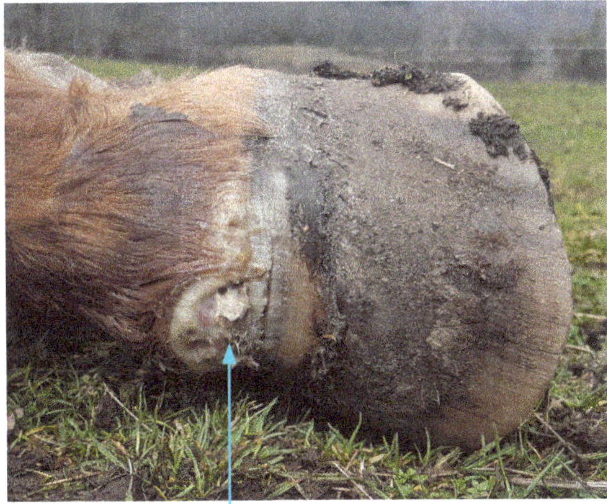

Coronary band abscess

> Many clinical signs are only or mainly visible in the front legs. This certainly does not mean that the hind hooves are not affected. The horse carries, at a standstill and in walk, about 65% of its weight on the forehand. As a result, the acute pain in the front hooves is more evident. The horse uses the hindquarters to push himself forward. This causes a much better functioning hoof mechanism, especially in canter, and therefore healthier hind hooves.

> The physiological characteristics described here are not constant and all present in the acute phase. For example, a strong pulse can come and go. Its absence is certainly no guarantee that there is no laminitis.

Abnormal stance of the horse

- Reluctant to move
- Leaning backwards
  - The hoof wall exerts leverage on the front of the hoof, the toe. In case of laminitis this is painful because the lamellae are inflamed and very sensitive. The horse tries to avoid weighting the front of his hooves by leaning backwards. This leaning backwards is also called laminitic stance.

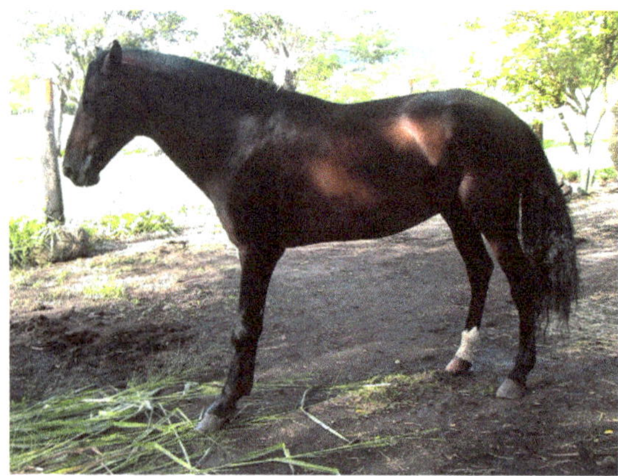

Laminitic stance
(photo: Advanced equine therapies)

- The laminitic stance gets worse when laminitis is more severe or when the horse stands on a harder surface.
- When laminitis is present in all four feet the laminitic stance is no longer possible or else the horse would fall backwards. The horse will then try to spare his hooves by placing all four feet close together under its belly. Some horses place their feet in a normal position again.

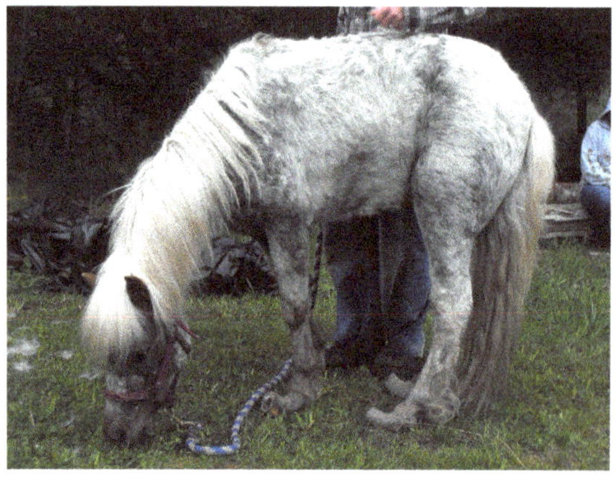

Four feet laminitic stance
(photo: Rose Kingery-Potter)

- Shifting of weight
  - Sometimes the feet are alternately lifted. This promotes the hoof mechanism and provides a moment's relief for one foot at the time.
  - This rhythmic motion is also considered distractive or even meditative behaviour. Also humans in considerable pain, can sometimes be seen doing this.
  - The intervals between the lifting of the feet is an indicator of the degree of pain experienced by the horse.
  - In rare cases, only the hind hooves are affected. The horse will then rock onto the hind legs, putting his front legs under the chest as far as possible while reaching forward with the head to stay in balance.
- Refusal to stand up. A horse that no longer wants to stand up often has laminitis in all four hooves.

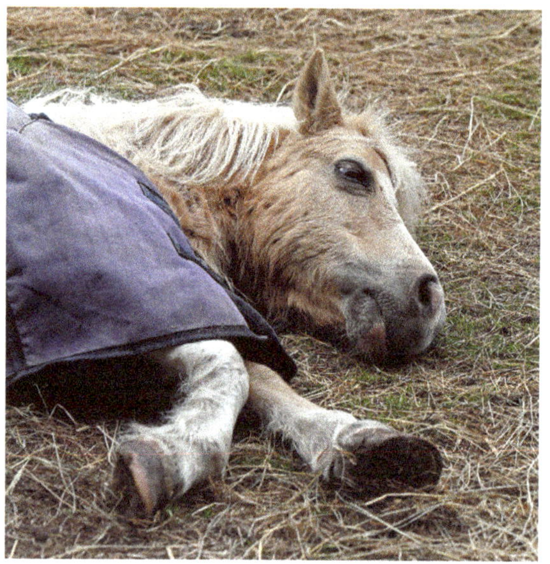

Refusal to stand up
(photo: Cathy Dee)

- Resuming the normal posture. Sometimes the horse become so desensitised to the pain that it stops leaning backwards, swaying, rocking or lying down. In case it gets this far, other signs will definitely be so clear you will know your horse has not made a full recovery.

ABNORMAL MOVEMENT OF THE HORSE

- The horse's movement is stiff and reluctant.
- The horse places the feet out in front of the body as far as possible trying to carry as little weight as possible on the toe.
- The horse tries to avoid turning. While turning more weight is carried by the leg on the inside of the turn. Furthermore the painful tissues inside the hoof are twisted when the horse turns.
- Strange quick steps with the front legs while the hind legs are lifted excessively high. This indicates all four feet are affected. By walking this way the horse tries not to break over the front of the hoof.
- Obviously when the horse is made to move on hard surfaces it will experience more discomfort.

ABNORMAL BEHAVIOUR OF THE HORSE

A horse in pain often shows one or more of the following behaviours:

- Irritable
- Anxious
- Withdrawn
- Tired
- Groaning or moaning

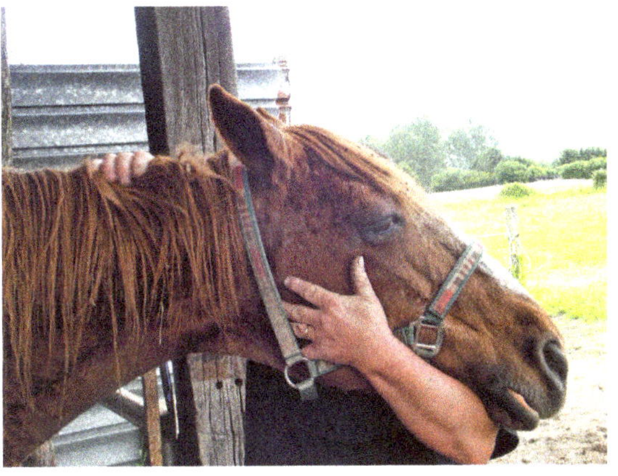

A horse in severe pain

CHARACTERISTICS ONLY VISIBLE ON RADIOGRAPHS

- White line separation.
    - Initially just an increase in the distance between the coffin bone and the hoof wall can be seen, while still remaining parallel.
    - Coffin bone rotation, which happens in chronic laminitis cases (more below), can occur together with the prolapse of the coffin bone (sinker). It is sometimes difficult to determine the extent to which these two phenomena occur with just one radiograph.
    - Bleeding
    - Swelling of the dermal lamellae
    - Oedema
    - White lines in the radiograph indicate the presence of gas in the space between the epidermal lamellae which were previously filled with dermal lamellae. This gas is nitrogen that is extracted from the blood by the resulting vacuum.

- Slight bone remodelling, in particular an excessive formation of bone tissue of the coffin bone.
- Sometimes demineralisation of the coffin bone can be seen.
- Early stages of coffin bone infection (osteomyelitis).

CHRONIC PHASE

In chronic laminitis, one, more or even all clinical signs of acute laminitis are present. Typically we see:

- Impairment of the normal anatomy of the hoof
- Abnormal stance
- Abnormal movement
- Characteristics only visible on radiographs

IMPAIRMENT OF THE NORMAL ANATOMY OF THE HOOF

This deterioration is visible in:

- The relation between the position of the coffin bone and the hoof wall
- The shape and condition of the coffin bone
- The shape and condition of the sole
- The shape and condition of the hoof wall

THE RELATION BETWEEN THE POSITION OF THE COFFIN BONE AND THE HOOF WALL

It is possible to look at the position of the coffin bone in relation to the hoof wall or vice versa. The commonly used term 'coffin bone rotation' can be debated. Essentially the angle between coffin bone and hoof wall has changed. In this book the term (coffin bone) rotation is used for convenience while (partial) hoof wall separation or something similar would probably be a better description. The space created by the rotation between the coffin bone and the hoof wall is filled by proliferating keratinocytes, blood and dead horn. Along the edges infection can occur and wound fluid (exudate) can be noticed. All of this material is called the lamellar wedge.

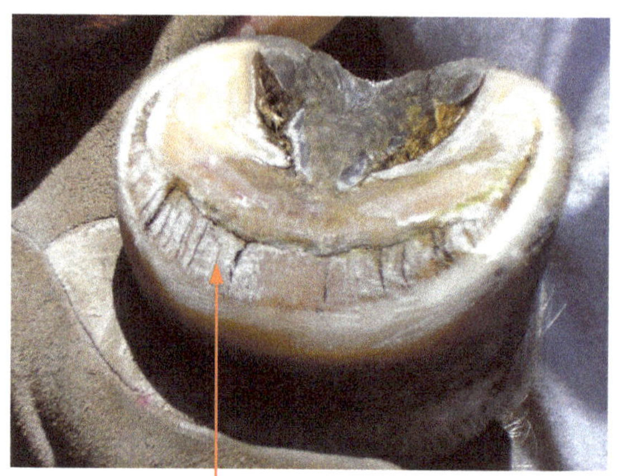

Lamellar wedge
(Photo: Cynthia Cooper)

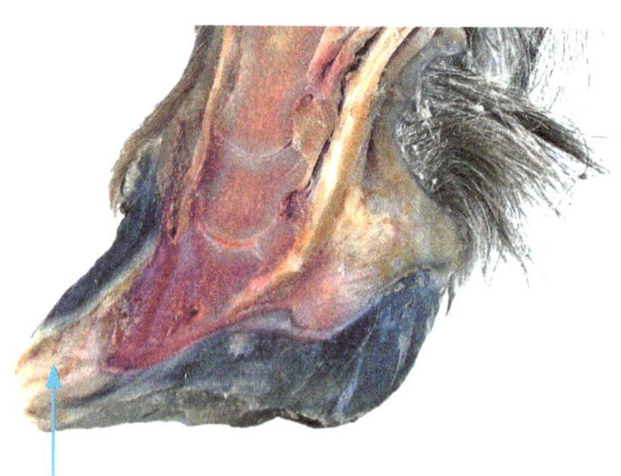

Lamellar wedge (cross-section)

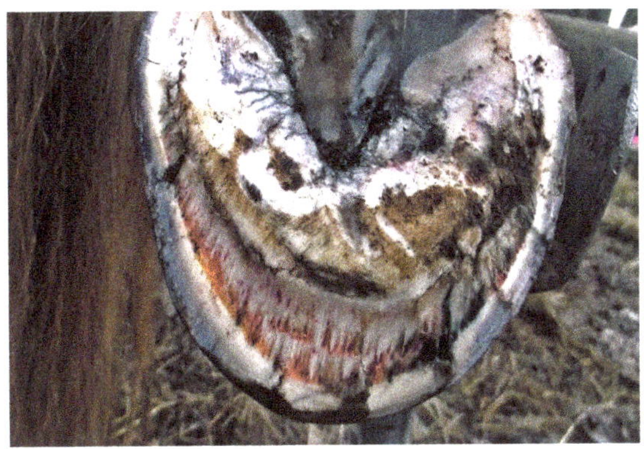

Blood and serum leaking
from the lamellar wedge

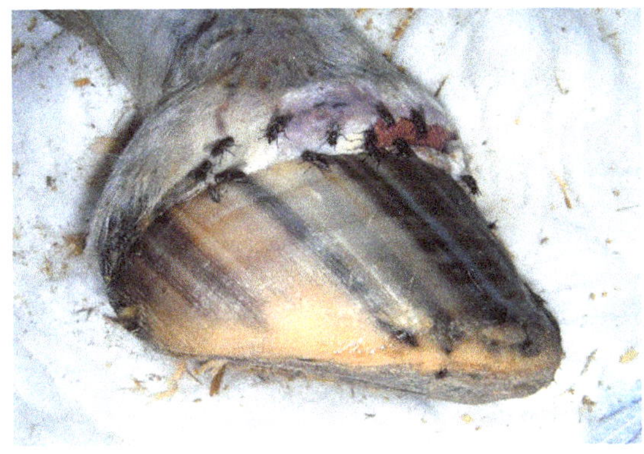

Coronary band prolapse
(photo: Kim Hillegas)

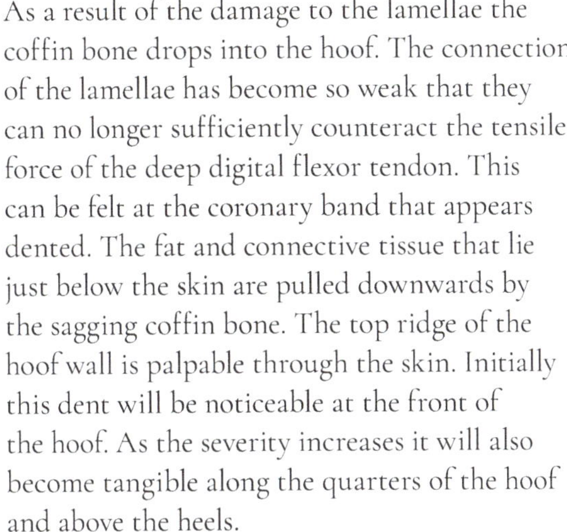

As a result of the damage to the lamellae the coffin bone drops into the hoof. The connection of the lamellae has become so weak that they can no longer sufficiently counteract the tensile force of the deep digital flexor tendon. This can be felt at the coronary band that appears dented. The fat and connective tissue that lie just below the skin are pulled downwards by the sagging coffin bone. The top ridge of the hoof wall is palpable through the skin. Initially this dent will be noticeable at the front of the hoof. As the severity increases it will also become tangible along the quarters of the hoof and above the heels.

CORONARY BAND SEPARATION

In more severe cases, the skin becomes detached. This phenomenon is called coronary band separation. A yellowish blood serum may emerge.

CORONARY BAND PROLAPSE

In even more severe cases the coronary dermis might start protruding from the coronary band. This is called a coronary band prolapse.

SINKER

The coffin bone can also sink completely. As mentioned before, this is called a sinker. A sinker is the result of breaking of the lamellar connection around the entire coffin bone instead of just in the toe section. When the coffin bone starts to sink, around the edge of the coronary band edge separation can be noticed. The coronary band lays down flat and feels empty.

In the stable chronic phase the coffin bone will stabilise, although in the rotated position. Hoof wall and sole start to grow again.

SHAPE AND CONDITION OF THE COFFIN BONE

Bone is living and active tissue. If pressure is exerted, changes will occur.

SKI-TIP

The tip of the coffin bone can deform under pressure. We call this bone deformation a ski-tip. This ski-tip can eventually break off. A ski-tip can also disappear after the hoof has healed. The pressure under which it developed

COFFIN BONE AND HOOF CAPSULE ROTATION

In the chronic phase of laminitis, the angle between the coffin bone and the hoof capsule changes: this change is due not only to the coffin bone tilting, but due also to rotation of the hoof capsule.

COFFIN BONE ROTATION

Initially, the coffin bone will tilt relative to the hoof wall. In that case, the lamellar connection is only damaged in the dorsal part of the hoof (the toe). The coffin bone turns (pivots) around the still-intact caudal (rear) part of the lamellar connection. This happens mainly due to the force resulting from the downward pressure of the horse's weight and, to a lesser extent, the pulling force of the deep digital flexor tendon during break over of the hoof. This phenomenon is called coffin bone rotation or, to be more precise, histological-mechanical coffin bone rotation.

HOOF CAPSULE ROTATION

In the next stage, the angle between the coffin bone and the hoof capsule will increase further. In addition to the continuing coffin bone rotation, there is now hoof capsule rotation. The hoof wall is hereby pushed away from the coffin bone.

There is a distinction between anatomical-mechanical and histological hoof capsule rotation. Anatomical-mechanical hoof capsule rotation is the result of incorrect biomechanical force distribution, which results in the hoof capsule being torn away from the internal foot. Toes or a hoof wall that are too long, or heels that are too high all contribute to this. Histological hoof capsule rotation is the result of the formation of a lamellar wedge. In many cases, anatomical-mechanical and histological hoof capsule rotation occur together.

TRIMMING

To increase the chances of recovery, it is important to realise that coffin bone and hoof capsule rotation are not the same. Apart from weight loss, nothing can be done to decrease the downward pressure of the horse's body weight. Even in an anatomically perfect hoof, where the strain on the lamellar connection is minimal and the heels have the correct height to align the coffin bone in its optimum position, the latter will still tilt as soon as the lamellar connection in the toe region breaks down. Hoof capsule rotation on the other hand, can be largely corrected with one or more trims. As soon as the coffin bone returns to its anatomically correct position, the hoof will be better balanced and the force distribution across all anatomical parts of the hoof will be optimal. This approach will also lead to a reduction in pain, a better hoof mechanism and thus a faster recovery.

LATERAL COFFIN BONE ROTATION

In some cases, X-rays show that the angle between the coffin bone and the ground also changes in a lateral direction. This medio-lateral coffin bone rotation deserves as much attention during the treatment (read: trim) as a 'normal' rotation.

This phenomenon is less common than the normal dorso-palmar coffin bone rotation, although it is seen more frequently since veterinarians ask more often for dorsal radiographs. These photos show that the coffin bone tilts medially inside the hoof capsule. In the rare cases that the coffin bone tilts to the other side, it is called a latero-medial coffin bone rotation.

The changed position of the coffin bone can also be observed in the joint space between the short pastern bone and the coffin bone, which then becomes wider on the lateral side than on the medial. On the medial side of the hoof the sole thickness is usually reduced.

A medio-lateral coffin bone rotation puts higher pressure on the medial side of the coffin bone. As a result, the risk of osteoporosis in this bone increases.

Without X-ray's, the following signs of lateral coffin bone rotation can be determined as well: there is reduced wall growth on the medial side of the hoof, the coronary band feels dented and the top of the hoof wall can be felt through the skin. These signs are less observable or entirely absent on the lateral side.

will then have disappeared. The new growth of a straight hoof wall will exert the necessary even pressure to force the bone back in the right shape. Again, bone tissue is dynamic and will adapt under pressure. This process takes time, the same amount of time it took to develop the ski-tip in the first place. Of course, all conditions must be right for this to happen.

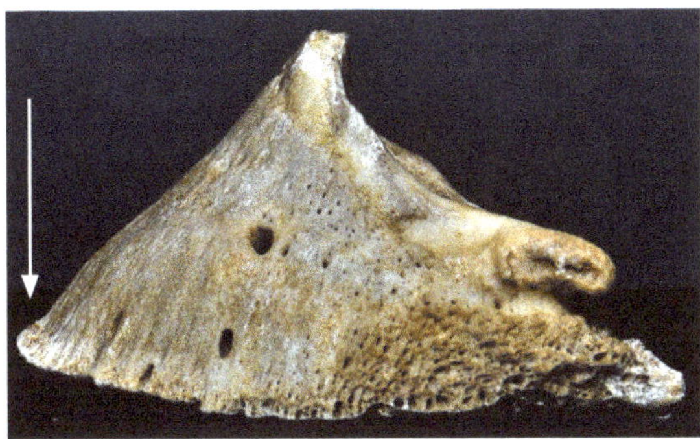

Ski-tip
(photo: Claudia Garner)

Coffin bone deformation and remodelling

When flaring of the hoof wall occurs for a long time, the body will in some cases try to fill the space between the coffin bone and the hoof wall by producing more bone tissue. At the level of the flare, the coffin bone takes the shape of the flare. This is called coffin bone remodelling. In more severe cases, the entire coffin bone deforms, which is what we call hoof bone deformation.

Coffin bone fractures

The edges of the coffin bone may also break under pressure. This is called a coffin bone fracture.

Bone demineralisation

The coffin bone can demineralise because of the decreased blood supply. The horse extracts magnesium and calcium from the bone. The density of the bone reduces, which increases the chances of the complications described above.

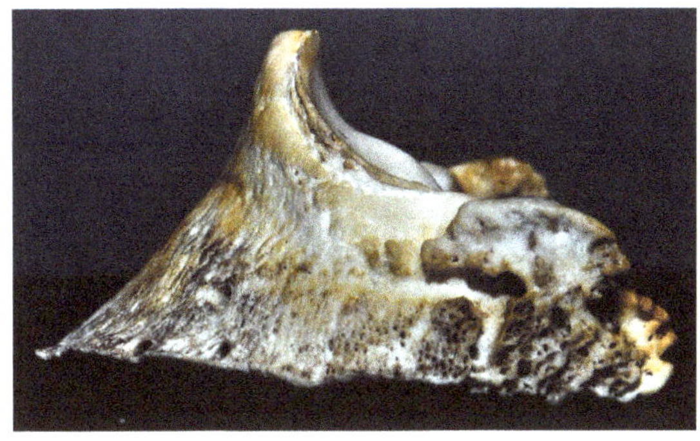

Demineralised coffin bone
(photo: Claudia Garner)

Osteomyelitis or osteitis

An infection in the (marrow of the) bone, usually in the tip of the coffin bone. The main complications of osteomyelitis in the coffin bone are deformity of the bone and inflammation of the hoof joint by spreading of the infection.

Shape and condition of the sole

- Deep collateral grooves.
- The sole is being compressed and thus becomes thinner and more sensitive.
- Black spots on the sole.
- Necrotic tissue as a result of compression of the sole and damage to the solar dermis and its blood vessels. The blood vessels that provide the sole with blood do not run through the coffin bone, but around the edge of the coffin bone. A rotated coffin

bone or sinker presses down onto these blood vessels thereby obstructing the blood supply to the sole.

- Flat or even convex sole in the front half of the hoof as a result of the pressure caused by the rotated coffin bone or sinker. This can already be seen after a few days and called a sole prolapse.
- Across the bulging sole dark lines or cracks may appear. This is a sign of the coffin bone that is about to break through the sole, which is called a sole perforation.

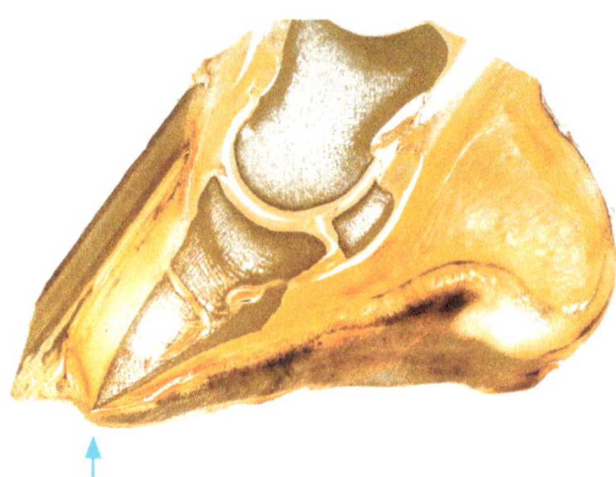

Sole perforation (cross-section)
(plastinate: Christoph von Horst)

- All of this may be accompanied by:
  - Sole abscesses
  - A moon shaped edge of red or purple sole bruises
  - Areas with leaking serum
  - Blood poisoning (septicemia)
  - A thrush-like infection, with or without the associated penetrating smell. The last bit of protection that the sole provides to the coffin bone is affected by this infection.
- All of these signs, with the exception of blood poisoning, will be more visible on a properly cleaned sole, possibly even carefully scraped clean with a hoof knife.

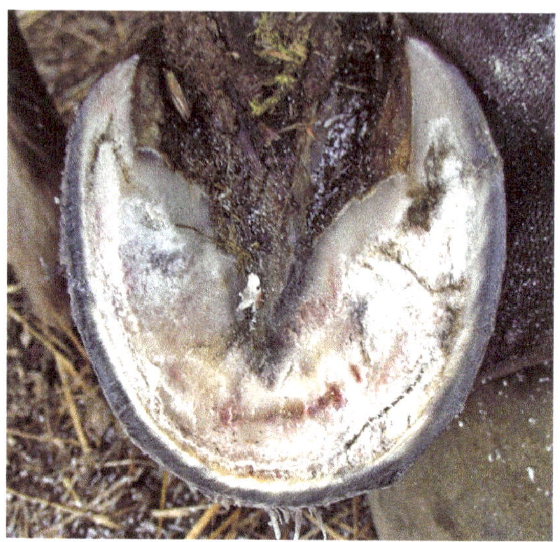

Moon shaped sole bruises

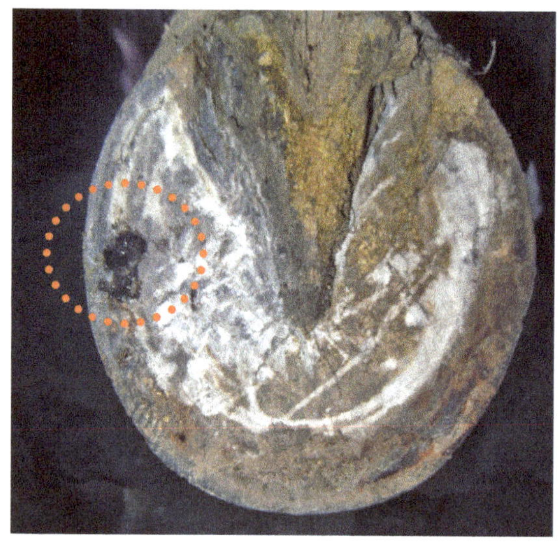

Sole abscess
(photo: Jamie Berning)

Shape and condition of the wall

At this stage the hoof wall often looks strange. The impaired blood flow in the hoof causes a shortage of sulphur containing amino acids. This slows down the horn growth in the toe section while the normal growth rate continues at the heels. A cup-shaped hoof with high heels is the result.

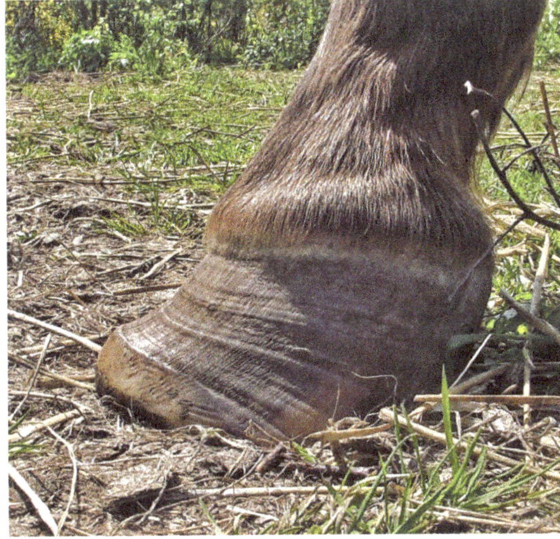

Cup-shaped hoof

Growth rings

Growth rings no longer run parallel to the coronary band, as is the case in a healthy hoof. As a result of the slower growth of the toe region, the rings there run closer together. The rings are also much more pronounced. This is caused by pulling forces from within by the sagging coffin bone.

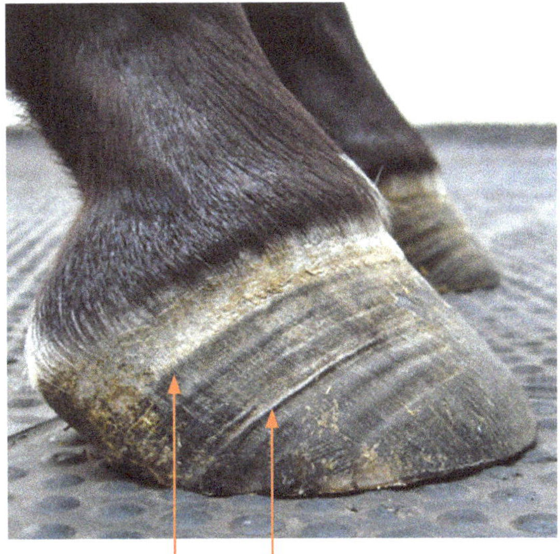

Disturbed growth rings
(photo: The Liphook equine hospital)

Laminitic rings

The dropping coffin bone pulls the dermal papillae of the coronary band downward. Meanwhile the papillae continue to produce the epidermal lamellae. As a result a deep laminitic ring becomes visible in the hoof wall.

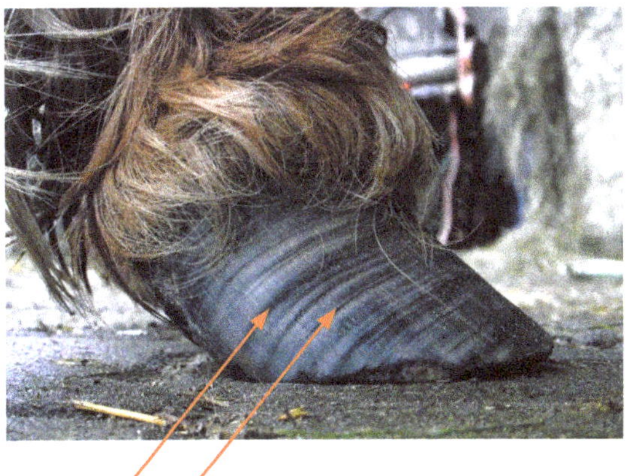

Laminitic rings

Bull nosed hoof

In severe cases the hoof deforms into a bull nosed shape hoof. In these hooves the horn is growing away from the coffin bone. This type of growth can be recognised by an extremely wide white line in the toe section. Bull noses are more common in sinkers than in hooves with coffin bone rotation.

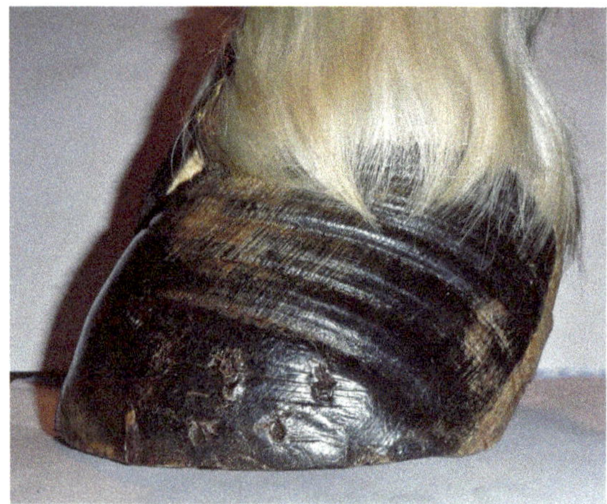

Bull nosed hoof

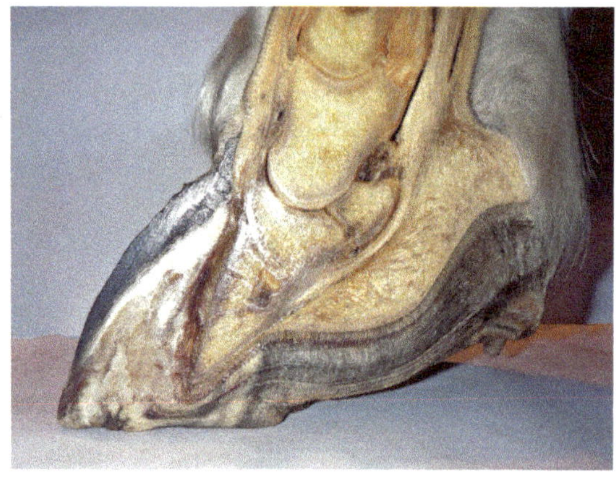

Bull nosed hoof (cross-section)
(photos: Lucy Priory)

Stretched white line

The hoof wall becomes (partially) separated from the coffin bone causing the white line to stretch. This can generate infections, like white line disease, as extra complication (see page 129 under 'Treating complications').

Flares

Flares will form. These are deformations of the hoof wall in which it fans outwards. The cause of flares is that the lamellar connection is not sufficiently capable of absorbing the mechanical forces acting on the hoof wall for a long time. In particular, but not exclusively, in case of flaring, the hoof wall may split and crumble.

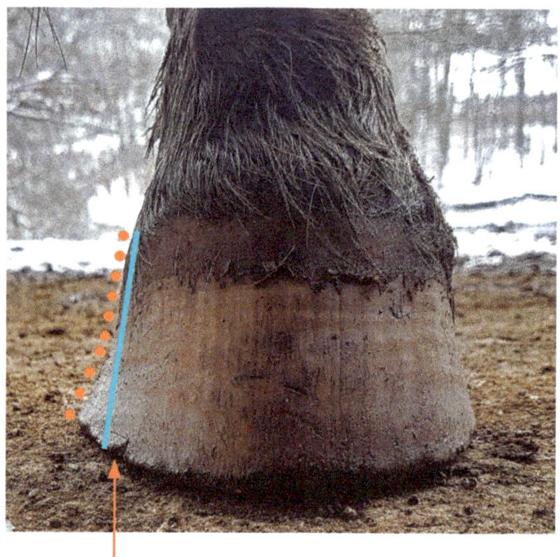

Flared hoof, with splits and crumbles

Slipper toes and duckbills

When the hoof is not correctly trimmed in time, the weakened lamellar connection is put under pressure during break over, creating the typical 'slipper toes' or 'duckbills'.

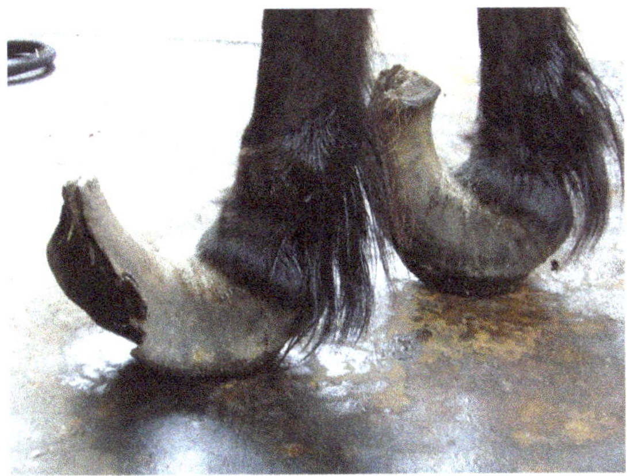

Slipper toes
(photo: Cynthia Cooper)

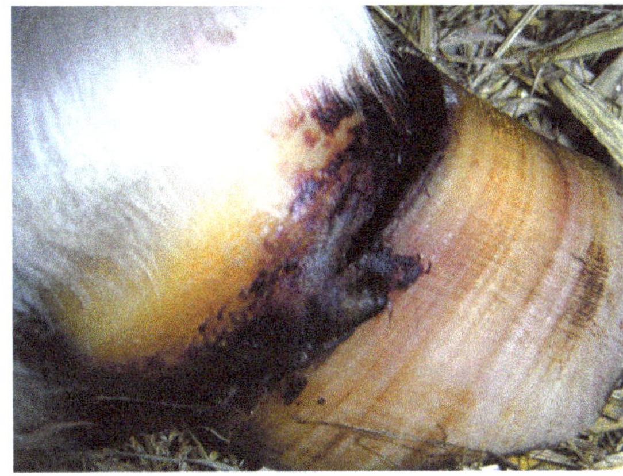

Hoof sloughing
(photo: Mike van Dijk)

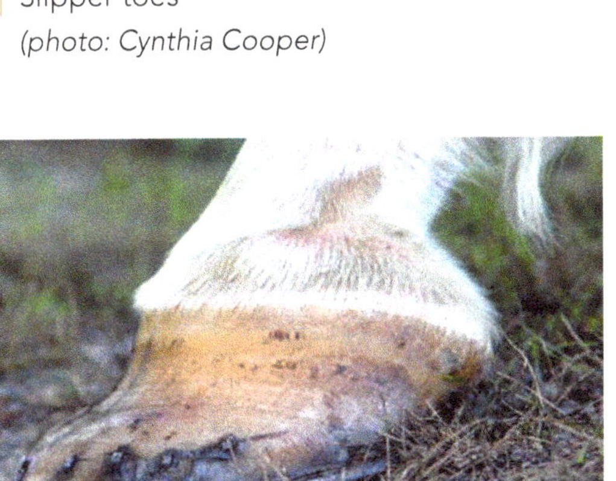

Duckbill
(photo: Gretschen Fathauer)

Hoof sloughing

In a worst case scenario, the entire connection between dermis and hoof capsule (wall, sole, frog and bulbs) fails. The horrible phenomena of a horse losing a hoof, is called hoof sloughing.

Abnormal stance

Similar to the acute phase, horses in the chronic phase adopt the typical laminitic stance to reduce pressure exerted by the tip of the coffin bone from the inside onto the sole. In case of a sinker the horse tries to place the affected legs as vertical as possible under the body.

Abnormal movement

The abnormalities of movement in the acute phase are often also present in chronic laminitis. Because of the altered position of the coffin bone and the sensitivity of the toe, walking becomes even more difficult. The horse shows an exaggerated heel landing to protect the toe and the sole area.

Because of this there is not enough time for the whole hoof to break over correctly. This causes the toe to slam on to the ground. This increases the chance of damage to the lamellae in the front of the hoof.

Characteristics only visible on radiographs

With radiographs (X-rays), the degree of white line separation and coffin bone rotation can be made visible. This may provide additional information in chronic laminitis cases, especially on the severity and duration of the disease so far. Based on these findings the hoof care provider, veterinarian and owner might be able to decide which treatment is most suitable.
In general, veterinarians and hoof care providers use the following rule of thumb:

- A 5.5 degree rotation or less has a hopeful prospect.
- A 11.5 degree rotation or more has a bad prospect.

There are many exceptions to these rules and they depend on the chosen treatment. A horse with a five degree coffin bone rotation, treated with therapeutic shoeing and heavy painkillers, without adaptations in movement, nutrition and housing, usually has a worse prospect than a horse with twice the amount of rotation that is treated as described in this book.

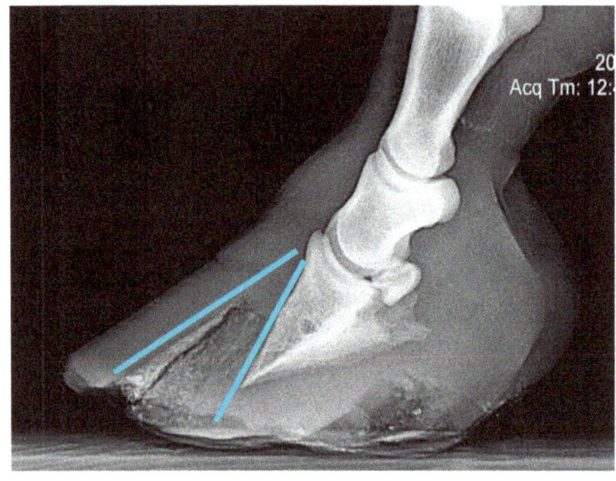

Coffin bone rotation
(photo: Myhre equine clinic)

The growing of a healthy, connected hoof wall will bring the coffin bone back into the previous, normal position, regardless of the degree of rotation. Naturally this can only happen with the right treatment and under the right circumstances. During the course of the healing process radiographs can give information regarding the progress that is made.

On the radiographs, one or more of the following characteristics may be visible:

- White line separation seen as dark lines.
- The degree of rotation or the occurrence of a sinker.
- In case the tip of a rotated coffin bone is already pressing against the sole, tissue of both may partially die off. This necrotic tissue is visible on radiographs.
- The shape and condition of the coffin bone:
  - Ski-tip
  - Coffin bone fractures
  - Bone demineralisation, including decalcification (osteoporosis) and disappearance of bone tissue by calcium deficiency (osteolysis).
- Bleeding, swelling, oedema and nitrogen gas can also be seen at this stage.
- Also gas and pus due to osteomyelitis or abscesses are visible.
- At a later stage signs of inflammation (a reaction of the body to tissue injury) and infections (caused by fungi and bacteria) can be verified using radiographs.

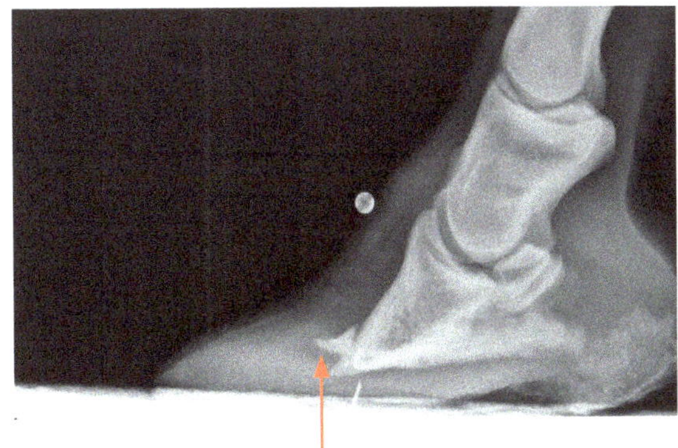

Broken off ski-tip
(photo: Elizabeth Fish)

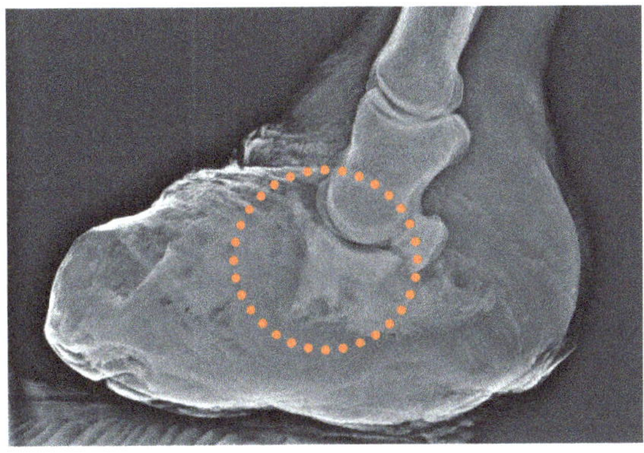

Demineralised coffin bone

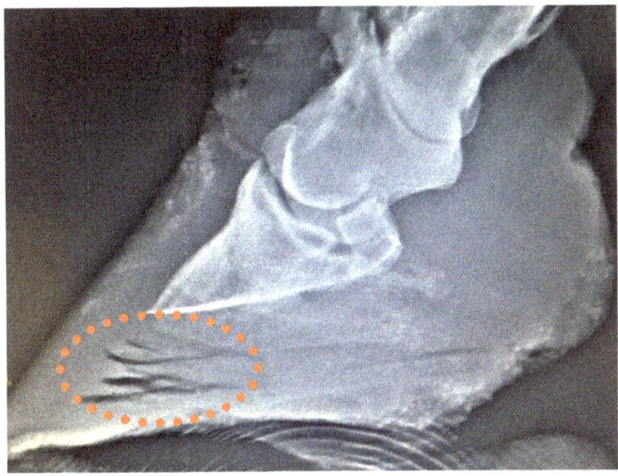

Sole abscess

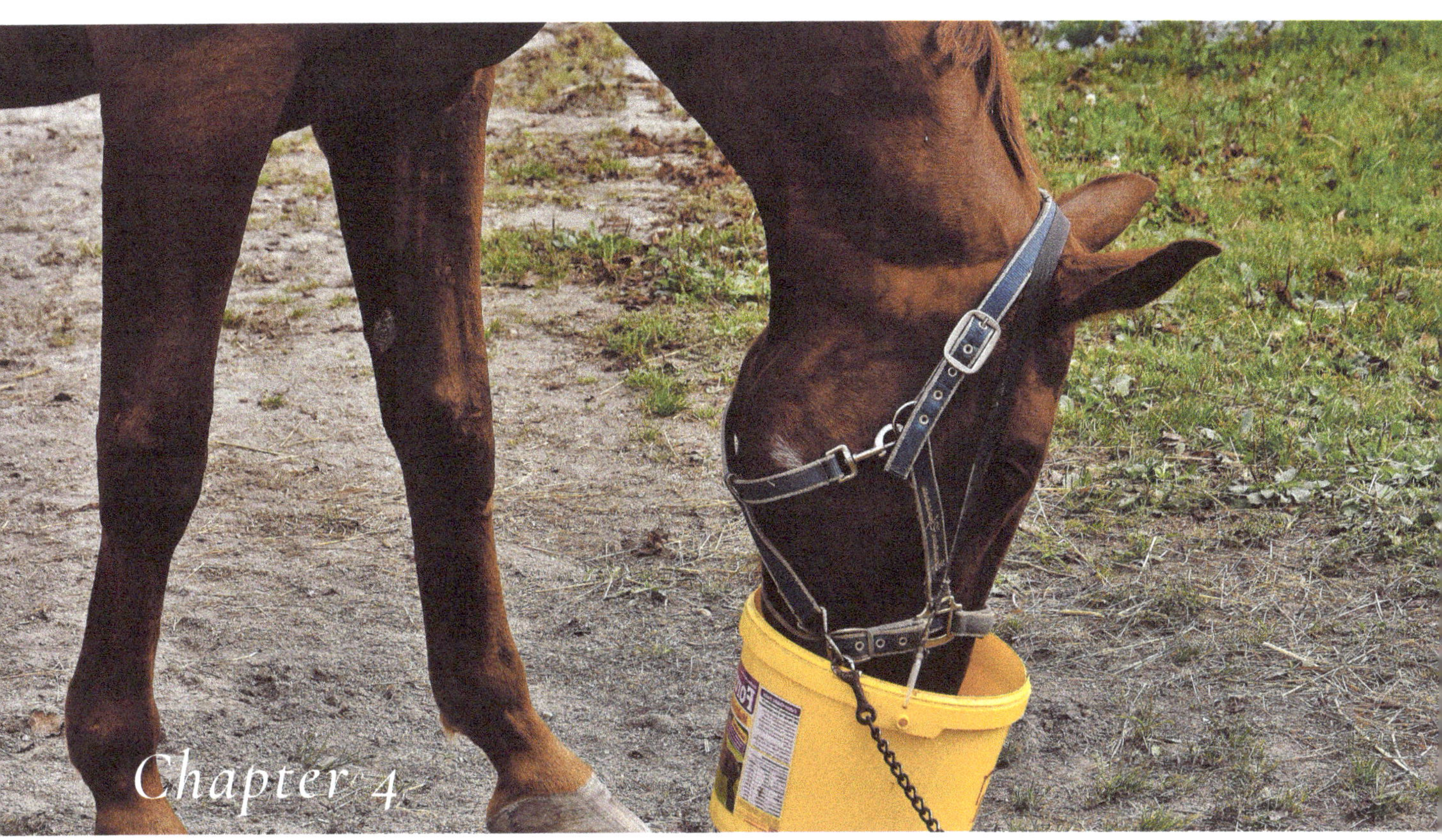

Chapter 4

THEORIES AND CAUSES

Dr. Chris Pollitt is one of the most leading and groundbreaking researchers on the subject of laminitis. He made the following, not very optimistic remark about scientific research on the disease: "One-half of laminitis science is incorrect but which half?"

Not so long ago every case of laminitis was regarded mainly as a circulatory problem. Fortunately, we now know better. Today at least five different theories exist about the cause and development of laminitis. The list of known and suspected causes is impressively long.

THEORIES

These current scientific theories regarding the development of laminitis partly overlap and are certainly not mutually exclusive. Often they clarify a particular phase or aspect of laminitis. The theories are all of a (patho)physiological nature. This means that the properties of cells, tissues, organs and the like are examined, both in healthy as in diseased state and under different circumstances.

These five theories look for the causes successively in the field of:

- Blood vessels and circulation
- Enzymes
- Inflammation
- Metabolism and hormones
- Trauma/overload

> Under the heading 'Conventional treatment', for each theory discussed, the same could be written about correct hoof trimming. From page 122, under 'Trimming a laminitic hoof', we will have a closer look at this subject.

After looking at the five theories, in this chapter we delve into the possible specific causes of laminitis. Below, however, lies the true 'origin'. It is found in the unnatural lifestyle the horse is subjected to while living with us. More about that will follow later in this book.

CIRCULATION THEORY

According to this theory, the horse's body is not able to maintain normal blood circulation inside the hoof. During the developmental phase, the blood supply is obstructed (ischemia). This can have several causes:

- Vasoconstriction
- Damaged capillaries
- Prolonged diversion of the blood supply to the hoof due to shunting (see page 33)
- High blood pressure in the hoof that hinders blood flow
- Microthromboses (blood clots)

These and others causes result in a lack of oxygen and nutrients that could lead to the destruction of the lamellae.

Oedema

Increased pressure in constricted and possibly damaged capillaries causes fluid to leak from those capillaries. This fluid accumulates in the surrounding tissue, as oedema in the lamellae. The lamellae are sandwiched between the hoof wall and the coffin bone and cannot move anywhere. The oedema compresses the blood vessels, which restricts circulation even more.

The reduced blood supply is apparent in a decrease in temperature of the hoof during the developmental phase, in contrast to an increase in temperature in the acute phase. Horses show little or no pain because the hooves are numbed by the lack of circulation. Once circulation resumes the pain becomes gradually noticeable.

Reperfusion injury

Reperfusion injury may occur when blood flow resumes. This is damage to hoof tissues caused by the return of the blood supply (with a corresponding higher temperature in the hoof). The renewed supply of oxygen and nutrients causes an inflammatory response and so-called oxidative stress. The presence of too many oxygen molecules result in cell damage.

Objections

Research has never found microthromboses and swelling during the developmental phase. Only at Obel 3 microthromboses have been observed. In this phase no necrotic lamellar tissue can be found either. As several studies contradict each other, an indisputable causal link between coagulation problems and laminitis remains unclear.

Decreased blood flow is definitely a problem, but more likely it is a consequence rather than a cause or else it is just one of the aspects involved. Other research data clearly show an increased blood flow just before the onset of laminitis. It seems that first there is an increased blood flow, then there is reduced blood flow with consequences as described above. Hence these research data are in agreement with the circulation theory rather than disproving it.

Conventional treatment

Treatment of laminitis based on the circulation theory focuses on:

- Stimulating circulation
- Anticoagulant, hypotensive and vasodilator drugs
- Burdening the horse as little as possible

ENZYME THEORY

The destruction and reconstruction of cells under the influence of enzymes is a common process in the body. When this process is disturbed many illnesses can occur. Cancer, osteoarthritis and fibrosis are well-known examples, as is laminitis.

The enzyme theory focuses on the basement membrane, the connective tissue located between the dermal and epidermal lamellae.

As mentioned before, the lamellar connection is subject to constant destruction and reconstruction. This allows the hoof wall, which consists of dead horn tissue, to grow downwards over the coffin bone but still to remain strongly attached.

Metalloproteases

This controlled destruction of the connective tissue takes place under the influence of a group of enzymes that break down proteins: (matrix) metalloproteases (MMPs). In fact, these MMPs are pro-enzymes. These are proteins, which remain inactive until they reach a place where their action is needed. After they have been activated their activity is controlled by a so-called TIMP (tissue inhibitor of metalloprotease).

The role of MMPs and other enzymes in the destruction of the basement membrane is still insufficiently known. For a long time the focus was primarily on MMP-9 and MMP-2, however recently science has changed this view. An improved research method and recognised gaps in previous research have contributed to this.

Hyperinsulinemia

In laminitis, as a result of elevated insulin levels (or hyperinsulinemia, discussed in more detail under 'Metabolism and hormone theory' on page 57) only an increase in MMP-9 can be seen. And only in the harmless, inactive form called pro-MMP-9. Furthermore, this increase is insignificant during the developmental phase. For this reason, the role of MMP-9 in the development of laminitis is nowadays considered negligible.

NSC overload

In laminitis caused by non-structural carbohydrate (NSC) overload, a rise of MMP-2 can be noticed. However, this is not the case before degradation of the basement membrane begins or when it is already in progress. Therefore we can conclude that MMP-2 does not influences the development of laminitis either.

The cause of MMP-2 overproduction is not yet known, however there is a strong assumption that toxins from the bacterium, Streptococcus lutetiensis (until recently known as Streptococcus bovis II/I), could trigger the rise in MMPs. This bacterium is present in large numbers in the intestines after for instance eating large amounts of cereals.

Other studies are showing that increased levels of MMPs are a result of inflammatory reactions, and therefor not a primary cause.

Although MMP-2 may not be involved in the onset of the destruction of the basement membrane, it cannot be ruled out as a contributing factor in the acceleration of the process. For this reason, further research is needed and treatment should aim to prevent activation of certain pro-enzymes. The function of other MMPs also gives sufficient reason to continue with both research and treatment.

ADAMTS-4

One enzyme of interest is the cartilage destroying enzyme ADAMTS-4. In the lamellae a protein is present that is degraded by this enzyme. Too much of this enzyme could lead to weakening of the lamellae and therefore weakening of the lamellar connection. The focus on MMP-2 and MMP-2 has now shifted to ADAMTS-4.

Hemidesmosomes and secondary epidermal lamellae

Searching for the cause of laminitis in a different direction does not change the fact that the hemidesmosomes and the secondary epidermal lamellae deteriorate. They change shape and start to slide over one another. Also the amount of hemidesmosomes decreases. The lamellar connection gradually disintegrates. This deterioration has been observed by researchers within 12 hours after the onset of laminitis. This is even before any clinical signs can be observed.

> ➤ Degradation of the basement membrane does not only take place in the hoof. Also, the skin and chestnuts suffer from it. However consequences are far less disastrous because these tissues are less structural compared to hoof tissues.

CARBOHYDRATES

Several types of carbohydrates (sugars or saccharides) can be distinguished:

- Simple sugars (monosaccharides) such as glucose (dextrose) and fructose (fruit sugar)
- Dual sugars (disaccharides) such as sucrose (beet sugar)
- Fructans such as inulin, levan and oligofructose
- Complex sugars (polysaccharides), such as starch and dietary fibres such as cellulose, hemicellulose and lignin
- Lignin is not considered to be a carbohydrate. It belongs to the non-carbohydrates. For convenience reasons, in this book the collective of dietary fibres are regarded as carbohydrates.

Carbohydrates can be grouped as follows:

- Ethanol-soluble carbohydrates (ESC): simple and double sugars
- Water-soluble carbohydrates (WSC): ESC and fructan
- Non-structural carbohydrates (NSC): WSC and starch
- Structural carbohydrates (SC): Dietary fibre

NSC occur in cells and saps of plants. SC occur in cell walls of plants.

Some types of fructan are regarded as ESC because of their relative simple chemical structure. In this book, to remain clear, all fructans are included to the group of WSC.

Hoof vasculature

The capillaries that provide blood to this area of the hoof get damaged as well. Blood is instantly transferred via the shunts from the blood supplying arteries to the blood draining veins. The foot itself is short-circuited by this.

Vasodilator and anticoagulant drugs

The damaged capillaries and short-circuiting of the hoof are the reasons veterinarians often prescribe vasodilator and anticoagulant drugs. Unfortunately, the latter are often erroneously called blood thinners. By inhibiting clotting of the blood a superficial wound will indeed bleed longer. This gave rise to the idea that these drugs made the blood thinner. However this is not the case. In addition, the thickness of the blood is not the problem, nor the width of the capillaries. In any case, these symptom controlling drugs hardly reach the hoof at all because of the occurrence of shunting.

Conventional treatment

Based on this theory, treatment of laminitis focuses on lowering enzyme activity. According to researchers that subscribe to this theory, during the developmental phase vasodilation takes place in the hoof, causing the supply of TIMPs. and MMP triggers to be higher than normal. The reduction of blood supply would therefore be helpful.

This is in stark contrast to the circulation theory (and the trauma theory, that will be discussed later) in which blood supply is stimulated. Blood circulation can be decreased by cold therapy (see sidebar 'Cold therapy' on page 116).

Decreasing the blood pressure, for example by using antihypertensive drugs or omega-3 fatty acids, also slightly reduces the supply of TIMPs and MMP triggers.

The administration of synthetic enzyme inhibiting drugs to reduce the MMPs (such as MMP-2 and ADAMTS-4) could be effective as well, however it is important to take potential harmful side effects of these drugs into account.

INFLAMMATION THEORY

Previously, the main focus was on the inflammation of the lamellae. Hence the suffix *-itis* that indicates inflammation: laminitis. In laminitis the inflammation of the lamellae is sterile. Neither bacteria or viruses play a role.

Inflammation is indeed present in laminitis, but nowadays the inflammation is no longer regarded as a cause but as a clinical sign or complication. This means the name laminitis is outdated.

SWELLING

Inflammatory fluid creates a swelling that breaks the lamellar connection. This might happen because the tissue is already weakened by increased enzymatic activity (as described above). In this respect the inflammatory theory and the enzyme theory coincide.

BLOOD PLATELETS

Blood platelets are a second aspect of inflammation associated with the onset of laminitis. When platelets are activated by infection they bind together and form microthromboses. These microthromboses can block the capillaries of the hoof. In addition, blood platelets also release the neurotransmitter serotonin, which acts as a vasoconstrictor.

> NEUROTRANSMITTER
> Endogenous chemical that transmits nerve impulses.

WHITE BLOOD CELLS

Infiltration is a phase of an inflammatory process, in which white blood cells (leukocytes) from the bloodstream infiltrate an infected area. In acute laminitis white blood cells infiltrate the dermal lamellae. Infiltration is a property of SIRS, the inflammation of the whole body (see sidebar 'SIRS-related laminitis').

During NSC overload many white blood cells are withdrawn from circulation. This has especially been proven in cases with starch or oligofructose overload. Activated white blood cells produce so-called inflammatory mediators (antibodies). One of these is cytokine, a protein that is able to increase the activity of MMPs.

Probably, the endotoxins released during NSC overload are responsible for the activation of the white blood cells. This will be discussed in more detail later in this chapter.

SIRS-RELATED LAMINITIS

SIRS is short for Systemic Inflammatory Response Syndrome. It is an inflammatory reaction of the entire body. In certain cases, laminitis can be seen as a local manifestation of SIRS. The tissue damage to the hoof - and in particular the lamellar connection - is a form of organ failure. If we take the focus off the hoof, we see that inflammatory mediators (antibodies) are also found in the liver, lungs and kidneys during the developmental and acute phase of laminitis.

SIRS can have many causes. In the first instance we think of infections and inflammations such as influenza, pneumonia or pleurisy, mastitis (udder inflammation), endometritis (inflammation of the lining of the uterus), a bacterial infection after placenta retention, nephritis (chronic kidney inflammation) or uveitis (eye inflammation). Also damage to the intestinal wall causes endotoxemia (the presence of toxins in the blood). This can happen, among other things, as a result of NSC overload. We will come back to these causes of SIRS and SIRS-related laminitis in detail, later in this chapter.

ENDOTOXIN
: Toxic component found in the outer membrane of gram-negative bacteria, that is released after the death of these bacteria.

GRAM-NEGATIVE BACTERIUM
: Bacterium that has an extra outer membrane around the cell wall. When this bacterium dies, endotoxins are released.

Some scientists suspect these inflammatory mediators contribute to the damage of the basement membrane and therefore the lamellar connection. On the other hand, the release of inflammatory mediators is seen by other researchers as a response to the degradation of the basement membrane and not as a cause.

SUPEROXIDE

White blood cells produce superoxide as well. This is a free radical (see also page 166 under 'Antioxidants') with a strong oxidising effect on cells (see also page 59 under 'Reperfusion injury'). Normally superoxide is cleared by the enzyme SOD (superoxide dismutase) before it can cause any major damage. Unfortunately, this enzyme is not present in the lamellar tissue.

FREE RADICAL
: Harmful molecular by-product of normal metabolism, inflammation, medication, residual pesticides in foods, strenuous exercise, stress, obesity and adiposity.

Conventional treatment

Treatment of laminitis based on this theory focuses on fighting the inflammation with anti-inflammatory drugs. Veterinarians who are also informed about blood platelets may prescribe vasodilator drugs and serotonin-antagonists as well. Veterinarians who assume that anti-coagulant drugs have a blood-thinning effect will possibly add them as well. When anti-platelet drugs are chosen for this purpose it is possible they could have a positive effect.

Metabolism and hormone theory

Insulin plays a very important role in metabolism. Unfortunately, the sensitivity of the body to insulin can be disturbed. This is called metabolic insulin resistance, or simply 'insulin resistance'.

> **Metabolism**
> The complex of physical and chemical processes that take place in living cells for the maintenance, breakdown and construction of tissue and the production of energy.

Insulin resistance

The hormone insulin is produced by the pancreas, a glandular organ located in the abdominal cavity, which opens into the duodenum. The regulation of blood sugar levels depend greatly on insulin. It is the only hormone that can lower blood sugar levels.

> **Hormone**
> Substance produced by endocrine glands that selectively alters functional activity of certain organs and tissues.

Carbohydrates

Food contains slow and fast carbohydrates, depending on the time the body needs to digest them. Simple and dual sugars and fructans, the so-called water-soluble carbohydrates (WSC, see sidebar on page 61) are examples of fast carbohydrates. A number of sugar molecules chained together form a carbohydrate that is slow to digest.

Fast carbohydrates enter the bloodstream quickly causing the blood sugar level to rise. Immediately the pancreas releases insulin into the blood. The cell walls of muscle, fat and connective tissue cells contain insulin receptors that respond to insulin. Insulin 'tells' the cells to absorb and burn the sugar. Any excess sugar is stored as fat or glycogen in the liver or muscles.

In case of insulin resistance the glucose metabolism in the dermal lamellae changes. This causes a risk of developing laminitis by degradation of the hemidesmosomes. On page 94 under 'Glucose problems' this will be discussed in more detail. Receptors become insensitive to insulin. More glucose will be stored as fat. Furthermore, regular and long-term high blood sugar levels result in damage, constriction or clogging of capillaries. This increases the risk to laminitis, as described in the section on the circulation theory.

The susceptibility of horses to develop insulin resistance can be found in the fact that they naturally live on a low sugar diet. Iron overload, for example from surface or bore water containing excessive iron, is regarded as a contributory cause of insulin resistance as well. More on this on page 178 under 'Iron'.

PPID, corticosteroids and EMS

In PPID cases and also in horses that have been administered long-acting corticosteroids over an extended period, insulin resistance is a complication that can trigger laminitis. In equine metabolic syndrome (EMS) insulin resistance is even the main disorder. Both syndromes will be discussed extensively later in this book.

EMS=INSULIN RESISTANCE?

EMS is a collection of disorders: insulin resistance, weight problems, high blood pressure and abnormal blood fat levels. The relationship between obesity and insulin resistance is entirely mutual. Obesity causes insulin resistance; insulin resistance causes obesity. Since insulin resistance is the main disorder, EMS is also referred to as insulin resistance syndrome. The distinction between EMS and insulin resistance is therefore mainly theoretical.

Two phases of insulin resistance

Insulin resistance can be divided into two phases. The first phase is characterised by impaired glucose tolerance. In this phase, which is also called hyperinsulinemia or pre-diabetes, the pancreas will release more and more insulin to stimulate muscle cells to do their job. The glucose levels remain under control but the amount of insulin in the blood will be much too high.

Vicious circle

The horse's over-productive pancreas will not be able to keep up when fed a diet high in fast carbohydrates. This is called hyperglycemia. Blood sugar levels spike temporarily, but due to the large amount of insulin in the blood too much sugar will be converted into fat. Because of this, blood sugar levels then drop too far below the limit. The body of the horse interprets this as being hungry and will then 'ask' for a new supply of fast carbohydrates. A vicious circle has been created.

In the second phase of insulin resistance, which is much less common than the first, the pancreas is no longer able to produce enough insulin. The blood sugar level rises but the cells are hardly capable of absorbing sugar anymore. The horse starves while getting enough food.

Insulin resistance and the vascular system

Insulin also regulates vasodilation and vasoconstriction. In vascular insulin resistance the vasodilatory effects of insulin are disrupted. This can lead to vasoconstriction, resulting in increased blood pressure and decreased blood flow. Sugar absorption will decrease which again leads to elevated blood sugar levels and insulin resistance.

Endothelin-1

Endothelin-1 (ET-1) is a peptide hormone produced by the endothelium, a layer of cells that cover the inside of blood vessels. This hormone has a strong vasoconstrictive action. Endothelium produces nitric oxide as well, that has a vasodilatory action. ET-1 and nitric oxide are each other's antagonists. This means they perform the opposite actions of the same function. In this case, the regulation of the width of blood vessels.

Insulin both stimulates the production of ET-1 as well as nitric oxide. Normally, production is in balance, but in insulin resistance this balance is disrupted. The production of nitric oxide decreases, while ET-1 levels remain the same. ET-1 becomes the dominant substance.

Venoconstriction

Veins in the hoof are more sensitive to vasoconstrictors than arteries. In particular, sensitivity to ET-1 is high. Increased ET-1 levels cause veins in the hoof to constrict more than arteries, creating a bottleneck effect. Blood will be able to enter the hoof more easily than it can flow back out, causing blood flow to stagnate. Therefore, ET-1 excess could result in a shortage of oxygen in the hoof tissue, with all the effects described earlier in this book in the section on the blood circulation theory.

Possible treatment consists of administration of ET-1 inhibiting drugs that stimulate nitric oxide production. Herbal medicine reports good results using jiaogulan to increase nitric oxide levels.

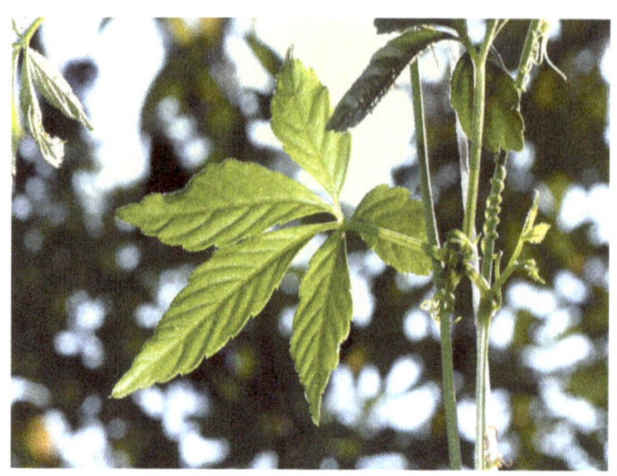

Jiaogulan
(photo: Petr Voboril)

Endothelium

Another problem caused by excess concentrations of insulin is damage to the endothelium, the layer of cells that covers the inside of blood vessels. The capillaries will become damaged even faster. Damage to capillaries has been discussed earlier in the circulation theory. In these last two points the circulation and hormone theory coincide.

Insulin resistance and inflammation

The occurrence of chronic inflammation is partly attributed to insulin resistance as well. Here the inflammation and hormone theory coincide.

Conventional treatment

Treatment of laminitis caused by insulin resistance, focuses on weight loss and controlled or reduced intake of NSC. In the case of PPID and EMS treatment aims to control these primary causes, as far as possible.

TRAUMA THEORY

Traumatic laminitis is caused by heavy, prolonged, repetitive strain on the hooves, often on hard surfaces. The hoof tissue is damaged because it is not able to cope with the excessive load. Capillaries are damaged or pinched, causing a decreased circulation. In this, the trauma theory coincides with the circulation theory.

Sole bruising and osteomyelitis of the coffin bone may be associated with it. In this, the trauma theory coincides with the inflammation theory, in particular with regard to the blood platelets.

Usually traumatic laminitis occurs due to a combination of several of the following conditions:

- Jumping, endurance, carriage driving
- Toe landing caused by chronic heel pain
- Incorrect trimming and shoeing
- Thin soles and hoof walls
- A long hoof wall that acts like a lever, pulling on the lamellar connection
- Long distance transport
- The horse is stabled at night and has practically no movement for more than 8 hours.

Horses at risk

Horses at risk are:

- Horses in moderate work that are suddenly overworked. For instance horses that are stabled all week and then taken out on Sunday for a long ride on rocky trails and roads.
- Shetland ponies because they gain weight quickly, are often insufficiently exercised and do not wear their hooves enough.
- Overweight horses in general. The horse hangs with his full weight in the hoof capsule. Each pound of excess weight increases the risk of traumatic laminitis.
- Large draft horses because they often have flat, thin soles.

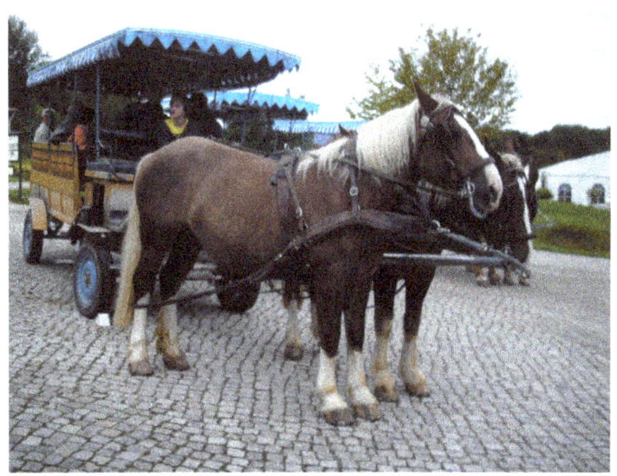

Quadruple risk
Large draught, overloading, not correctly trimmed, shod (photo: Inka Piegsa-Quischotte)

Avoiding pain

Overstraining of one or more legs may also be caused by an attempt to relieve pain in another body part, for example as a result of nerve damage, a bone fracture or a bacterial joint infection.

> This specific cause of laminitis can often be encountered in donkeys. Their high pain threshold, combined with their susceptibility to hoof problems, means that problems often remain unnoticed. More on donkeys in chapter 8.

> The results of three different studies vary considerably. But if we take the average outcome it still means there is a more than 11% chance that a horse with one immobilised leg (cast or pins) will get laminitis in the hoof of another leg.

The leg that is constantly weighted experiences a constant pull of the deep digital flexor tendon to the coffin bone and therefore to the lamellae at the front of the hoof. This can damage the lamellar connection. In some cases the overloaded foot, that has now become laminitic, will cause so much pain that the horse will start loading the leg with the initial problem again to unload the laminitic foot. This may create the false illusion that the leg with the primary problem has improved.

> Scientific data, knowledge and progress with regard to this theory lag behind those of the other theories. This is because it is difficult to reproduce traumatic laminitis for a scientific study in a humane way. It is not ethically acceptable to mechanically overload a horse's hooves to that extent, for research purposes.

Conventional treatment

Based on this theory, treatment of laminitis aims to reduce the overload. In case of a problem somewhere else in the body, the main focus is on treating that issue and pain medication. Box rest is often prescribed but will only make laminitis worse. If the horse is able to move freely, circulation is at least stimulated in the healthy legs. Obviously there are situations where box rest is inevitable to recover from the primary problem. Consult your veterinarian about how to keep the period of box rest to a minimum.

A form of overload, fortunately, long gone

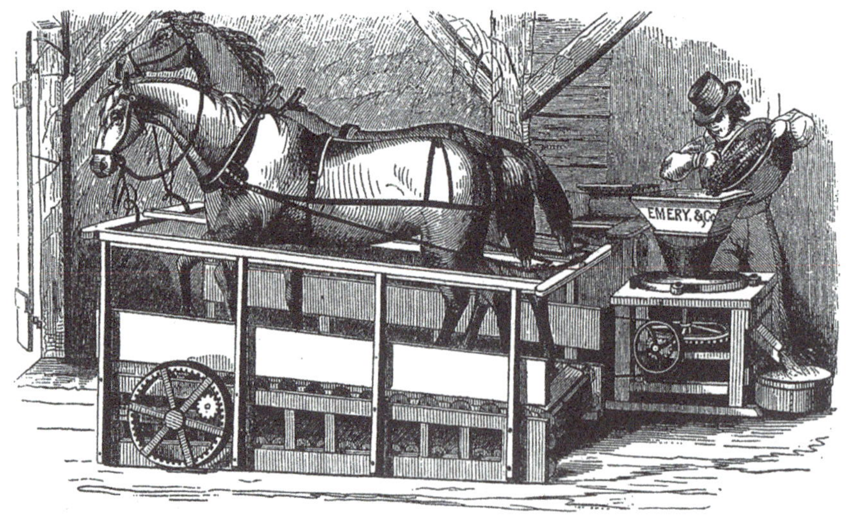

CAUSES

Primary cause

Now we know the different theories we will look at specific causes. Laminitis is hardly ever the result of one cause, but often a main culprit can be identified. However, the elimination of just this primary cause will often not be effective when all the other (unnatural) aspects and (partial) causes remain unchanged.

Unfortunately, there are still care providers who focus on their specific solution without looking at the entire problem. Like the veterinarian that prescribe analgesic, anticoagulation and anti-inflammatory drugs to a horse that remains stabled 23 hours a day and gets fed a bucket of concentrates twice a day.

Facilitative causes

Sometimes causes have been stacking up over a long period of time. Adding a new (partial) cause can tip the balance towards the wrong side. This (partial) cause could facilitate laminitis. That is the reason why we speak of facilitative causes.

For example, a horse with chronic liver disease, such as hepatitis, or liver damage caused by piroplasmosis (see page 97) is more likely to have an adverse reaction to toxins than a horse with a healthy liver. When the existence of liver disease is unknown it is easy to conclude that the resulting laminitis was caused by a poison. For example, a worm treatment is blamed, while it is just a facilitative cause. This often complicates treatment because the owner and care providers focus on the wrong cause.

Facilitative causes are divided into:

- Digestive problems
- Circulatory problems
- Toxins
- Hormonal problems
- Glucose problems
- Stress
- Hyperlipidemia
- Tick-borne diseases
- Genetic abnormalities

DIGESTIVE PROBLEMS

Usually digestive problems are related to one or more of the following aspects:

- Bacteria in the digestive tract
- ESC and starch
- Damage to the intestinal wall
- Ammonia and ammonia compounds

Bacteria in the digestive system

The large intestine (or colon) plays a crucial role in digestion. A good bacterial balance and a healthy gut are essential requirements. An excessive supply of NSC causes acidification of the colon.

Acidosis

A horse is a grazer-browser that normally eats for about 18 hours a day. The NSC enter the digestive system at regular intervals, without hardly any surges.

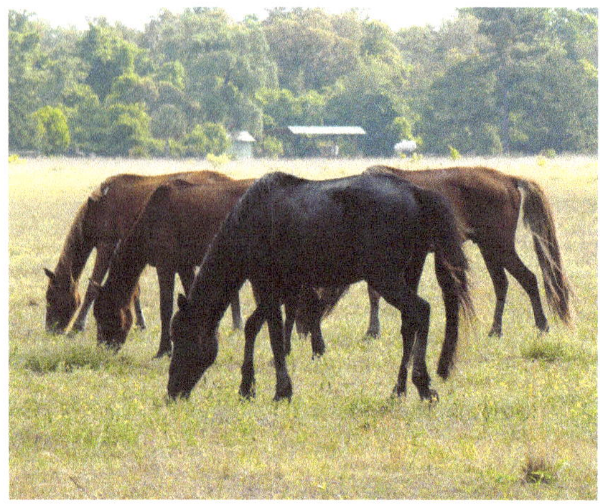

A horse is a grazer-browser
(photo: Rebekah Wallace)

Food containing high levels of NSC cannot be sufficiently digested by the horse, due to the absence of sufficient enzymes and a lack of absorption capacity by the small intestine. The undigested NSC enter the large intestine and the bacteria in there multiply rapidly to ensure predigestion. This multiplication causes the formation of lactic acid and therefore a decrease in the pH level (increase of acidity) of the large intestine.

At a pH level of five or lower the most important gram-negative bacteria and the cellulose-processing single celled microbes are destroyed. Toxins and genetic material are released: endotoxins, exotoxins, and DNA of the single celled microbes.

> pH
>
> The pH is a measure of the acidity. The more acidic the environment, the lower the pH.

Low pH levels damage the intestinal mucus layer and the intestinal wall itself. The harmful germs, yeasts and fungi that dominate the resulting imbalanced intestinal flora also contribute to the damage of the intestinal wall.

Microthromboses

Excessive amounts of endotoxins can cause blood clotting inside blood vessels (microthromboses) and result in a reduced blood flow to the hooves.

> ➤ The increased concentration of endotoxins can be reduced by administering drugs. But this does not prevent laminitis from occurring.

Bacteria and lactic acid

The amount of so-called gram-positive bacteria (Streptococcus lutetiensis) and lactic acid bacilli increase enormously. As discussed before under 'Enzyme theory', a link seems to exist between the Streptococcus lutetiensis and the occurrence of laminitis

> ➤ The higher the fibre content, for example in coarse hay, the slower the process of digestion. The slower the digestion, the less carbohydrates pose a risk. Obviously this only applies if all other circumstances are in order.

Water-soluble carbohydrates (WSC)

WSC concentrations (ESC and fructans) in grass change throughout the day and throughout the year. They depend on the amount of sunlight and its intensity, the temperature, availability of water and nutrients (natural or artificial) and growth stage of the plant.

Photosynthesis

Photosynthesis is a biochemical process in plants that takes place under the influence of daylight, converting water and carbon dioxide into oxygen and sugars.

Cellular respiration

The reverse of photosynthesis is a process called cellular respiration which occurs at night, in the absence of light. The plant then uses the sugar produced during the day to grow. Therefore grass has a lower sugar level early in the morning.

Stressed grass

When growing conditions are good (sunny, 5 °C/40 °F or more, sufficient water and nutrients) the plant uses WSC for growth. When one or more growth factors are insufficient, respiration will stop earlier than photosynthesis. Consequently, the plant's WSC levels will increase. At that stage, grass is referred to as stressed. Sunny days combined with night frost will cause grass to become stressed. Abundant sunlight combined with low day temperatures or insufficient nutrients also creates stressed grass.

Fructans

Fructan is a type of WSC that has received a lot of attention in recent years. Fructans are water-soluble, non-structural carbohydrates that belong to the group of fructose-containing composite sugars.

If more sugar is available than needed for growth, C3 grasses (see sidebar 'C3 and C4 grasses and starch' on page 72) store it as fructan to use for growth when conditions have improved. All major growth factors, such as appropriate temperature and sufficient water and nutrients need to be available. In short, when grass is stressed fructan is stored.

Antifreeze

Besides this, fructans are produced by grass as a kind of antifreeze. When the temperature is below -10 °C (14 °F) fructans are converted into sugar. Because sugar water freezes at lower temperatures than pure water, the plant will be better protected against frost. The conversion of fructans into sugar and vice versa can take place continuously throughout the day.

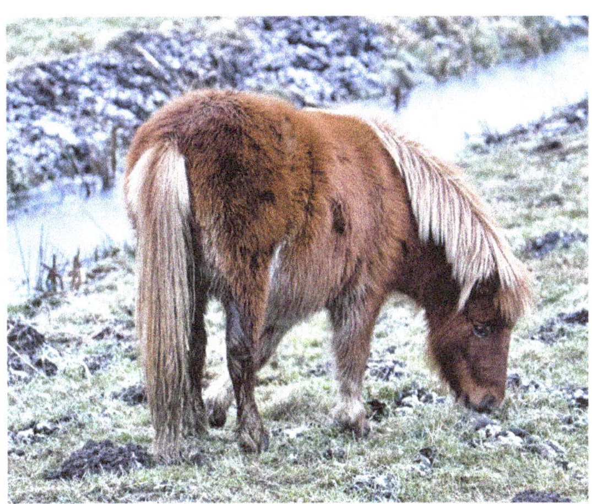

Fructan acts as antifreeze
(photo: Matthias Zomer)

Early in the year, when the days are getting longer and sunlight hours increase, it is often still frosty at night. Grass with a high fructan content will already begin to grow. This is one of the reasons (in addition to high nutritional value, palatability, and rapid growth) why this

C3 AND C4 GRASSES AND STARCH

Grass species can be divided into two groups: C3 grasses that thrive especially in colder climates and seasons and C4 grasses that grow well in hot, humid climates and seasons. This classification is based on the different ways photosynthesis takes place in these types of grass. C4 grasses need more light and warmth to transform atmospheric carbon dioxide into organic compounds and are therefore better adapted to warmer climates and seasons. More differences are found in water requirements, frost sensitivity, nutritional value and yield of the grass.

Stems and leaves of C3 grasses contain hardly any starch. Only when C3 grass is in full bloom, the plant can contain up to 4% starch. The seeds of C3 grass plants do contain starch. C4 grasses usually do contain starch. Starch is the way C4 grasses temporarily store excess sugar, the same way C3 grasses use fructans as a means of storage. However, starch content in C4 stems and leaves is low. Most starch in C4 grass can be found in the seeds, just like in C3 grass.

In Europe, pasture predominantly or entirely consists of C3 grasses such as timothy grass, brome grass and orchard grass. In America, Australia and New Zealand both C3 and C4 grasses grow, but also in these countries C3 grasses are the majority. Sometimes C4 grasses such as sorghum and sudan grass are added to existing pasture.

It is tempting to suggest that starch concentration in grass from these continents may be higher. However, differences in starch concentrations largely depend on the amount of seed a grass sample contains.

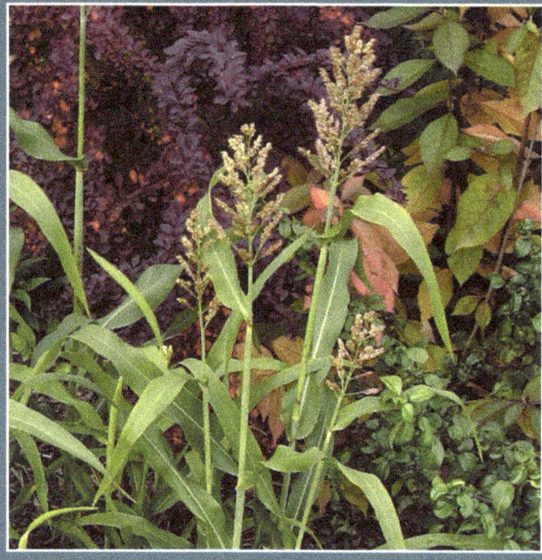

Sorghum
(photo: Michael Kesl)

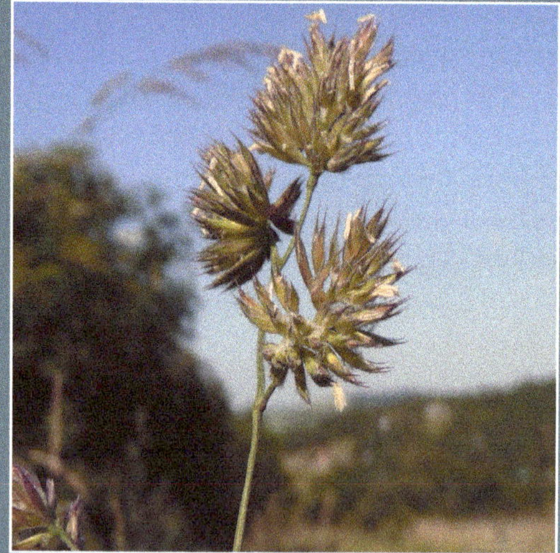

Sudan grass
(photo: Pavel Šinkyrík)

grass is cultivated. Nowadays grass is being genetically engineered to generate even higher fructan levels. Also during fall, when frost returns and the sun shines during the day, the risk of high fructan levels increases. On average, the months of April, May, October and November, are the months when grass contains the highest fructan levels.

Objections

Despite all the available information about fructans, their role in the development of laminitis is still not entirely clear. The importance attached to that role has decreased in recent years and scientific evidence is being questioned as well. The research that indicated that fructans can cause acute laminitis used a different type of fructan than naturally occurs in grass. This type of fructan, an oligofructose called raftilose, has a very short chain length, and thus a low degree of polymerisation (see sidebar). Also the dosage used was so high that it is highly unlikely a horse would be able to consume such a quantity while grazing. Furthermore, the total dose of fructan was inserted at once into the stomach by a hose. The resulting acidification of the colon would probably not occur in a horse that consumed the same amount of fructans gradually while grazing for 24 hours. In all honesty it needs to be said that the researchers would not deny this as research often magnifies examined causes to test hypotheses.

In raftilose induced laminitis clinical signs occurred that are attributed to SIRS such as fever, diarrhoea, infiltration of white blood cells and other changes in blood values. However, in the majority of horses that become laminitic after grazing this is not the case.

DEGREE OF POLYMERISATION AND ACIDOSIS

Carbohydrates consist of one or more sugar molecules. Several sugar molecules joined together form a chain. The chain length differs for each type of carbohydrate. Simple and double sugars are examples of carbohydrates with a so-called short chain length. Fructans and complex sugars have a greater chain length. Chain length can be expressed as the degree of polymerisation. Different fructan types have various degrees of polymerisation. The lower the degree of polymerisation, the more lactic acid it causes in the hind gut. Therefore some grass species are more harmful to laminitic horse than others. For example, degree of polymerisation of brome grass is ten times lower than that of timothy grass.

What fructan does

The current hypothesis is that it is unlikely that a healthy horse would get acute laminitis by grazing on a spring or autumn morning in a meadow with high fructan levels. However, a large amount of fructans can give the final push to an already insulin-resistant horse. If a horse gets laminitis for the first time under these circumstances it would be a good reason to have it tested for PPID and EMS. Both syndromes have insulin resistance as an important characteristic.

In addition, PPID horses have higher levels of the hormone ACTH in late summer and early autumn. This causes larger quantities of the hormone cortisol to be released, which results in fats and proteins being converted into glucose more rapidly. This glucose, combined with the increased fructan supply, elevates blood sugar levels. The pancreas will then release more insulin. As you now know this could mean serious trouble for the insulin-resistant horse. (Both EMS and PPID will be discussed extensively, later in this book.)

Insulin resistance

Do not forget that a high fructan diet can eventually cause or worsen insulin resistance. Avoiding high levels of all NSC in the diet remains important in the fight against laminitis.

> For a long time the overconsumption of proteins was thought to be the main problem. Excess protein however is broken down and disposed of via urine. It is true that ammonia is then released, which increases the acidity of the intestines. This causes the liver and kidney to overload and disturbs the bacterial culture in the large intestine. But protein is certainly not a main cause.

ESC and starch

ESC and starch play a role in causing laminitis early in the digestive process, in the small intestine. Glucose is one of the ESC that is responsible for causing hyperinsulinemia. In the small intestine starch is converted to glucose as well, therefore contributing to this effect.

Incretins and hyperinsulinemia

In the gastrointestinal tract, specialised cells secrete incretins after the ingestion of food. Two important incretins are GIP and GLP-1:

- GIP stands for glucose-dependent insulinotropic polypeptide
- GLP-1 stands for glucagon-like peptide-1

These hormones are produced in the small intestine shortly after the intake of ESC, starch, proteins and fats. They cause the pancreas to secrete more insulin. This prevents blood sugar levels rising too much. As you have read earlier in this chapter, increased insulin levels are undesirable and harmful, especially for insulin-resistant horses. They can cause laminitis or worsen the condition. This type of laminitis is called pasture-associated laminitis.

Why some horses are more prone to increased insulin levels than in others is not exactly known. The reason might be found in the genetic make-up of different animals.

Damage of the intestinal wall

A damaged intestinal wall makes it easier for the MMP triggers to enter the bloodstream. As discussed in the previous section, the intestinal wall may become damaged by acidification. Other possible causes of damage:

- Salmonella bacteria stimulate the intestine to create the protein zonulin. Zonulin prevents the cells of the intestinal wall lining from attaching properly to each other.
- Gluten stimulate the production of zonulin as well. This is another reason not to feed grain to your horse.

NSC AND THEIR EFFECTS

ESC and starch	Fructans
Digestion in the small intestine	Digestion mainly in the hind gut
Surplus causes hyperinsulinemia	Surplus causes, along with undigested ESC and starch coming from the small intestine, hind gut acidosis and death of large numbers of micro organisms
Related to a hormonal problem	Related to a digestive problem
Possible results: • Insulin resistance • Hyperglycemia • Vasoconstriction • Damage to the blood vessels • Increased blood pressure • Poor circulation of hoof tissue • Microthromboses • Oxygen deficiency in hoof tissue • Impaired glucose metabolism • Destruction of hemidesmosomes • Chronic inflammation • Increased fat storage	Possible results: • Endotoxins, exotoxins and DNA are released • Proliferation of bacteria, yeasts and fungi • Intestinal wall damage • Microthromboses • Poor circulation of hoof tissue

- Enteroviruses that live in the gastrointestinal tract and faeces can cause various diseases in horses. One of their signs is damage of the intestinal wall.
- A significant inflammation of the intestines could potentially cause intestinal perforation.
- Colic. A twisted colon causes blood flow to the bowel wall to stagnate. The quality of the wall deteriorates allowing toxins to pass through more easily.
- Gram-positive bacteria produce certain proteins (exotoxins) that cause harm to the body. The intestinal wall gets 'burned' and can no longer prevent lactic acid and toxins entering into the bloodstream. This can already take place as early as 24 hours after an excessive intake of NSC. A classic example is the horse that manages to get access to the feed bin or a Shetland pony living under an apple tree. Lush green meadows are a problem as well. The horse

hardly moves while eating. It is literally standing ankle deep in its food. Another common example is the horse that has only eaten grass and hay from spring to autumn. Suddenly, when winter arrives, his diet changes to grains, concentrates and cereals. Some owners feed their horses these products with the best intentions, worrying their horse has or will get deficiencies.

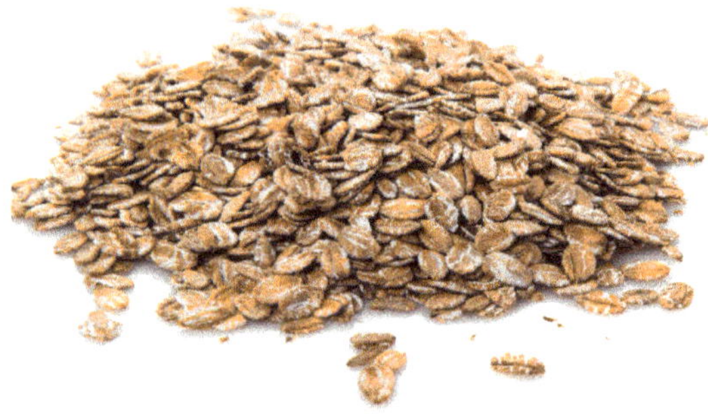

Ammonia compounds

Out of boredom or in need of more crude fibre some horses eat sawdust or straw in their stable. This raw fibre consists mainly of cellulose but also hemicellulose and lignin, the three types of so-called structural carbohydrates. When large quantities of sawdust or straw are digested ammonia compounds are formed that can overload the liver. A horse that has been turned out in spring and summer and then stabled again in autumn will suffer from a disturbed bacterial balance in the intestines when it suddenly starts eating straw. This is one of the many reasons not to stable a horse.

Surface or bore water may also contain too many ammonia compounds (see more on page 179 under 'Drinking water').

CIRCULATORY PROBLEMS

The lamellae have a continuous need for good circulation. Blood flow allows for the delivery of oxygenated blood, nutrients, and hormones on one hand and the removal of carbonated blood and waste products on the other.

Circulatory problems can be a result of:

- High pressure in the hoof that pinches off the blood supply. For example caused by a swelling due to inflammation.
- Sudden diet change that affects the intestinal flora and causes a massive bacterial death. With this death toxins are released from the intestines into the bloodstream where they cause microthromboses that get stuck in the capillaries of the hoof dermis. These clots are called endotoxin microthromboses. A sudden diet change can also be the drinking of *too much* water and not *too cold* water, as is often suggested.
- Damaged capillaries caused by overactive enzymes.
- (Heat) exhaustion can result in circulatory problems and cause high concentrations of lactic acid to disrupt the bacterial balance in the intestines. Metabolism and mineral balance are under pressure in the exhausted body.
- Shock
- Low blood pressure, for example caused by general anaesthesia
- Immune thrombocytopenia. This is an abnormal immunological reaction that is mainly found in young horses and often after the occurrence of strangles or a respiratory infection. It causes the inflammation of blood vessel walls.
- The breakdown of red blood cells
- Coagulation diseases

- Some types of drugs have a vasoconstrictive side effect. For example the drug Prostaglandin, administered to mares in order to bring on oestrus. Corticosteroids are also known for disturbing the blood circulation.

TOXINS

The following toxins can be distinguished:

- Bacterial toxins
- Non-bacterial toxins
- Poisonous plants
- Contamination and chemical toxins
- Drugs
- Endogenous toxins
- Muscle pigments

BACTERIAL TOXINS

What we discussed about the death of bacteria in the intestines is also true for bacterial toxins originating from other parts of the body. In the same way influenza, pneumonia and pleurisy, sometimes caught during transportation, may result in laminitis as a complication.

Also mastitis (udder inflammation), endometritis (inflammation of the lining of the uterus) or placenta retention after foaling may produce a similar complication.

Sepsis, fever and allergy all cause increased toxin levels in the body. Again, this will not cause laminitis by itself but may contribute to its occurrence.

NON-BACTERIAL TOXINS

Moulds, fungi and yeasts release mycotoxins. These are toxic by-products. Food can be contaminated by improper storage or already be contaminated during cultivation. For example in rye and wheat this could be the case, although chances are minimised by the use of disinfected seed.

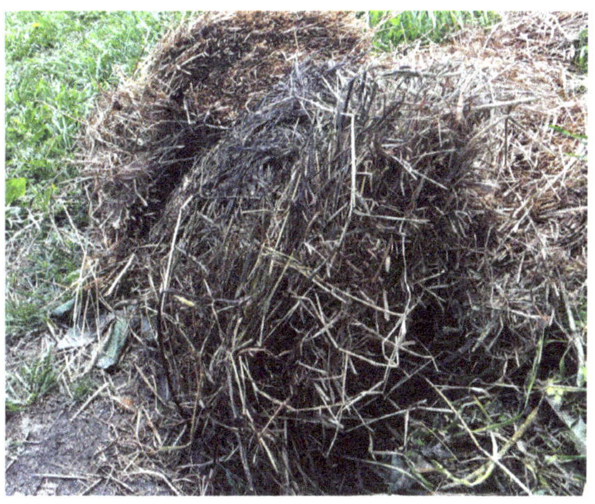

Mouldy hay bale
(photo: Kate Light)

ENDOPHYTE

Rye grass and fescue grass may be contaminated with an endophyte (symbiotic fungus), that protects the plant against insects, but releases a mycotoxin that is associated with laminitis.
In times of stress, illness or excitement blood vessels constrict under influence of this toxin. The risk of endophyte contamination is higher in soil that contains high levels of potassium (see sidebar 'Potassium' on page 193).

For lawns and sports fields these types of grass are often used because of their resistance to insect damage. Horses could ingest these toxins when fed their clippings.

Silage

Grass silage gets mouldy very easily. A bale of silage needs to be finished within a week. After that, especially when temperatures are high, the risk of mould is too high. Mouldy silage should absolutely be discarded. Sometimes condensation is visible in places where bales have been touching each other. If the plastic is still intact, the part that has been exposed to moisture can be removed. The rest of the bale is still usable.

> Even when fungi are not visible they can definitely still be present.

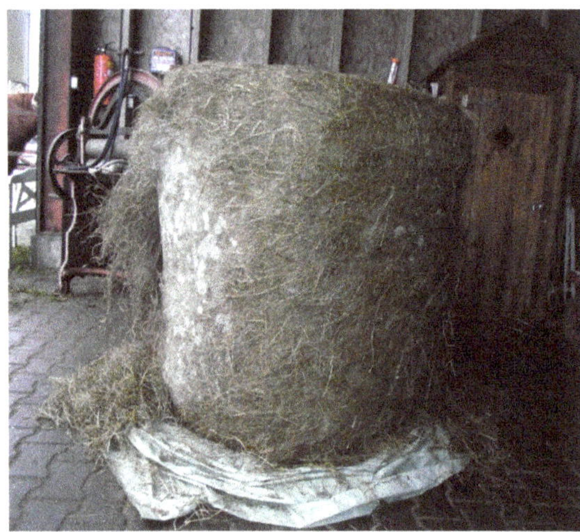

Mouldy grass silage

Poisonous plants

Toxins in plants can damage the body or cause disorders that could facilitate laminitis. For example beechnuts, green acorns and oak bark contain high levels of tannic acid (tannin). Ingestion of large quantities may cause damage to the intestinal wall and overload the liver and kidneys.

Also sawdust of black walnut and butternut, sometimes used as stable bedding, contains a toxin, that is probably absorbed through the skin.

Contamination and chemical toxins

Contaminated water

Both surface water, pumped groundwater (bore or well water) and rainwater can be contaminated. Besides contamination with heavy metals, levels of nitrite, nitrate, ammonia compounds, iron or salt can be above acceptable limits as well (see further on page 179 under 'Drinking water').

Pesticides, fungicides and herbicides

Pesticides, fungicides and herbicides may be present in non-organic feed (grass, hay, hard feed), nutritional supplements, stable bedding, groundwater and surface water.

Fertilisers:

Artificial fertiliser that has not broken down yet can be ingested by the horse when grazing. Horses have no problems with residual nitrogen in grass or hay. However, if the content rises very quickly, it affects metabolism. The liver suffers, resulting in high concentrations of toxins. A rapid increase of nitrogen can be caused by:

- A growth spurt in spring
- Fertilising
- Lots of clover in the pasture, especially on calcareous clay soils.

Drugs

The administration of certain types of drugs have been linked to the incidence of laminitis, although this risk seems to be low. Exceptions are long-acting corticosteroids.

The next chapter explores the use of drugs. We will limit ourselves here to drugs that can contribute to the development or worsening of laminitis. These are:

- Corticosteroids
- Vaccinations
- Anthelmintic drugs
- Analgesic drugs

Corticosteroids

Corticosteroids are chemical versions of cortisol. They are used to fight inflammation and infection. Just like cortisol, which is produced by the body under stress, it increases blood sugar levels because corticosteroids reduce insulin sensitivity. If this takes place over a longer period it can lead to or contribute to insulin resistance.

Apoptosis

A second effect of corticosteroids is so-called apoptosis. Normally this is programmed cell death or the death of cells that exhibit an abnormality. Apoptosis is considered suicide of cells. Corticosteroids may force the occurrence of apoptosis and thereby contribute to a weakening of the basement membrane.

Catabolism

Besides this, corticosteroids trigger a process called catabolism. This is a type of metabolism in which body tissue is broken down, in particular proteins derived from connective tissue, for use elsewhere in the body. The basement membrane is weakened by this process.

Vasoconstriction

Finally, corticosteroids have a vasoconstrictive effect. By now we know how vasoconstriction contributes to the onset of laminitis. Corticosteroids are a good example of a facilitative cause. They will never cause laminitis out of the blue but a horse that is teetering on the brink of insulin resistance could get the last push in the wrong direction by the administration of corticosteroids. Unfortunately horses with navicular syndrome are sometimes injected with the corticosteroid triamcinolone into the coffin joints, which results in a higher sensitivity to laminitis.

Corticosteroids are sometimes given to prevent SSRD (summer seasonal recurrent dermatitis or 'sweet itch').

In cases where corticosteroids cannot be avoided, it is best to administer them in the morning. The day-night rhythm of the body's cortisol is then the least disturbed.

Vaccinations

A healthy horse in healthy living conditions has enough antibodies to resist diseases. Consider only vaccinating against tetanus. Inform yourself well about this controversial issue.

> Chronically laminitic horses can develop stronger allergic reactions than healthy horses. This may also be the case with reactions to vaccinations that could lead to more pronounced clinical signs of laminitis.

Anthelmintic drugs (worm treatment)

A healthy horse in healthy living conditions is able to resist parasites quite well. Only use wormers to treat against parasites that are actually present. Have manure samples tested for worms at regular intervals.

> ➤ Laminitis caused or facilitated by worm treatment is extremely rare.

Analgesic drugs

Analgesic drugs (painkillers) mask the pain of inflammation, making horses move more or differently than is good for them. The lamellar connection is already affected and will get damaged more by overload, especially combined with an inadequate trim. Analgesic drugs burden the liver and kidneys.

Endogenous toxins (produced by the body)

A normal metabolism releases toxins which are broken down by the kidneys. A reduced renal function, for example as a result of a chronic kidney inflammation (nephritis), causes toxins to stay present in the body longer than is healthy. The toxins could then facilitate the occurrence of laminitis.

Muscle pigments

The muscle spasms or cramps of exertional myopathies like ER (equine exertional rhabdomyolysis, tying up), AM (atypical myoglobinuria, Monday disease) or PSSM (polysaccharide storage myopathy) can damage muscle cells. As a result, the muscle cells release their muscle pigments (proteins). This can cause kidney damage. The pain and stress caused by exertional myopathies and the resulting increase in cortisol levels in their turn contribute to an increased risk of laminitis. The effect of stress will be discussed later in this book.

HORMONAL PROBLEMS

The most important hormonal problems that are associated with laminitis are:

- Equine Metabolic Syndrome
- Malfunction of the pituitary gland or adrenal glands
- Winter laminitis
- High oestrogen concentrations
- High IGF-1 concentrations

Endocrinopathic laminitis

Laminitis that occurs as a result of hormonal problems is called endocrinopathic laminitis (endocrine = related to the release of hormones into the bloodstream, pathos = suffering). We also use this term when the administration of long-acting corticosteroids (see page 79) is the main cause of laminitis. It is also simply referred to as hormone-related laminitis.

Research of case histories in a large veterinary clinic showed that about 80% of all laminitis cases could be linked to hormonal problems.

Equine Metabolic Syndrome

Type 2 diabetes in humans is an incurable metabolic disorder in which blood sugar levels are repeatedly elevated. Because the body does not respond well to the presence of insulin, not enough energy from sugar can be utilised. Equine Metabolic Syndrome (EMS) is the equine variety of this disease.

Clinical signs

- Insulin resistance with an increased risk of laminitis
- Difficulties with weight regulation
  - Overweight (obesity)
  - Sometimes underweight
- Abnormal fat deposits (adiposity)
  - Cresty neck: CNS>3 (see sidebar)
  - Behind the shoulders, over the rump, above the tail implant and in the area of the sheath or udder
- Increased blood pressure
- Abnormalities in the fat levels of the blood
- Increased levels of leptin in the blood.
  - Leptin plays a role in the regulation of appetite. Elevated leptin without elevated insulin levels can be seen as a warning sign. There is a real chance that the horse will develop EMS. Leptin will be discussed later in this book.
- Blood sugar levels are elevated but remain just within acceptable range
- Sometimes slight tying up
- General listlessness.

Complications

- Damage to blood vessels
- Thrombosis
- Oxidative stress
- The fat tissue itself may become infected which releases toxins as well
- Reduced fertility

Thyroid gland

For a long time clinical signs were attributed to decreased thyroid function. Increased production of endogenous glucocorticoids (steroids) disturbs the function of the pituitary gland which influences the thyroid gland in a negative way. However, the thyroid gland itself is working correctly.

CRESTY NECK SCORE (CNS)

1. No palpable crest.
2. No visual appearance of a crest, but slight filling felt with palpation.
3. Noticeable appearance of a crest that can easily be bent with one hand. Fat evenly deposited from poll to withers.
4. Crest enlarged and thickened, more difficult to move from side to side. The crest has a mounded appearance.
5. Crest grossly enlarged and thickened and can no longer be cupped in one hand or bent from side to side. Crest may have wrinkles or creases perpendicular to the topline.
6. Crest is so large it permanently droops to one side.

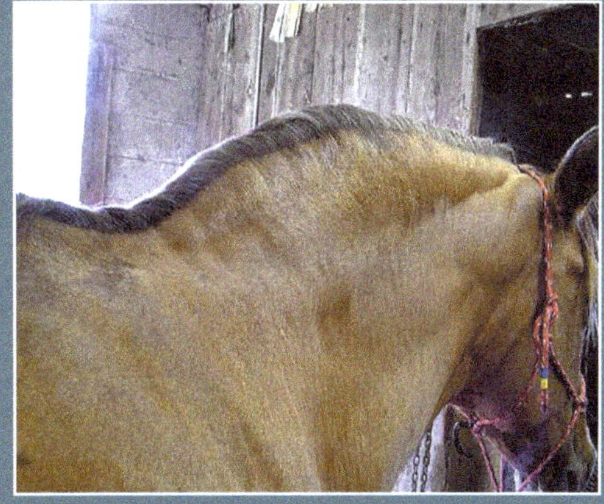

A cresty neck score of 5
(photo: Gretschen Fathauer)

Adipokines

Fat tissue acts similarly to glands, releasing substances which play a role in the immune system. These substances are called adipokines. Some stimulate the onset of inflammation, as inflammation is necessary to ward off foreign bodies. Unfortunately these adipokines reduce insulin sensitivity as well, acting as vasoconstrictors and causing damage to blood vessels.

Adipokines are cell signaling proteins that are activated by receptors on the cell wall. Subsequently they take care of the communication within the cell.

The production of adipokines is disturbed in horses with obesity or adiposity. Fatty tissue of a cresty neck produces more adipokines than subcutaneous fat. Adiposity is a worse sign than regular obesity.

Leptin

An important adipokine is the peptide hormone leptin. Leptin is transported via the blood to the brain where it connects to leptin receptors on the cell walls of the hypothalamus. Lots of fat cells in the body mean high levels of leptin. Subsequently the hypothalamus induces a decrease of the food supply and an increased metabolic rate. Vice versa, when little leptin connects to the receptors, a message will be given that more food needs to be eaten to maintain a stable body weight and metabolic rate is slowed down. In this way leptin monitors the balance between hunger and satiety.

Leptin resistance

The more body fat a horse has, the more leptin is circulating in the blood. When leptin levels remain high for a long time, leptin receptors will become less sensitive to the hormone. In this state, which is called leptin resistance, leptin still circulates in the blood, but the hypothalamus no longer responds adequately to it. The horse then eats more than it can utilise. This results in (aggravation of) obesity, as well as adiposity and insulin resistance.

Research on rats shows that a long-term high intake of fructose can lead to leptin resistance. The rats that were given food with a higher content of fructose but the same amount of energy became leptin-resistant.

Leptin levels in stallions and geldings are higher than in mares. This is notable since leptin levels in humans are higher in women. In addition, in summer leptin levels are higher than in winter.

Adiponectin

Adiponectin is another type of adipokine. This hormone enhances the insulin sensitivity of the body. It is one of the hormones that is responsible for keeping blood sugar at the right levels. Obese horses secrete less adiponectin. This contributes to the worsening of insulin resistance or its occurrence. A vicious circle occurs when insulin-resistant horses have to deal with lower adiponectin levels as well. Besides this, adiponectin seems to suppress oxidative stress and inflammation.

> **Oxidative stress**
> Cell damage caused by excess reactive oxygen compounds.

BODY CONDITION SCORE (BCS)

	NECK	WITHERS	BACK AND LOIN	RIBS	HIND QUARTERS
1. VERY THIN	Bone structure easily felt. No muscle shelf where neck meets shoulder.	Bone structure easily felt	Three points of vertebrae easily felt	Each rib can be easily felt	Tailhead and bones projecting
2. THIN	Bone structure can be felt. Slight muscle shelf where neck meets shoulder.	Bone structure can be felt	Top point of the spine can be easily felt	Slight fat covering but can still be felt	Hip bones can be felt
3. FAIR	Fat covering bone structure	Fat deposits over wither	Fat covering the spine	Can't see ribs, but ribs can still be felt	Hip bones covered with fat
4. GOOD	Neck flows smoothly into shoulder	Neck rounds out withers	Back is level	Layer of fat over the ribs	Can't feel hip bones
5. FAT	Fat deposits along neck	Fat padded around withers	Positive crease along the back	Spongy fat over and in between ribs	Can't feel hip bones
6. VERY FAT	Bulging fat	Bulging fat	Deep positive crease	Pockets of fat	Pockets of fat

CAUSES

- Hereditary. Appaloosas, Welsh, Exmoor, New Forest and Shetland ponies, cobs, Icelandic horses and certain bloodlines in other breeds. In some horses the hereditary component makes it very difficult, sometimes impossible, to keep the weight under control with diet and exercise.
- Prolonged and regular high blood sugar levels caused by a diet with too much WSC, like grains and concentrates.
- Insufficient exercise.

DIAGNOSIS

- History of the horse.
- Physical examination including cresty neck score (CNS) and body condition score (BCS, see sidebar).

> Originally the BCS was developed for quarter horses. In assessing other breeds, especially pony breeds, some flexibility should be maintained. For donkeys a modified BCS has been created (see sidebar 'Body condition score - Donkeys' on page 202).

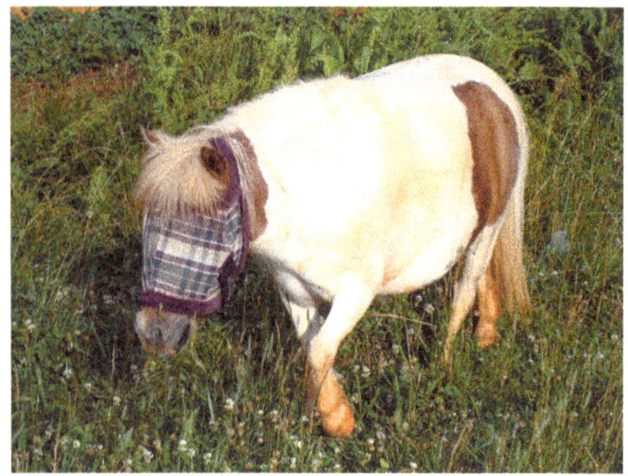

A body condition score of 5
(photo: Liz Jaynes)

- Insulin testing. A single reading is unreliable. 'Dynamic' testing is preferable.
- During stress or when in pain, for example caused by laminitis, horses produce more cortisol and catecholamines (the hormones epinephrine, norepinephrine and dopamine), which influence the test results. Wait until pain has decreased before taking the test.
- Leptin blood test. A test to measure the level of the appetite regulating protein leptin.
- Glucose tolerance test. This test determines if hormonal problems occur in the processing of sugar by the body. The value of these test results is limited.

Treatment

Addressing EMS is a good example of treating the primary cause of laminitis.

- Dietary modifications. Keep an eye on NSC levels of grass when horses are grazing on pasture (see more on page 187 under 'NSC prevention'). Do not feed concentrates or grains. Do not feed in portions, this makes the blood sugar levels spike.
- Modifications in movement.
- Modifications in housing. Allow horses to move 24 hours a day, 7 days a week to make them burn calories.
- Fatty acids. Omega-3 fatty acids and vitamin A and D can have a beneficial effect.
- Minerals. Chromium, vanadium and magnesium have been said to have a beneficial effect because they are suspected to be able to increase the sensitivity of muscle cells to insulin.

> ➤ There is no clear scientific evidence for this, other than from human medicine or research on rats. The only relevant scientific research on this subject actually shows that these minerals do *not* have this effect. However, there is so much anecdotal evidence that they will still receive attention in this book.

- Drugs and hormones. Some drugs and synthetic hormones can have a beneficial effect. We will discuss these later.
- Minimising exposure to toxins. Breaking down toxins (discussed on page 77) burdens the liver. Because of this it will be less able to break down insulin. Therefore make sure to minimise toxins in the body.

Malfunction of the pituitary gland or adrenal glands

The terms PPID, Cushing's disease and Cushing's syndrome are often confused or used interchangeably. However, these are three different problems, one of which hardly ever even occurs in horses.

Cushing's disease

The pituitary gland is a small gland at the bottom of the brain that secretes stimulating hormones. These hormones control the action of hormone glands elsewhere in the body. In Cushing's disease, described by Harvey Williams Cushing in 1912, a usually benign adenoma (tumour of glandular origin) is formed in the anterior lobe of the pituitary gland. This tissue secretes too much ACTH (corticotropin), which results in over-activity and enlargement of the adrenal glands, that secrete too much cortisol as a result.

The clinical signs of Cushing's disease are primarily attributed to the effect of elevated cortisol levels. In contrast to dogs and humans this disease hardly ever occurs in horses.

Cushing's syndrome

Cushing's syndrome was first described in 1943 by Fuller Albright. It is the umbrella term for all problems caused by prolonged exposure to excess cortisol in the blood. This excess can be the result of Cushing's disease, however, long-term administration of synthetic long-acting corticosteroids also increases cortisol levels in the blood. A tumour or other disorder of the adrenal glands could also be the cause, although these problems are very rare in horses.

Pituitary Pars Intermedia Dysfunction

PPID is short for Pituitary Pars Intermedia Dysfunction. This neurodegenerative disorder is markedly different from Cushing's disease. In PPID the intermediate lobe of the pituitary gland is enlarged. This causes an increased release of melanocortins. Melanocortins are a group of hormones that ACTH also belongs to. The ACTH that is released by the intermediate lobe is biologically less active than the ACTH secreted by the anterior lobe of the pituitary gland as in Cushing's disease. On average, only one third of PPID horses have overactive and enlarged adrenal glands due to increased ACTH.

The essential problem in PPID is the increased level of melanocortins circulating in the bloodstream. The specific clinical signs of PPID are partly attributed to this.

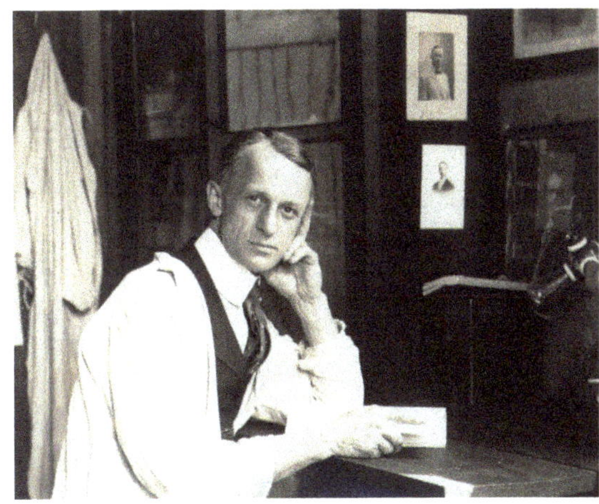

Harvey Williams Cushing

Cause of PPID

The hypothalamus is located directly above the pituitary gland. From this part of the brain dopamine producing nerves lead to the pituitary gland. This dopamine controls the production of melanocortins in the intermediate lobe of the pituitary gland. In PPID horses, the quantity of these nerves gradually decreases and therefore less dopamine is produced.

Because of the lack of adjustment or inhibition, production of melanocortins increases enormously. Over time, the intermediate lobe of the pituitary gland swells by the enlargement and multiplication of cells. Eventually one or more (usually benign) tumours may form. The pressure of the enlarged pituitary gland on the surrounding brain tissue causes some of the clinical signs of PPID as well.

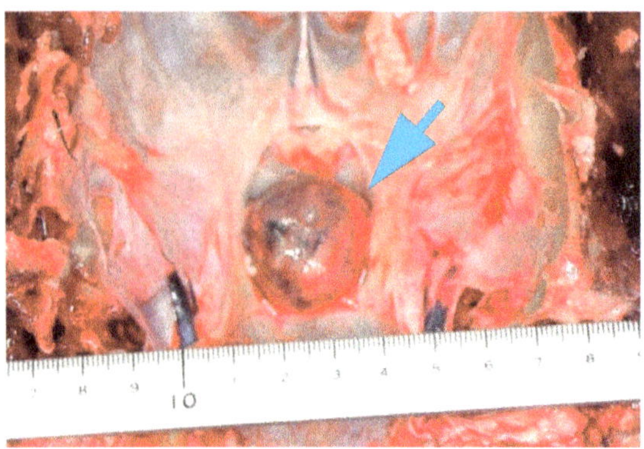

Enlarged pituitary gland
(photo: The Japanese society of equine science)

Neurodegradation

The cause of the nerve degeneration, or the degradation of dopamine-producing nerves is attributed to:

- Oxidative stress
- Toxins (see page 77)
- Stress (see page 95)
- EMS

Since some horses have a genetic predisposition to develop EMS, you could argue that, indirectly, there is a genetic predisposition to develop PPID. However, there is no scientific evidence yet for EMS being a cause.

Clinical signs

The clinical signs are:

- Abnormally thick curly hair (hypertrichosis)
- Difficulty shedding the winter coat
- Coat discolouration
- Excessive or too little sweating (hyperhidrosis or hypohidrosis, resp.)
- Excessive drinking (polydipsia) and urinating (polyuria, see sidebar 'Polyuria and polydipsia' on page 88)
- Adiposity, in particular fat deposits on the abdomen or above the eyes
- Weight loss
- General listlessness (apathy)
- Loss of stamina
- Decreased musculature
- Poor wound healing
- Milk production in unbred mares
- Irregular oestrus
- Infertility
- Swollen sheath (due to adiposity), often prior to a bout of laminitis
- Excessive smegma production
- Blindness
- Seizures
- Susceptibility to sole abscesses
- Disturbances of the immune system, infections. In particular, sinus inflammation (sinusitis) with yellowish, foul-smelling nasal discharge is common.
- Osteoporosis
- Dental problems
- Increases susceptibility to worm infestation, higher egg count in manure
- Hyperglycemia
- Insulin resistance with increased risk of laminitis
- Enlargement of the adrenal glands (adrenal hyperplasia)

HYPERTRICHOSIS OR HIRSUTISM?

Human medicine distinguishes between hypertrichosis and hirsutism. Both terms refer to a condition associated with excessive hair growth. Hirsutism is characterised by excessive hair growth in those parts of the body where hair normally is absent or minimal. In humans, hirsutism is usually caused by excess male hormones (androgens) or hair follicles that are oversensitive to these hormones. Hypertrichosis is characterised by increased hair growth in areas of skin that are normally already covered with hair. The condition is usually hereditary or caused by certain types of drugs.

Hirsutism is a clinical sign of Cushing's disease in humans. For a long time veterinary science did not distinguish between Cushing's disease and PPID so the term hirsutism was used for the clinical sign of excessive hair growth in horses.

The cause of excessive and abnormal hair growth in PPID horses is also hormonal, however not by problems with androgens but with cortisol. The typical discoloration of the hair that occurs in hypertrichosis is absent in hirsutism.

In recent years, excessive hair growth in PPID horses is preferably referred to as hypertrichosis.

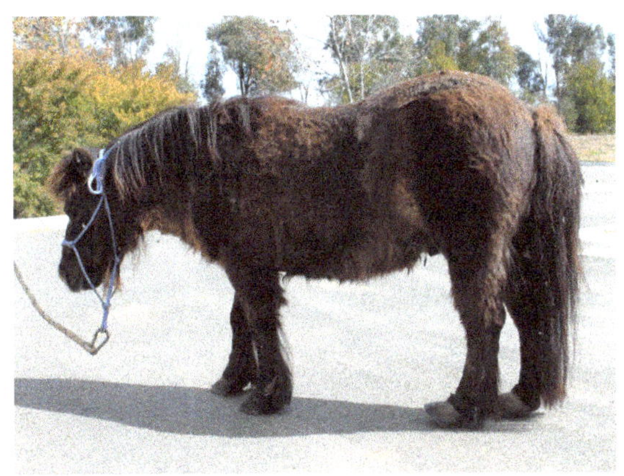

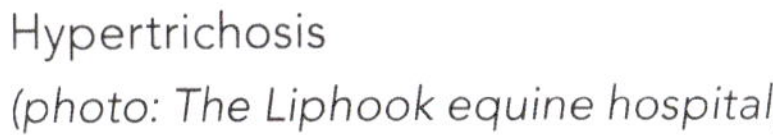

Hypertrichosis
(photo: The Liphook equine hospital)

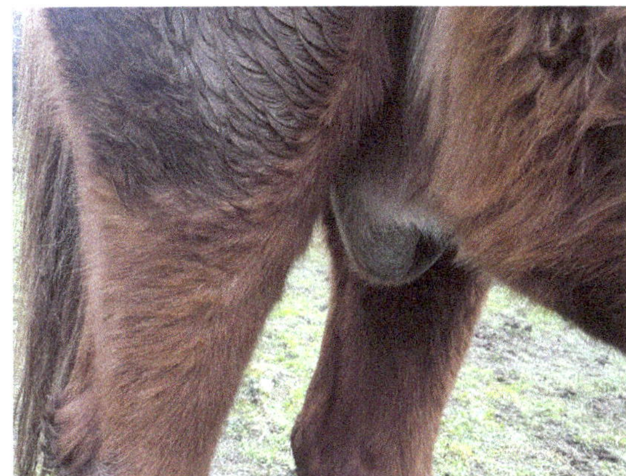

Swollen sheath

OSTEOPOROSIS AND PPID

Osteoporosis (and the precursor osteopenia) is decalcification of bone tissue that deteriorates the quality of the bone tissue. The risk of bone fractures increases. Osteoporosis can occur as a complication of PPID. Available figures indicate an increased risk for PPID horses being euthanised because of fractures of the ribs, jaws, coffin bones or pelvis.

Osteoporosis causes another problem: the surface of the coffin bone becomes smaller leaving less space for each individual lamella. The bonding surface between dermal and epidermal lamellae decreases and the quality of lamellar connection deteriorates. On page 47 under 'Shape and condition of the coffin bone' you can read more about problems of the coffin bone.

POLYURIA AND POLYDIPSIA

One of the consequences of insulin resistance is an increased level of glucose in the blood (hyperglycemia). Normally the kidneys are able to remove glucose from the pre-urine before it becomes urine. However, if the amount of glucose in the pre-urine is higher than the maximum absorption capacity of the kidneys (the renal threshold), glucose will end up in the urine. This phenomenon is called glycosuria. The glucose retains water, causing the horse to urinate more (polyuria) and as a result, drink more (polydipsia). Polyuria and polydipsia are clinical signs of PPID and EMS/insulin resistance.

The increased cortisol level that we can find in the blood of horses with PPID also has an inhibitory effect on the antidiuretic hormone (ADH). By stimulating water resorption by the kidneys, ADH ensures that less water ends up in the urine. An inhibition of ADH is therefore the second cause of polyuria in horses with PPID. Moreover, less ADH is produced. This is because the enlarged intermediate lobe of the pituitary gland presses on the part of the posterior lobe (pars posterior, neurohypophysis) where ADH is stored and from which it enters the bloodstream.

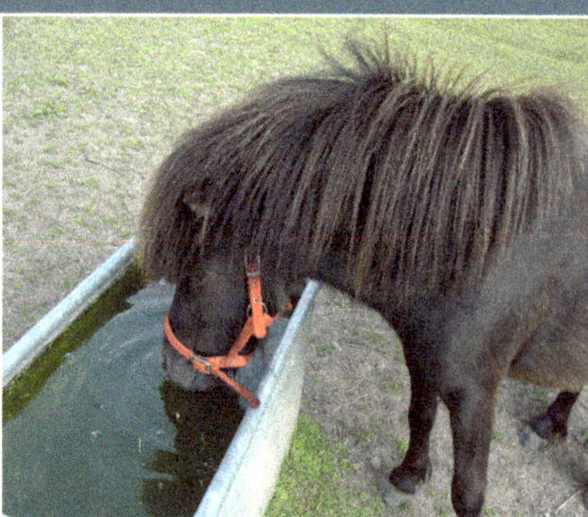

(photo: Triton barns)

CATABOLISM

Excess cortisol causes a process that is called catabolism. On page 79 you can read how the basement membrane is damaged by this process. It also causes other connective tissues to weaken as well, with chronic pain as result. Partly for this reason it can often be difficult to trim a horse with advanced PPID. They simply have too much pain to cooperate.

DIAGNOSIS

To diagnose PPID, veterinarians can perform a clinical examination, take blood tests or use MRI scans.

Clinical examination

Initially a diagnosis will be made by observing the clinical signs. In particular, hypertrichosis gives a clear indication, although hypertrichosis occurs at an advanced stage of the disease.

To diagnose the syndrome in an earlier stage is more difficult as the clinical signs are less clear. Unfortunately, this often hinders early intervention.

Blood tests

Besides clinical diagnosis the veterinarian has the following tests at his disposal:

- ACTH test
- Dexamethasone-suppression test (DST)
- TRH stimulation test
- Domperidone response test
- Glucose and insulin concentration test.

ACTH test

This test determines the quantity of ACTH in the blood. It should be noted that ACTH produced in the intermediate lobe of the pituitary gland is biologically less active than ACTH produced by the anterior lobe of a healthy pituitary gland. Therefore the test shows the quantity of ACTH but not its effectiveness. Some horses with high ACTH values do not develop PPID.

> Age should not be a factor in weighing the necessity to perform this test. Horses can have PPID as early as six years old.

Seasonal rise

From roughly July through November, ACTH levels are elevated in all horses, usually peaking in September/October. this is called the seasonal rise. In horses with PPID these values are significantly higher than in healthy horses. The seasonal rise often lasts longer for them, especially in older horses and horses that have been dealing with PPID for a longer period of time. If your horse becomes laminitic during this period, have it tested for PPID immediately.

> Food intake increases ACTH levels. Ask your veterinarian if they want your horse to be sober before taking a blood sample.

Alpha-MSH and beta-endorphin test

Alpha-MSH and beta-endorphin are two other melanocortins secreted by the intermediate lobe of the pituitary gland. Both are elevated in horses with PPID. Some veterinarians will therefore want to test the blood levels of these two hormones as well.

Dexamethasone suppression test

Another available test to determine the presence of PPID is the dexamethasone suppression test (DST). Dexamethasone is a synthetic version of cortisol. Administering this medicine makes it possible to determine if the adrenal glands produce less cortisol. In a healthy horse that will be the case, but not in a PPID horse.

> The DST may cause laminitis, although the risk is relatively small. Besides, the test is not always accurate in early stages of the disease.

TRH stimulation test

Some cells in the intermediate lobe of the pituitary gland secrete ACTH under the influence of TRH (thyrothropin-releasing hormone). When administering TRH, PPID horses will produce significantly more ACTH than healthy horses. This test can be used in case the ACTH test as well as the DST give questionable results. This test is suitable to detect PPID in an early stage.

Domperidone response test

Domperidone has an inhibitory effect on dopamine. When administered, the pituitary gland of PPID horses will produce much more ACTH. In healthy horses this will hardly ever be the case.

Glucose and insulin concentration test

In addition to the above tests, the veterinarian may decide to take a glucose tolerance test or an insulin reading. They would do this to confirm the common clinical sign of insulin resistance.

Unsuitable tests

Measuring cortisol levels in blood, saliva or urine is not sufficient, because not all PPID horses have too much cortisol in their bodies. Furthermore, a variety of other and diseases can affect cortisol levels, such as:

- Stress
- Pain
- Other diseases
- Heavy exercise
- Drugs
- Sedation
- Use of a twitch
- Season

PPID A HYPE?

A lot more horses are now diagnosed with PPID than there were ten years ago. So many more that some people label PPID as a hype. Yet this is not justified.

Firstly, the clinical signs of PPID are no longer attributed to the normal ageing process. The willingness of horse owners to monitor and improve the health of older horses has increased considerably in recent years. Veterinary care for older horses has improved in line with this. Veterinary science is giving more and more attention to PPID. Research results are now accessible to a wide audience. Finally diagnostic methodology has improved.

Previously, an ACTH stimulation test was also used to detect abnormal cortisol levels in the blood throughout the day. Neither of these types of cortisol tests are used very often anymore.

> ➤ Changes in the pituitary gland are already developing before a blood test can detect PPID.

MRI-scan

An MRI-scan can be used to visualise the enlargement of the pituitary gland. This diagnostic tool is only needed in rare cases. Usually evaluation of clinical signs combined with one or more blood tests will be sufficient to diagnose PPID.

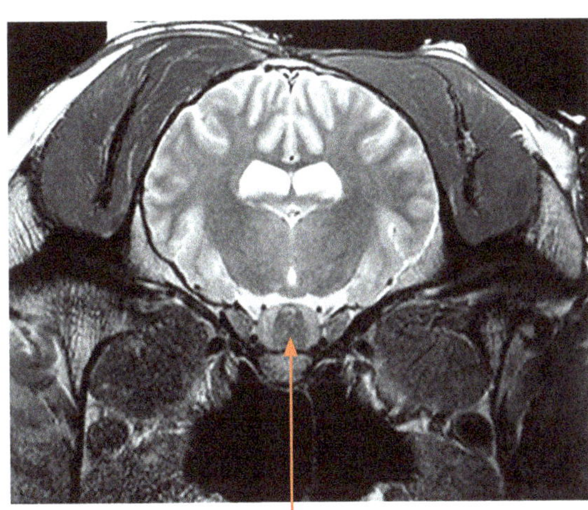

MRI showing an enlarged pituitary gland *(photo: University of Veterinary Medicine Hanover, Clinic for horses)*

Treatment

- Removing a tumour in the pituitary gland is not an option.
- Avoiding stress.
- Dietary modifications suitable for insulin resistance.
- Horses that have not had PPID for a long time can benefit greatly from administration of pergolide (see page 160), a drug that limits production of ACTH. Approximately 75% of these horses show clinical improvement within 8 weeks. Diarrhoea, general lethargy and anorexia are known side effects.
- Serotonin-antagonists such as cyproheptadine also appear to be effective in suppressing production of ACTH. This drug also inhibits the histamine receptors. Histamine seems to play a role in the production of ACTH as well. In PPID horses this side effect is undesirable.

EMS OR PPID?

Adiposity, insulin resistance and laminitis are clinical signs of both disorders. They can be distinguished as follows:

- EMS usually starts at an earlier age, PPID usually at a later age.
- Clinical signs typical for PPID are missing in EMS.
- Testing positive for PPID means increased ACTH levels have been detected while the horse was not in pain or under stress. The test should not be performed in late summer or early fall when ACTH levels are usually higher

Horses can have both disorders as well. EMS horses seem to have an increased risk of developing PPID.

- The use of bromocriptine, a drug with an active substance similar in effect to dopamine, is not recommended because of its side effects. It is prescribed in order to suppress production of ACTH.
- The herbal therapist can prescribe chaste-tree berry (or monk's pepper). Scientific studies on the effectiveness of this herb are contradictory.

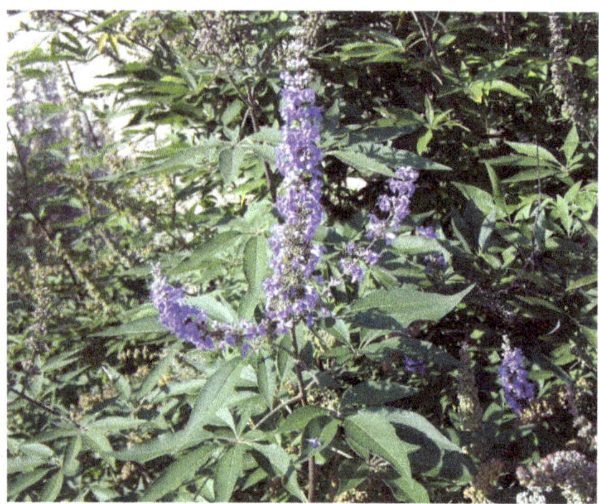

Chastetree berry
(photo: Karan Rawlins)

WINTER LAMINITIS

Insulin-resistant horses, whether as a result of PPID or not, can suffer from aching feet in winter. This is known as winter laminitis, though in fact no laminitis is present. Something like 'winter-related hoof pain syndrome' would be a better name. Suddenly plummeting temperatures make the body produce more cortisol. This has not only a negative effect on insulin resistance in general, but also has a vasoconstrictive effect on blood vessels.

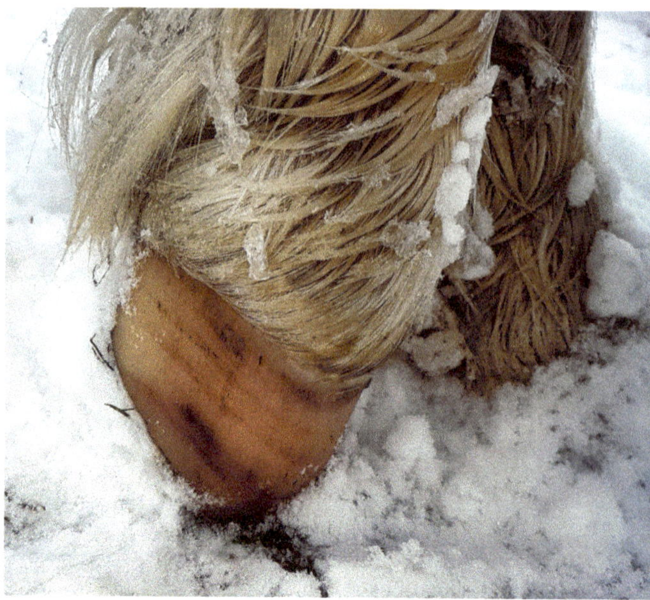

Winter laminitis

In addition, a healthy body produces more thyroid hormones to fight the cold. In insulin-resistant horses this production will be too low (see also page 81 under 'Thyroid gland'). Blood flow to the hoof reduces even more because of this, on top of the often already existing reduced blood flow that results from damaged blood vessels, microthromboses and oedema.

This poor circulation causes pain that gets worse when the horse has to walk over frozen, bumpy surfaces. Because pain and the associated stress cause an increase in cortisol production, this creates a vicious circle.

> Walking on hard, frozen ground can give the last push to horses that already have a compromised lamellar connection, causing the horse to develop traumatic laminitis.

Horses at risk

Especially horses with PPID or EMS often suffer from winter laminitis. Horses with damaged blood vessels because they have been laminitic in the past also run a higher risk. All preventative and curative measures that you take for these types of horses will by definition turn out to be beneficial with regard to winter laminitis.

Treatment

Although under normal circumstances most horses will do well without blankets, you could consider making an exception in this situation. A winter laminitic horse will definitely benefit from being kept warm. A good wind- and waterproof blanket with a fleece underneath, transport protectors with fleece lining and hoof boots can make a difference. A good water- and windproof shelter, with the entrance facing southwest, is indispensable. Keep an eye on the body temperature of your horse during the day. When the sun breaks through and the wind stops, the horse can suddenly become too hot under its blanket.

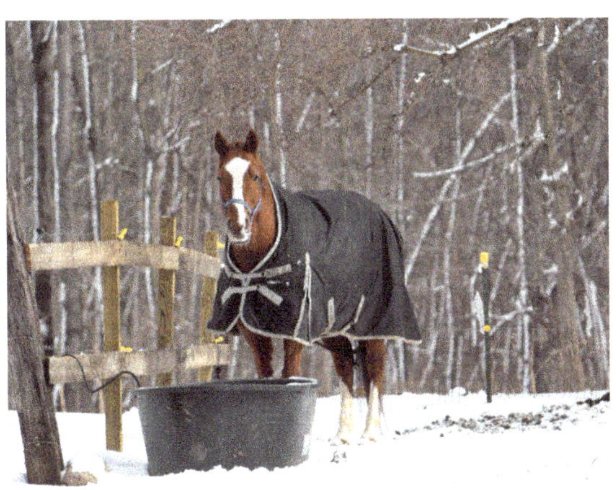

Keep your winter laminitic horse warm

Hay

Hyperlipidemia (the presence of elevated fat concentrations in the blood) causes vasoconstriction and thereby contributes to winter laminitis. Food shortage – even if it is brief – can lead to hyperlipidemia. All the more reason to provide enough hay.

Movement

If you can provide your horse a soft surface (for example an indoor riding arena) it is good to let the horse move around there quietly, optionally on hoof boots. This stimulates circulation to, and in the hooves.

Stress

Avoid any form of stress. The body produces more cortisol in times of stress.

Medications, supplements and therapies

The veterinarian may prescribe L-arginine. This amino acid has a vasodilatory effect and is therefore not advisable for horses with acute laminitis.

The herbal therapist can prescribe cinnamon, rhodiola (golden root), ginger root, or jiaogulan. These herbs have vasodilatory properties as well. Ginger root also inhibits the production of cortisol and has both a stress-reducing and an analgesic effect. Jiaogulan also supports vascular nitric oxide production, which improves blood delivery to the extremities and hooves. Do not start using these herbs at random without an herbal therapist telling you the correct dosage and informing you about possible interactions with any other medications your horse receives.

Manual lymphatic drainage (MLD) stimulates blood circulation. You can also give your horse a massage yourself. Because of his aching feet his entire body may be tensed. The relaxation and improved circulation that a massage brings, will have an overall positive effect.

Time may help to heal the ill of winter laminitis too; the clinical signs and the suffering will gradually decrease when weather conditions get better. Circulation improves and pain will be reduced.

High oestrogen concentrations

Excess oestrogen, whether endogenous or derived from food can cause:

- Excessive fat storage (obesity)
- Higher concentrations of endogenous histamine

The effects of corticosteroids are greater when oestrogen levels in the body are high.

High IGF-1 concentrations

Insulin-like growth factor 1 (IGF-1) is a hormone which, among other things, is responsible for the growth of cells and tissues. As the name suggests IGF-1 is very similar to insulin. Both have their 'own' receptors in the body. When large quantities of IGF-1 are present in the body, they could bind to insulin receptors. This hinders the binding of insulin which could result in insulin resistance. In return, insulin will bind to the IGF-1 receptors. These are, in contrast to the completely absent insulin receptors, present in large numbers in the dermal lamellae. IGF-1 receptors respond to insulin as if it is IGF-1. A growth impulse makes the dermal cells multiply and live longer. The secondary dermal lamellae become longer and narrower, causing them to disconnect from the secondary epidermal lamellae.

Hormone blocking drugs

A solution is being sought in the development of hormone blocking drugs. This should prevent insulin from binding to IGF-1 receptors. The major disadvantage is that these drugs must be administered during the developmental phase of the disease, or perhaps even before that, preventively. This is not very realistic, partly because of the high cost of this type of drug.

GLUCOSE PROBLEMS

The connection between the epidermal lamellae and the basement membrane depends on glucose. The hormones glucagon, epinephrine and cortisol play an important role in relation to glucose. Glucagon regulates glucose production in the liver. Glucose is absorbed from the intestinal contents, and transported to the liver to be converted and stored as glycogen. Cortisol stimulates the conversion of proteins and fats into glucose during times of stress and decreases glucose uptake by skin and hoof tissue. Epinephrine promotes the conversion of glycogen into glucose and also decreases glucose uptake by skin and hoof tissue.

Besides the degradation of the basement membrane under the influence of MMPs disturbances in the production of one or more of the hormones mentioned above can also have a negative effect on the lamellar connection. For example, disturbed sugar metabolism causes the degradation of hemidesmosomes. This happens in horses with PPID, liver disease, obesity, infections and toxic overload.

> ➤ Just like brain and retina cells, the basement membrane cells need a high and constant glucose supply. To ensure this, the basal cells have their 'own' enzyme, GLUT-1, that regulates this supply. Insulin takes no part in this. Contrary to what was long assumed, insulin resistance does not disrupt glucose uptake by basal cells.

STRESS

Prolonged and increased stress causes hormonal, blood sugar level and circulatory problems. It disturbs production of the adrenal hormone cortisol, which stimulates conversion of proteins and fats into glucose under stressful conditions. This increases blood sugar levels.

The production of catecholamines (the hormones epinephrine, norepinephrine and dopamine) increases under stress as well. This results in reduced insulin sensitivity and increased blood sugar levels, which causes the blood vessels to constrict.

Possible causes of stress are:

- Pain
- Transportation
- Competition
- Chronic worm infestation
- Veterinarian consultation, rushed or angry farrier, dentist
- Badly fitting saddle. Saddles can irritate the withers. In the wild the withers are the place that often get attacked by predators.
- Weaning too young. Stress for both the mare and the foal.
- Starting young horses under saddle or teaching them to drive too early
- Monotonous training
- Lack of social interaction. No herd, solitary stabling, or too many changes in the herd.
- Restless living environment. For example, a busy livery yard or a meadow next to a highway.
- Mourning. When two horses that have grown up together or bonded closely are suddenly separated.
- Predisposition. Some bloodlines produce stress sensitive horses.
- Radiation
- Transmission towers and power lines

> ➤ Note how many of these stressors are related to domestication.

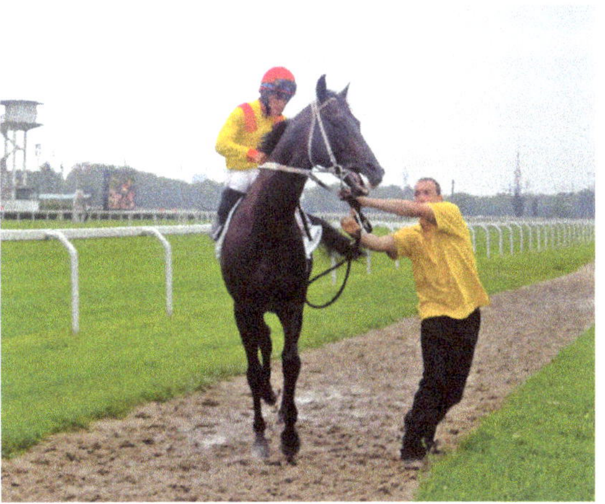

Severe and prolonged stress
(photo: Maria Alexandra)

HYPERLIPIDEMIA

Hyperlipidemia is the presence of elevated fat concentrations in the blood.

When (late) pregnant or lactating mares do not have enough food at their disposal to compensate for the gestation or milk production hyperlipidemia may occur, resulting in vasoconstriction in the hooves.

When a horse suddenly has nothing or much less to eat this problem can also occur. For example when sudden heavy snowfall makes grazing impossible.

Horses at risk

Horses at risk are:

- Ponies, donkeys and miniature horses
- Mares
- Obese horses
- PPID horses

Clinical signs

The clinical signs of hyperlipidemia are:

- Overall listlessness
- Lack of appetite
- Decreased bowel sounds
- Reduced stool
- Difficulty breathing
- Trembling
- Coma

TICK-BORNE DISEASES

There are some so-called tick-borne diseases that could result in laminitis as a complication or clinical sign. Two tick-borne diseases are:

- Lyme disease
- Piroplasmosis

Lyme disease

Lyme disease is an infectious systemic disease caused by a bacterium that is transmitted by deer and sheep ticks.

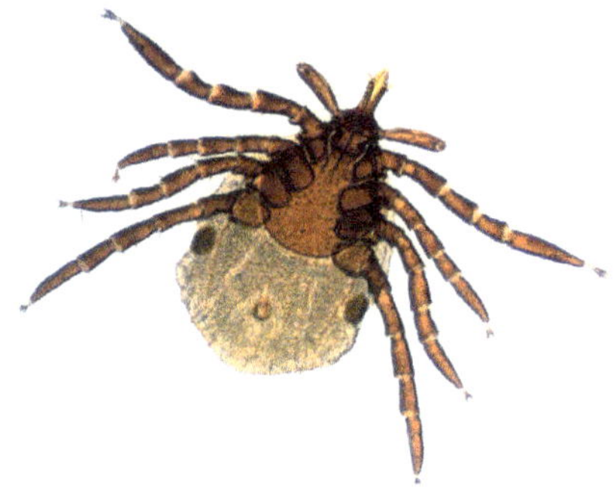

Sheep tick
(photo: Vladimír Motycka)

Lyme can contribute to the onset and especially the worsening of existing insulin resistance. The cause of this can be found in infections in the body. These infections may arise when the immune system is affected by the parasite. The presence of the bacteria that causes Lyme's disease contributes to the aggravation of insulin resistance as well.

The fever that sometimes accompanies Lyme disease leads to higher quantities of toxins in the body. These will not cause laminitis by themselves but may contribute to its occurrence.

> The clinical signs of Lyme disease can be quite similar to those of laminitis. Especially in autumn they are more pronounced than in other seasons. Well known signs are lameness, joint-pain, fever, muscle aches and fatique.

PIROPLASMOSIS

All of the above is also true for piroplasmosis, apart from the fact that it is caused by a single-cell organism (protozoan) rather than a bacterium. More tick species are able to transmit this disease. Piroplasmosis may cause liver damage which makes the liver less able to convert excess glucose into glycogen.

> In horses treated with cortico-steroids, the clinical signs of piroplasmosis, including laminitis, are more pronounced.

> Not only the number of ticks, but also the percentage of ticks that are infected increases every year.

GENETIC ABNORMALITIES

Sometimes Belgian or French horses (in particular the Belgian draft horse, the Comtois, and the Breton) are born with a rare genetic disorder called epidermolysis bullosa junctionalis, which causes the connection between the hoof wall and coffin bone to malfunction, as an essential protein in the tissue is missing. Usually, these horses are euthanised instantly. If this does not happen the foal dies within a month after birth due to infections.

The cause is an inborn error in the skin proteins, as a result of which the different skin layers are not properly attached to each other. This causes the epidermis to detach, resulting in extreme blistering. 'Bullosa' is the scientific name for blister and 'lysis' for release. 'Junctionalis' refers to the location of the blistering, which is the junction between the epidermis and the dermis.

A test to identify carriers of the mutated gene has been available since 2002. The test is done on a sample of mane or tail hair. Breeders are trying to reduce the occurrence of this nasty incurable disease with the help of this test.

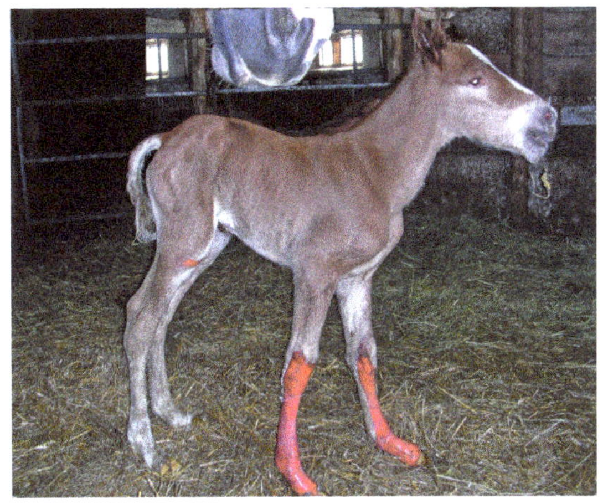

Belgian foal with epidermolysis bullosa junctionalis
(photo: Dr. John D. Baird)

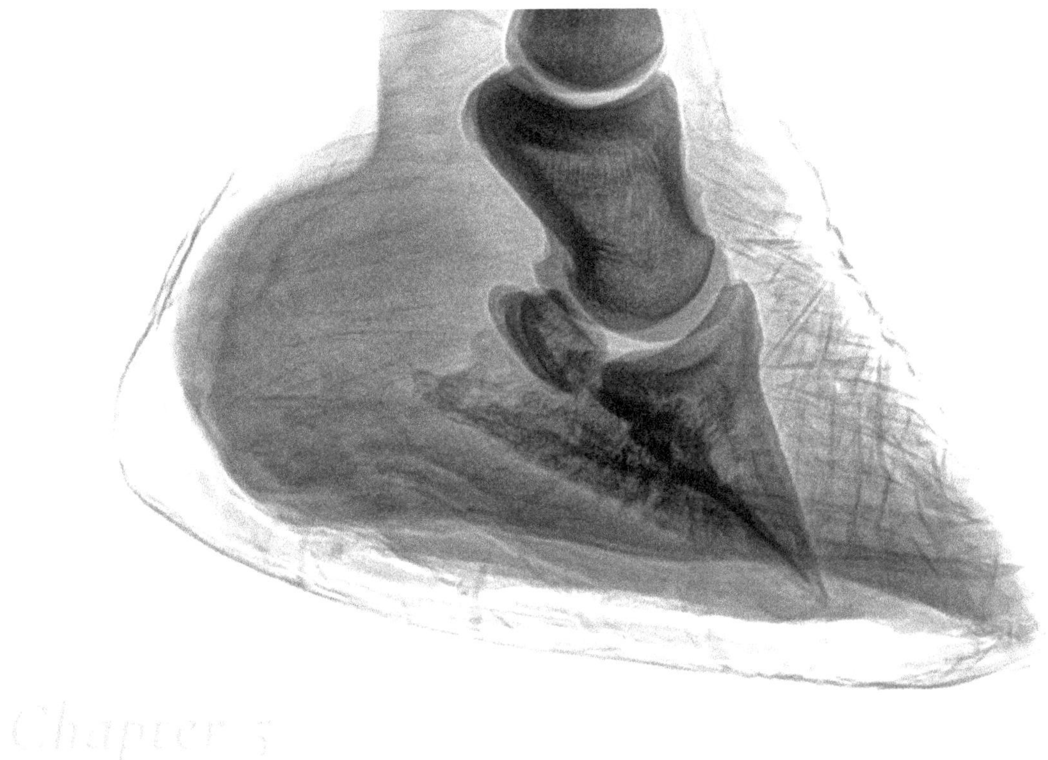

Chapter 5

DIAGNOSIS AND PROGNOSIS

THE TREATMENT OF A DISEASE CAN ONLY BEGIN AFTER DETERMINING WHAT THE DISEASE IS, WHAT ITS SEVERITY IS, AND WHAT THE PRIMARY CAUSES AND COMPLICATIONS ARE. TO MAKE A CORRECT DIAGNOSIS REQUIRES SPECIALIST SKILLS AND KNOWLEDGE. THEREFORE WHEN YOU HAVE EVEN THE SLIGHTEST SUSPICION YOUR HORSE HAS LAMINITIS THEREFORE, IT IS IMPORTANT TO CALL YOUR VETERINARIAN IMMEDIATELY. THEY WILL TRY TO GIVE YOU A PROGNOSIS, AS CORRECT AND FAIR AS POSSIBLE, TO PREDICT THE FURTHER PROBABLE COURSE AND THE CHANCES OF RECOVERY FROM THE DISEASE.

Even when it is obvious that a horse has laminitis, the diagnosis should still be made by a veterinarian. They are the right person as well to interpret the results of, for example, a blood test. In interpreting the results of X-rays, they can call in the help of a radiologist. A good veterinarian will gratefully make use of the knowledge, expertise and insight of the hoof care provider. After all, the latter is a specialist, where the vet is a generalist. You can also identify certain characteristics well. The ideal veterinarian is a good listener and asks questions of the horse owner.

If your veterinarian and hoof care provider disagree, ask a second opinion from another expert. Follow your own common sense, experience and intuition as well. You know your horse like no one else. But don't overestimate yourself. A 2017 study showed that horse owners failed to recognise 45% of laminitis cases.

The diagnosis will include at least two, but preferably more, of the following:

- Anamnesis
- Clinical examination
- Medical imaging
- Differential diagnosis

ANAMNESIS

Ideally, veterinarians will look extensively at the (recent) past of the horse. They will ask many questions to get the most complete picture of the situation. Together with the owner, they will try to gain insight into factors that may have played a role in the development of laminitis. They will also need information to form a prognosis. What are the factors promoting and hindering the recovery at the moment? All information that you as the owner can provide is important here. Therefore, don't be hesitant or shy to share your vision with your vet.

The following points may be addressed in the anamnesis:

- Living conditions:
  - How long has the horse been with you?
  - Nutrition. Is the horse overweight and what are the causes of this?
  - Housing and movement/exercise. Pasture quality and size.
- Hereditary predisposition
  - Breed
  - Bloodlines
- What expectations does the owner have about both the course of the disease and the future use of the horse?
- Appearance. Are there any clear signs of PPID or EMS?

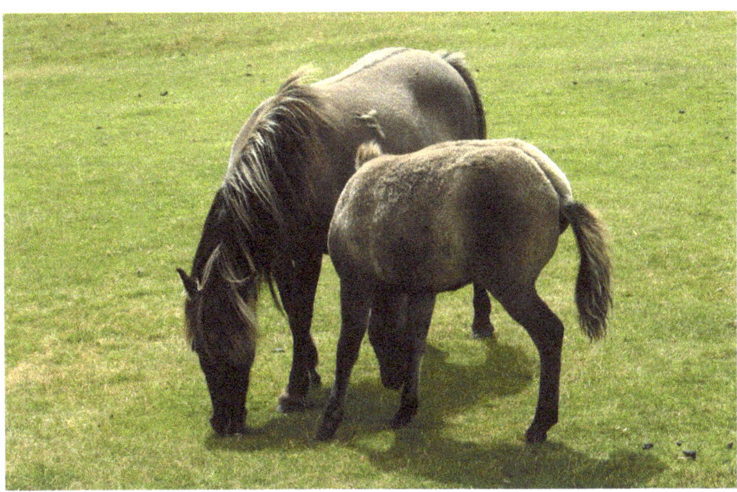

Dartmoor ponies have a genetic predisposition to develop EMS *(photo: Ruth Steele)*

- Hoof care:
  - Who has been the hoof care provider and since when?
  - Who was his predecessor? Why did you switch hoof care providers?
  - Shape and condition of the hooves, hoof maintenance or quality of shoeing
- Veterinary history:
  - Is this a new case of the disease or has the horse never fully recovered and has another bout of laminitis?
  - Has a diagnosis been made before? What was this diagnosis? Are pathological anatomical reports, medical imaging results, blood tests or treatment plans available?
  - Is the horse receiving any medication or supplements for laminitis or related conditions? Which are these? Have they proven to be effective? Are these remedies still given today?
  - The same for therapies.
  - Does the horse have other non-laminitis related disorders? Is it getting any medication or therapies for this?
  - Is the horse, whether or not for its laminitis, seen and treated by other specialists? Are pathological anatomical reports and treatment plans available?

> Mild cases of laminitis are often mistaken for sole bruises, arthritis, or trimming or shoeing errors.

> Tell your veterinarian and hoof care provider clearly what you think is the cause. You see the horse every day, so you know all its peculiarities and what is normal behaviour for your horse. You are able to see things that nobody else will notice. Your input is an essential component in the healing process.

CLINICAL EXAMINATION

CLINICAL SIGNS

It is important to determine the clinical signs, as described on page 41, as precisely as possible, to determine what phase the laminitic horse is in. Write them down in a log (Later in this book you will read more about creating a log).

PHYSICAL EXAMINATION

A physical examination should be performed by your hoof care provider or veterinarian. It usually comprises one or more of the following components:

- Knocking on the front of the hoof wall, possibly with a small hammer. Sometimes a hollow sound can be heard when tapping the hoof because the damaged blood vessels behind the hoof wall no longer contain blood.
- Rotating the hoof or twisting it laterally. The dermal lamellae are twisted by this movement. In the acute phase, the horse will show signs of discomfort.
- Pressing the sole in the toe section with hoof testers or by hand.
  - The coffin bone presses down onto the toe section. The laminitic horse will usually react strongly to pressure on it.
  - Some horses have so much damage in this area that they hardly respond to the hoof testers. The horse has become numb for the pain. It is also possible the horse cannot feel the pressure because of the amount of dead tissue in this area.
  - If the horse does not respond to the hoof testers it does not guarantee it is not laminitis.
- Walking on a circle or lunging. In the developmental or sub-acute phase of laminitis, the horse will show a slight lameness on a circle but not while walking in a straight line.
- Observing movement on both hard and soft surfaces. Hard surfaces give pressure on the lamellae but when the horse walks better on soft ground it probably has sole bruises or (sole) abscesses. Soft surfaces give more pressure to the sole and the possibly rotated coffin bone.

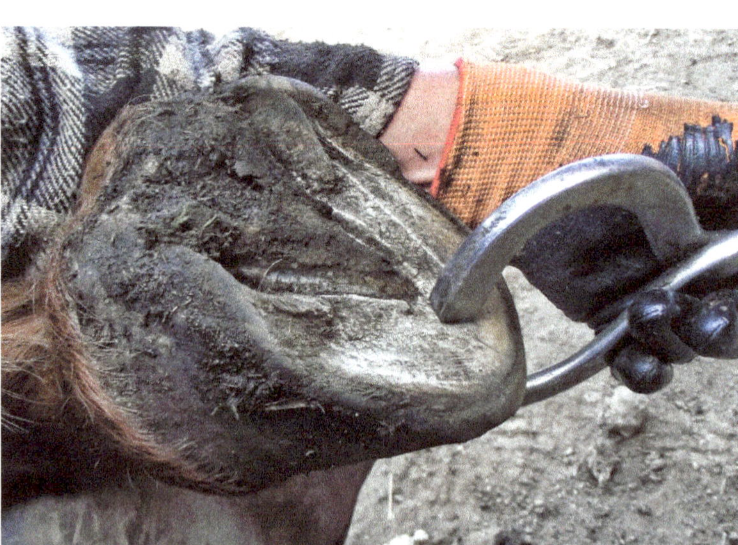

Pressing the sole with hoof testers

MEDICAL IMAGING

Techniques and processes used in medical imaging are:

- Radiography
- Venography
- Thermography

RADIOGRAPHY

Radiographs may be useful:

- As a starting point for a series of photos to compare to later in the process.
- To see any evidence of previous laminitis, for instance dead tissue or the condition of the coffin bone (ski-tip, fractures and bone demineralisation).
- To determine the severity of laminitis and the phase the disease is in.

Radiographs required of each laminitic hoof:

- From the side (lateromedial), while the hoof is loaded
- From the side, unloaded
- Front and rear (dorsal and palmar/plantar)
- Top and bottom (proximal and distal)

By using a metal strip or a thin layer of barium paste at the front of the hoof and a short thumb tack in the frog, the position of the coffin bone can be determined accurately.

Having radiographs taken is quite expensive and their significance should not be overestimated. Even without them the healing process can be put in motion and assessed over time.

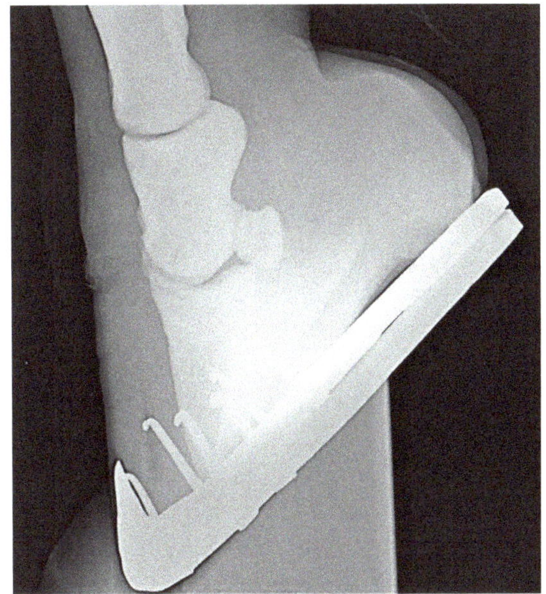

Radiograph showing a sinker
(photo: Alfons Geerts)

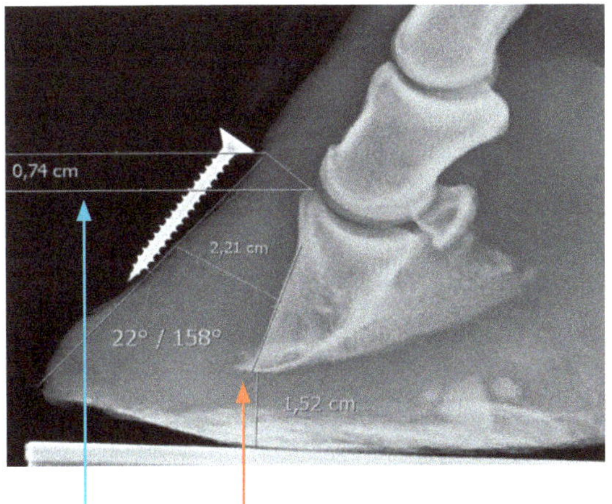

Radiograph showing a ski-tip (red arrow) and a sinker (blue arrow)
(photo: Carlton veterinary hospital)

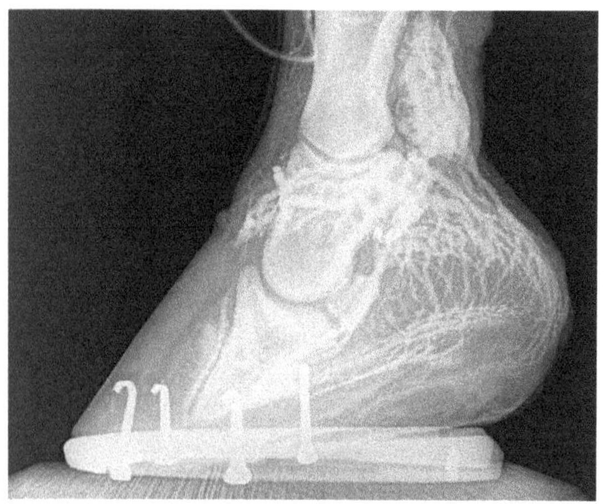

Venogram showing the absence of blood in the veins in the toe section *(photo: Alfons Geerts)*

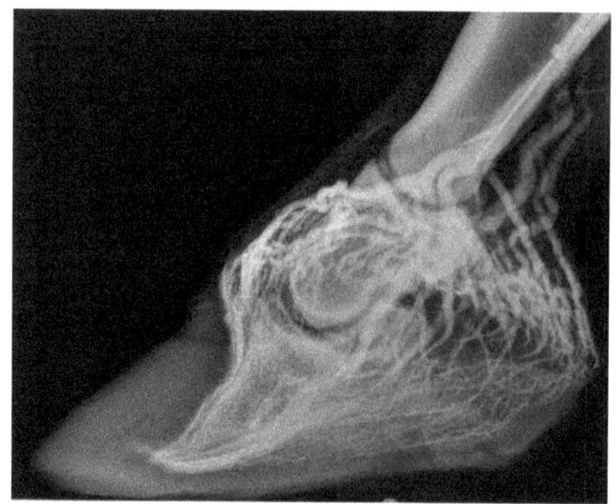

Venogram showing a ski-tip *(photo: Michael Porter)*

VENOGRAPHY

Venography (or scintigraphy) is a procedure in which a radiograph of the veins, a venogram, is taken after a iodinated contrast agent is injected into the veins in order to visualise the circulation. Based on venograms the severity of laminitis can be determined in the acute phase. Damage to blood vessels can be assessed before it would be visible on radiographs.

Venography may have the following complications:

- Formation of microthromboses
- Blood vessel inflammation (vasculitis)
- Allergic reaction to the tracer

Incidentally, venograms also appear to have unexpected but positive side effects:

- Reduced oedema
- Dissolved microthromboses
- Improved circulation as a result of the injection of contrast dye under pressure

Other methods of vascular research can be done by means of ultrasound (ultrasonography) or laser. These methods are typically only used in scientific research and are beyond the scope of this book.

THERMOGRAPHY

A thermographic image or a laser thermometer, are able to assess hoof temperature. A temperature of 30 °C (86 °F) or more, for at least 24 hours, is a clear indication of laminitis. An increase in hoof wall temperature, while the temperature of deeper hoof tissue remains normal, is also a clear sign of laminitis.

In the acute phase, thermographic images of the sole show hot areas underneath the location of the coffin bone. In the chronic phase, a decrease in temperature can be noticed along the coronary band and at the front of the hoof. This is caused by poor circulation as a result of the rotation of the coffin bone, and the

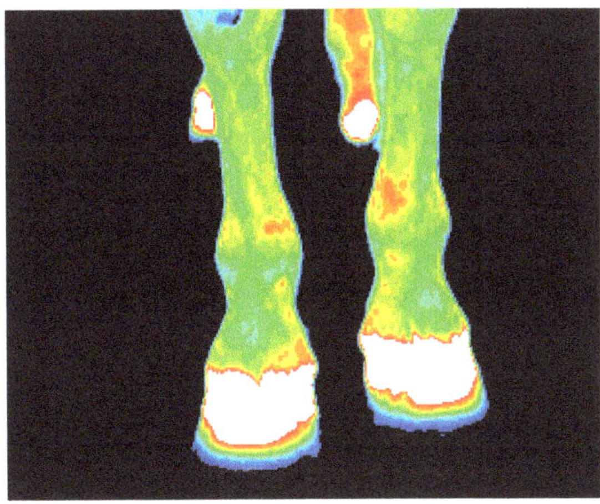

Four hooves with a 33 °C (91 °F) temperature in the acute phase of laminitis
(photo: Sophie Gent)

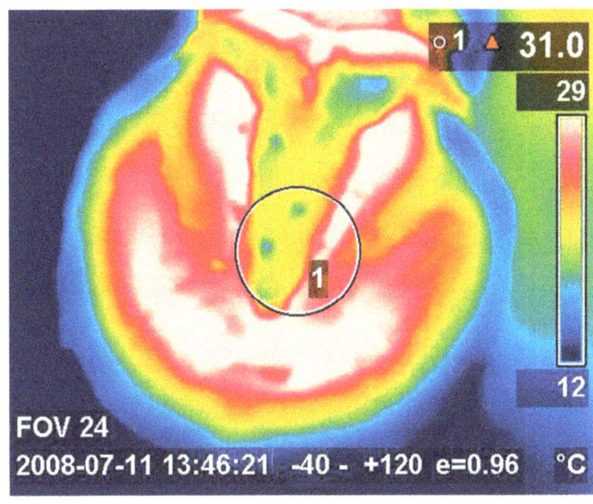

29 °C (84 °F) areas on the sole underneath the, not yet rotated, coffin bone
(photo: Heidi Billing)

damage to the lamellae. At the same time, the pressure of the tip of the coffin bone results in a high temperature at the front of the sole. These two thermographic images together can provide an indication as to the degree of coffin bone rotation.

Thrombosis and oedema cause disturbances in the blood circulation as well and are therefore likewise traceable with thermography. Inflammation can also be made visible, both in the acute and chronic phase. That way laminitis can be excluded in case of a sole abscess that was misdiagnosed at first.

Thermography is only reliable if the ambient temperature is lower than the temperature of the hoof that is being measured. And as mentioned previously, the temperature of a laminitic hoof rises and falls during the day. A thermographic image can therefore give a distorted view when taken at a time when the hoof had a relatively low temperature. Even a very slight draught can have a big impact on the outcome of a thermal image. Just having a thermographic camera is therefore not enough. The skills and experience of the photographer are vital for taking and interpreting the thermographic images.

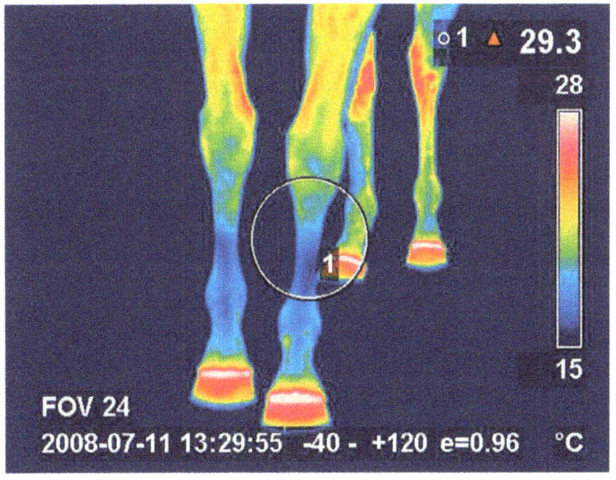

Four hooves with a 28 °C (82 °F) temperature in the sub-acute phase of laminitis
(photo: Heidi Billing)

DIFFERENTIAL DIAGNOSIS

Differential diagnosis is a method to determine a disease by exclusion, where multiple alternatives may be possible. In addition to the abovementioned (differential) diagnostic methods and techniques blood test, and sometimes, local anaesthesia, are being used.

BLOOD TEST

A blood test is a good starting point when obvious causes like overeating are excluded. Blood tests provide clear and factual information on:

- Impaired hepatic and renal function
- Vitamin and mineral deficiencies
- Hormone and blood sugar levels:
  - ACTH, insulin, cortisol and glucose in order to diagnose possible PPID or EMS/insulin resistance.

> To take random blood tests in search of abnormal blood values is not useful. A blood test should be only be used in order to confirm or disprove an existing suspicion.

LOCAL ANAESTHESIA

Occasionally local anaesthesia is used to diagnose laminitis. Nerves in the lower leg or foot are numbed, after which the horse will walk reasonably well. This diagnostic method will only provide a reasonably reliable result in the acute phase of laminitis. Furthermore, this method unnecessarily burdens the body with anaesthetic drugs.

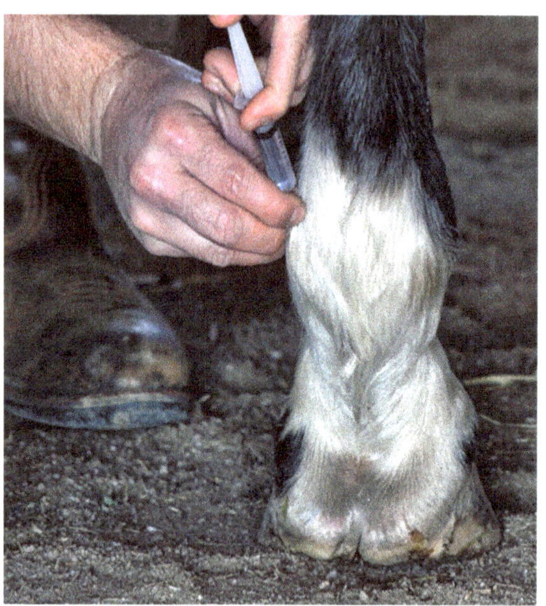

Local anaesthesia
(photo: Leslie Potter)

PROGNOSIS

Every horse owner would like to hear the most accurate prognosis from his vet. The three most important questions are: will my horse survive this and if so, will he be back to normal and how long will it take? These questions can never be answered with certainty. Sometimes even the effect of a treatment is not the same for two hooves of the same horse.

The veterinarian will try to answer as correctly and honestly as possible. They will consider the following factors:

- Whether or not the horse belongs to a risk group (we will come back to this in the next chapter)
- The degree of lameness (Obel) and pain
- The level of leukocytes (white blood cells) in the blood (see page 62)
- The degree and type of overweight
- Whether two or four hooves are affected
- The presence and degree of coffin bone rotation or a sinker. Veterinarians attach great importance to this factor. A study conducted in 1993 with 591 horses shows that this is unjustified. Radiographic findings should therefore not be the only or main decisive factor in making a prognosis or in the choice of euthanasia.
- Primary and facilitative causes.
  - Single or multiple
  - The seriousness of them
  - The treatment options and to which extent the horse will be likely to respond to them.
- The presence and severity of complications.
  - The treatment options and to which extent the horse will be likely to respond to them
- The owner's dedication and practical, financial and emotional ability to support treatment and improve living conditions.

The prognosis can be adjusted up or down during treatment. Overall, you can assume that a horse that shows unmistakable progress after six months of treatment and for which the living conditions have been optimized, has a high chance of recovery. In the next two chapters, we'll take a detailed look at existing treatment methods and possible improvements with regard to living conditions.

MORTALITY RATE AND THE OBEL GRADING SYSTEM

A study showed that the Obel grading system defined a clear prognosis of the survival chances of laminitic horses that were admitted to a specialised clinic. It should be noted that the nature and severity of both primary and facilitative causes and complications, as well as the treatment of choice, are not taken into account in these figures.

	OBEL			
	1	2	3	4
MORTALITY RATE	11%	31%	61%	76%

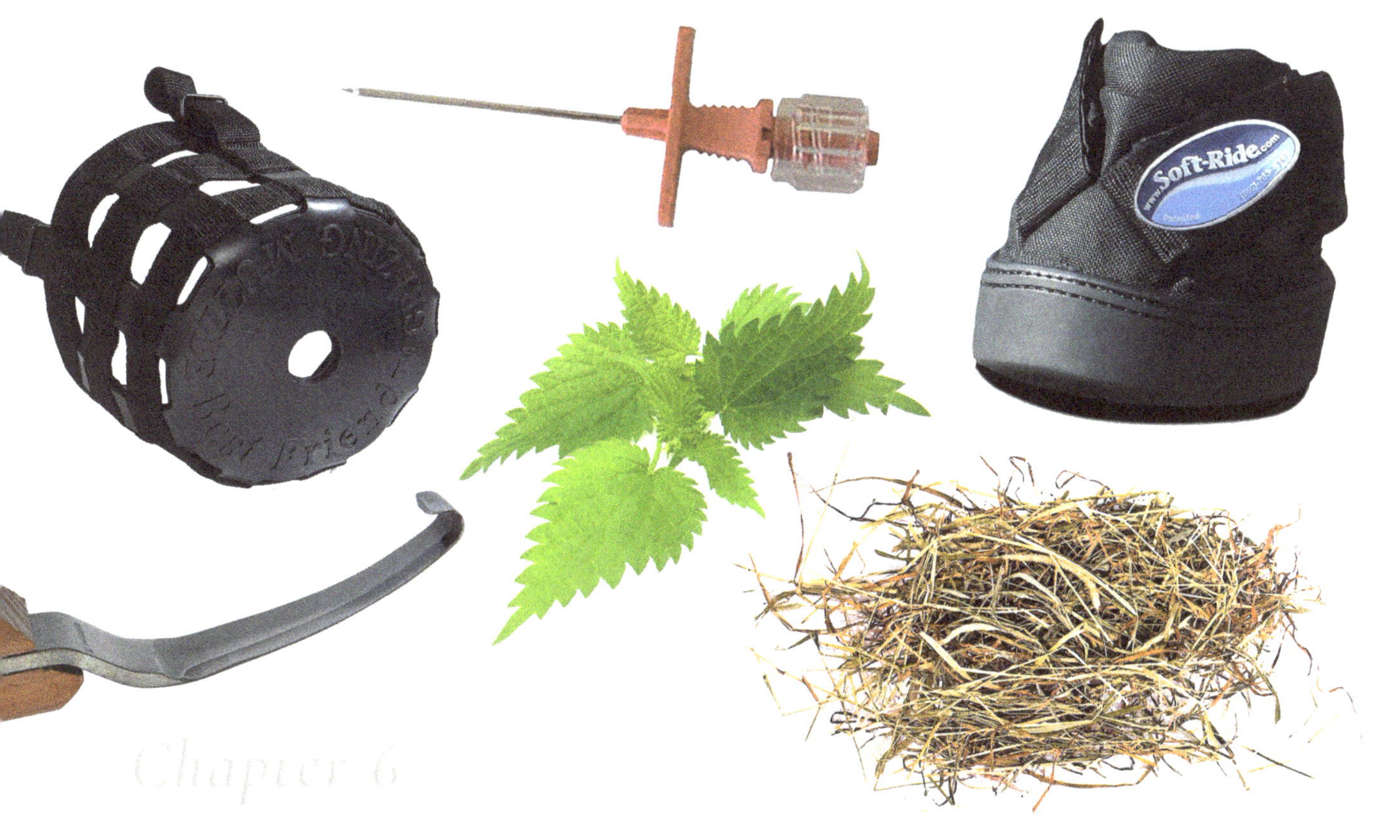

Chapter 6

TREATMENT AND PREVENTION

To prevent laminitis and enhance the chances of recovery, the primary causes of the diseases will have to be eliminated effectively. Facilitative causes and complications need to be thoroughly addressed. Correct trimming is essential for the horse to move properly, possibly supported by hoof protection. Additionally, many kind of medications, supplements and therapies are available to aid the healing process.

As described in previous chapters, the opinions on the cause of laminitis are divided, so you will not be surprised about the multitude of opinions, views and sentiments with regards to the treatment of the disease. It is simply impossible to give an objective overview. Researchers contradict each other, horse owners want the best for their horse without knowing exactly what that is and manufacturers and pharmaceutical companies want to make money. For each statement in this chapter it is easy to find someone who claims the opposite. Experience shows that it is definitely worthwhile to take the contents of this chapter to heart. And, as is true in all medical situations, horse owners need to remain objective about care providers, treatment options and their own choices.

TREATMENT

Before we are going to discuss the various kind of therapies, surgeries, supplements, hormones and medications, we will clarify a number of important principles for treatment and prevention of laminitis.

The chance of resolving laminitis by just focussing to the hooves is very limited. But when broadening your vision, it is important not to get stuck on the (patho)physiological approach of cells, tissues, organs, enzymes and so on. In a worst case scenario this will just lead to symptom control (for example, only therapeutic shoeing or mainly pain or inflammation suppression). In a slightly better scenario the importance of making changes in the horse's living conditions to address systemic problems, might still be overlooked.

Eliminate as many possible causes. Both the obvious primary causes and the less obvious facilitative causes. Laminitis will only be able to heal when the underlying disease, or causative issues are thoroughly addressed.

> ➤ Focus on more than just one cause. For example, because a clear and strong relationship exists between insulin resistance and laminitis, chances are insulin resistance, combined with EMS or not, will be seen as the first and only possible cause, while other causes remain overlooked.

Establishing an adequate diagnosis can be difficult and expensive while the question remains whether the identified causes are treatable.

The cost, duration and success of treatment will depend amongst other things on:

- The severity of laminitis
- The nature and gravity of the primary causes (for example inflammatory bowel disease)
- The nature and severity of the facilitative causes (for example ER/tying up after an endurance ride that was too much)

- The nature and the seriousness of complications (for example white line disease)
- The living conditions as described in the next chapter
- The dedication and consistency of both owner, veterinarian and hoof care provider
- Whether or not the shoes have been removed
- The trimming method
- The use of emergency insoles or hoof boots

Traditionally, a distinction is often made between treatment and prevention. In this book they are seamlessly integrated. The guidelines can be used to prevent healthy horses and horses at risk of developing laminitis from getting the disease. The same guidelines are used to treat horses that already have the disease. Of course additional treatment may be required to treat complications.

Treat wisely

Base the treatment on common sense and sound knowledge. In case you don't have this knowledge yet, find experts who do. This is true for horse owners as well as the experts and professionals that are involved. Although veterinarians and hoof care providers might have successfully treated dozens of laminitic horses, they could potentially come across a case where their expertise falls short. Pride and honour should then not stand in the way. They will have to call upon the assistance of a colleague who does have the required knowledge or experience. Collaboration or referral will then be the right decision. Excessive treatment can be just as damaging as insufficient or unsuitable treatment.

Do what you can and don't get frustrated when some things are beyond your capabilities. Find help to increase what's possible. For example, a neighbour might be willing to walk your horse daily while you are at work.

Progress of healing

Each horse has a different pain threshold, a different response to changing circumstances and a different self-healing ability. Give the horse the time it needs to heal. Observe carefully how he responds to treatment. Keep these observations in mind when listening to the views and opinions of others. Be observant and don't be fooled by suppressed clinical signs.

> ➤ The clinical signs, especially the amount of pain, are not always a reliable indicator of the degree of damage to the hoof tissue. Do not let this influence you in a positive or negative sense.

Prepare yourself to be criticised by other horse owners, veterinarians and hoof care providers. Remain open minded but do not get dissuaded too quickly. If you choose a barefoot approach it is because you are convinced it is the right approach.

Take into account that it takes between nine and fifteen months to grow a completely new hoof wall. During this period a relapse could occur. This downturn could cause doubt as to whether the chosen treatment is the right one. Feel free to discuss this doubt with your

EMPATHY AND POSITIVE REINFORCEMENT

For you, this might be the two hundred and fiftieth case of laminitis. For your client, it is often a first time confrontation that concerns their dearly beloved horse.

Never lose your empathy. An overly theoretical explanation of what is happening at the cellular level in the hoof may appear cold hearted. The horse is more than just a case.

Mind your words, especially when children are present. Adults are more able to understand the seriousness of the situation and to put it into perspective than a young girl who sees her pony is very sick. However, do remain realistic. Don't say it will be all right until you are almost certain.

Positive reinforcement supports the owner to faithfully keep on soaking the hay, walking the horse, administering medications or treating complications.

hoof care provider or veterinarian. If they are true professionals they will always be happy to explain what they do and why. They will also ask the right questions to discover the cause of the relapse.

- Recovery from hoof tissue damage in laminitis is relatively slow compared to other types of tissue damage, as no evolutionary pressure has occurred. This is because laminitis is primarily a domestication disease.

In case the horse experiences bouts of laminitis again and again, despite all good care, there might be one aspect that you, the hoof care provider and the veterinarian have still overlooked. A log, as described on page 171, is then even more valuable.

In some cases the highest achievable is partial cure. You have halted the development of the disease and there are no complications. If you, your vet and your hoof care provider agree on this, you'll have to settle for it. Even be proud that you have been able to achieve this result.

Keep a humane perspective. You may wonder about the quality of life of a pony with a completely deformed coffin bone, that struggles to walk and no longer responds to treatment. For whom is he still alive? We will return to this sad topic at the end of this chapter.

OVER- AND UNDERTREATMENT

Not every horse recovers equally well from laminitis. Therapies, medication, dietary changes, modifications in housing, exercise and hoof care are not always successful. Effective treatment of the underlying problems is not

WE MUST BLEED HIM!
HIS ARTERIES NEED AIR! WE'D BETTER BLOW SOME INTO HIM!
WHERE ARE THE CUCURBITULAE? *
YOU DON'T KNOW A THING! MIX UP SOME GROUND IVORY WITH TORTOISE AND PIGEON BLOOD! IF THE PATIENT LIVES...
* CUPPING-GLASSES

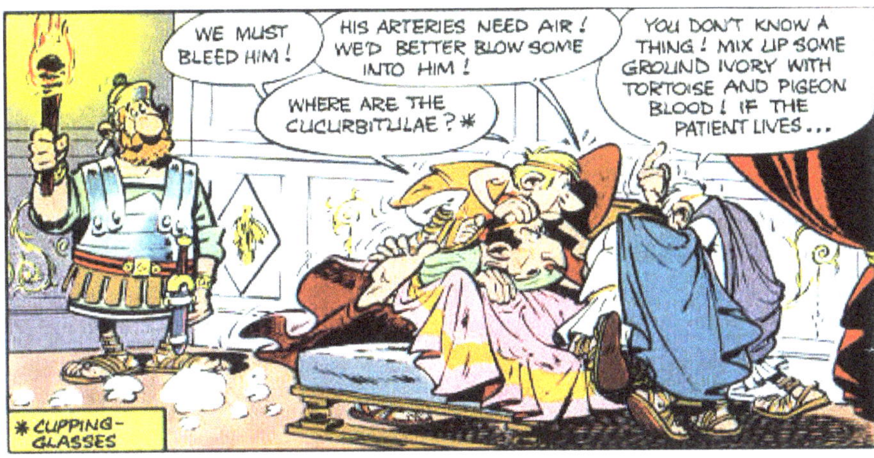

The perils over overtreatment
(illustration: Albert Uderzo)

always possible either. In many cases though, it would help to have another critical look at whether all conditions for a reasonable chance of recovery are being met. However, some horse owners will first look at the possibilities of other, new therapies or try to intensify the current treatment. This approach involves a risk of both over- and undertreatment. Both can be harmful to the horse.

In the first case, we bombard the horse with diagnostic methods, drugs, herbs, needles, magnets or over-engineered therapeutic horseshoes. In case of undertreatment, on the other hand, the horse does not receive the care it needs. Over- and undertreatment often go together. For example, by opting for the promising, radical therapy X (overtreatment), we discontinued therapy Y, which did not deliver the quick results we hoped for (undertreatment). The damaging side effects of a new, revolutionary drug can be more significant even than the relief it offers. Or the results of unproven diagnostic methods, which were used to prove the veterinarian wrong, might give the owner hope, but can cause the horse to keep on limping unnecessarily long. The same applies to complementary therapies for which there is not more than some anecdotal evidence.

Placebo effect

Another risk of over- or undertreatment arises where the personal and professional interests of a therapist stand in the way. On the internet you will find many websites of people who claim to have had the most incredible successes in treating laminitic horses. Any lack of success would endanger their reputation. They will try to prevent this happening at any cost and continue treatment until they (or the horse) drop. The credibility of the therapy and the associated positive expectations contribute to the well-known placebo effect that the owner of the horse is subject to.

Pygmalion effect

Then there is the ego-boosting admiration for the therapist and his status. Not every therapist can disengage from this and admit that his therapy did not produce the long-awaited (and expensively-paid) positive results. If the perception of the horse owner is blurred by this admiration this is called the Pygmalion effect.

Akrasia

Veterinarians and hoof care providers can continue for too long with an unsuccessful treatment in an attempt to prevent the horse owner from seeking help from someone else. This can be a noble goal if they are convinced that the horse will be worse off with that other caregiver. Acting against one's better judgment in this way is called akrasia. Unfortunately, the horse will ultimately be the victim of this. Let's have a look at an example. A hoof care provider who does not manage to change a client's behaviour, while this is essential for the recovery of the horse, will never be able to perform miracles with trimming alone. If, in that case, giving up means that the horse will end up with an unexperienced, shoe-happy farrier, there is a fair chance that the hoof care provider chooses to proceed working in this far from ideal situation to at least prevent worse. Understandable, but a clear case of undertreatment.

Let's be honest – there are also many horses that were given up on by both the veterinarian and the farrier, who were then cured, because their owners chose not to listen indiscriminately and instead seek a good and proven alternative. Indeed, a large part of the readers of this book consists of such horse owners. However, we cannot just say when we cross the line to over- and undertreatment. It can differ on a case-by-case basis. The bottom line is that a sensible horse owner strives to provide the best possible care and will thereby keep both eyes open for the perils of over- and undertreatment.

TREATMENT

Creating an effective treatment plan to cure laminitis is not always easy. Many aspects are involved. No fail proof treatment yet exists, nor indisputable evidence of the origins of the disease.

Consult an experienced hoof care provider or a veterinarian that is familiar with the latest insights on laminitis. They will, preferably together with the owner and as far as circumstances allow, take the following steps:

- Determine the severity of laminitis and identify the primary causes. When a sole perforation or a coronary band prolapse have occurred at Obel 3 or 4 (see sidebar 'The Obel grading system' on page 38), the veterinarian will probably prefer to admit the horse to a clinic. Because a horse with these complications needs intensive treatment and supervision during the healing process, this is a good idea in most cases.

- As the horse's owner you need to define your goals and expectations clearly. Enjoying a pain-free retirement is different than being able to compete at Grand Prix level.
- Estimate costs:
  - Thermography, radiography, venography
  - Blood tests
  - Drugs, supplements
  - Hoof boots
  - Soil, grass and forage analysis
  - Adaptations to the environment
- Make agreements about communication. Pass on any news, both good and bad. You are able to notice things the hoof care provider and veterinarian can't see and vice versa.
- Create a log (see page 171).

FIRST AID

These instructions apply mainly in case of acute laminitis. Take the horse out of the pasture. Do this as gently as possible (see page 197 under 'Social interaction'). Put the horse in the paddock or arena. Sand supports the entire underside of the hoof. Keep the horse away from very soft grounds. This could put too much pressure on the sole. Cool the hooves and lower legs (see sidebar 'Cold therapy' on the next page).

Provide the horse with a place to lie down comfortably. Make sure the horse doesn't eat the straw he is lying on. Make sure the horse has clean drinking water (see page 179 under 'Drinking water'). Feed the horse coarse hay, preferably soaked in hot water to drain out as much NSC as possible (see sidebar 'Soaking hay' on page 117). Do not feed anything else but this for at least 72 hours during the acute phase. Do not give any food containing NSC. No handful of grain or a piece of apple. Make sure the horse has access to a salt lick.

In case of laminitis caused by excessive NSC intake the veterinarian could administer paraffin or vegetable oil to prevent colic. Activated carbon or probiotics may help as well. More on this subject on page 155 under 'Supplements, hormones and remedies'.

Give magnesium to increase insulin sensitivity. In case later in the process diagnosis shows that there is no insulin resistance then magnesium will certainly not be harmful to the horse. However, be careful not to supplement magnesium to horses with kidney problems.

If the horse is shod, call a hoof care provider to remove the shoes as soon as possible. Ask the hoof care provider to trim the horse as described from page 122 on. A hoof care provider that has kept up to date with recent developments in his field will certainly already trim this way. Keep your horse away from hoof care providers that are reluctant to shorten the hoof wall or propose to solve problems by shoeing or other old fashioned methods. Create emergency insoles if necessary.

COLD THERAPY

Cold therapy (cryotherapy) would be very useful in the developmental phase when no clinical signs are visible yet. In the acute phase cold therapy can also be used as a first aid measure.

Cold therapy provides the following:

- Decreased metabolism in the lamellar cells
- Reduced need for sugar by the lamellae
- Decreased circulation causing a decreased supply of MMPs, MMP triggers and TIMPs
- Reduction of inflammation by a reduced production and activity of antibodies
- Protection of tissue against damage from reduced circulation (ischemia)
- Pain relief

Place the hooves in buckets or soaking boots with ice water. The deeper the hooves are in it, the better. Keep adding crushed ice and replacing the warmed-up water to keep the temperature low. A lower limit of 2 °C (35.5 °F) for a minimum of 24 and a maximum of 72 hours is safe. In consultation with your vet you can cool longer than 72 hours.

Cooling with a garden hose, cold therapy compresses (gel packs) or cooling ointment is not effective enough to achieve the goals mentioned above.

When infection is suspected inside the foot (abscesses, septic osteitis) cold therapy should be avoided because hypothermia reduces the natural anti-inflammatory response to infection.

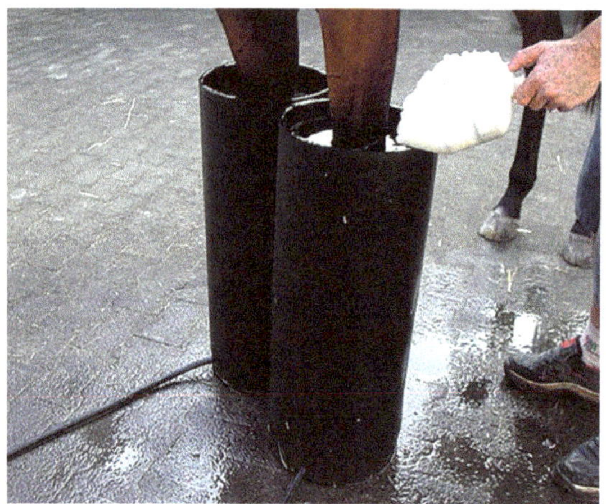

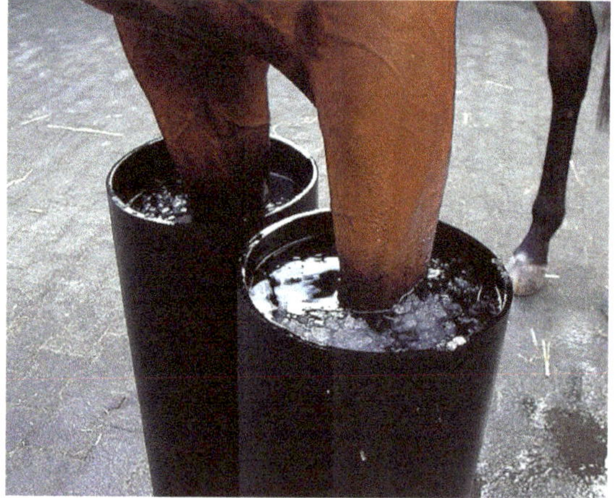

Cold therapy with ice water
(photo: Polyplas)

SOAKING HAY

Water-soluble carbohydrates (WSC), can be partly removed from hay (and beet pulp) by soaking and rinsing. Approximately 50% of the WSC drain out in one hour's time. Soaking for longer is not more effective. However, rinsing in larger volumes of fresh water does remove more WSC. Warm water removes sugars twice as fast as cold water.

Unfortunately, soaking also removes important minerals and vitamins from the hay. Soaking for 15 to 30 minutes results in the best balance between WSC reduction and mineral and vitamin retention. Hay soaked for more than 12 hours potentially puts horses at risk of phosphorus deficiency.

Ethanol soluble carbohydrates (ESC) wash out more easily than fructans. Starch is not water soluble and therefore remains in soaked hay. As described on page 72 under 'C3 and C4 grasses and starch', starch in grass is a relatively small risk.

Soaked hay will stay in the stomach only for a very short time, allowing bacteria to reach the small intestine and cause abdominal pain or colic.

Do not soak more hay than the horse can eat in one day. Wet hay turns mouldy quickly.

Keep wet hay clean. For instance, soak in a wheelbarrow, drain the residual water and let the horse eat out of the wheelbarrow. Needless to say, do not allow the horse to drink the residual water.

Soaking hay should be an emergency solution when low NSC hay is temporarily unavailable.

Silage and haylage should not be soaked. A second fermentation could set in, leading to an increase of undesirable bacteria. Given the low level of WSC soaking is not necessary.

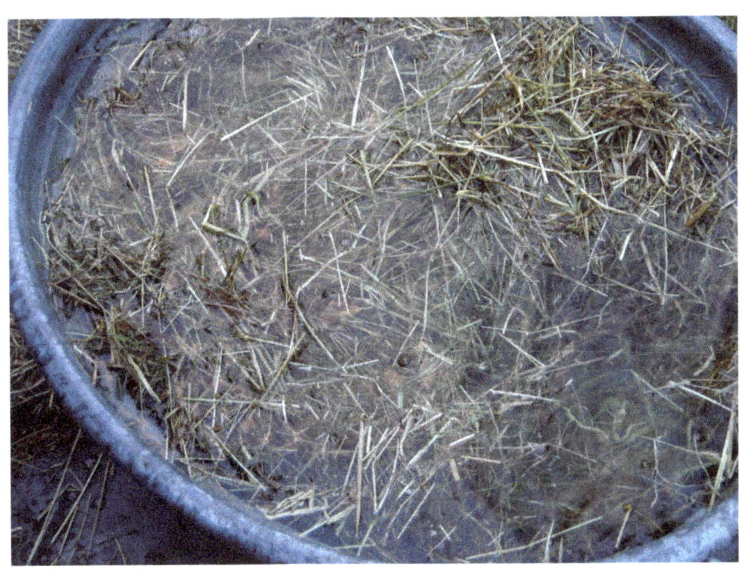

Soaking hay
(photo: Marlou van Blitterswijk)

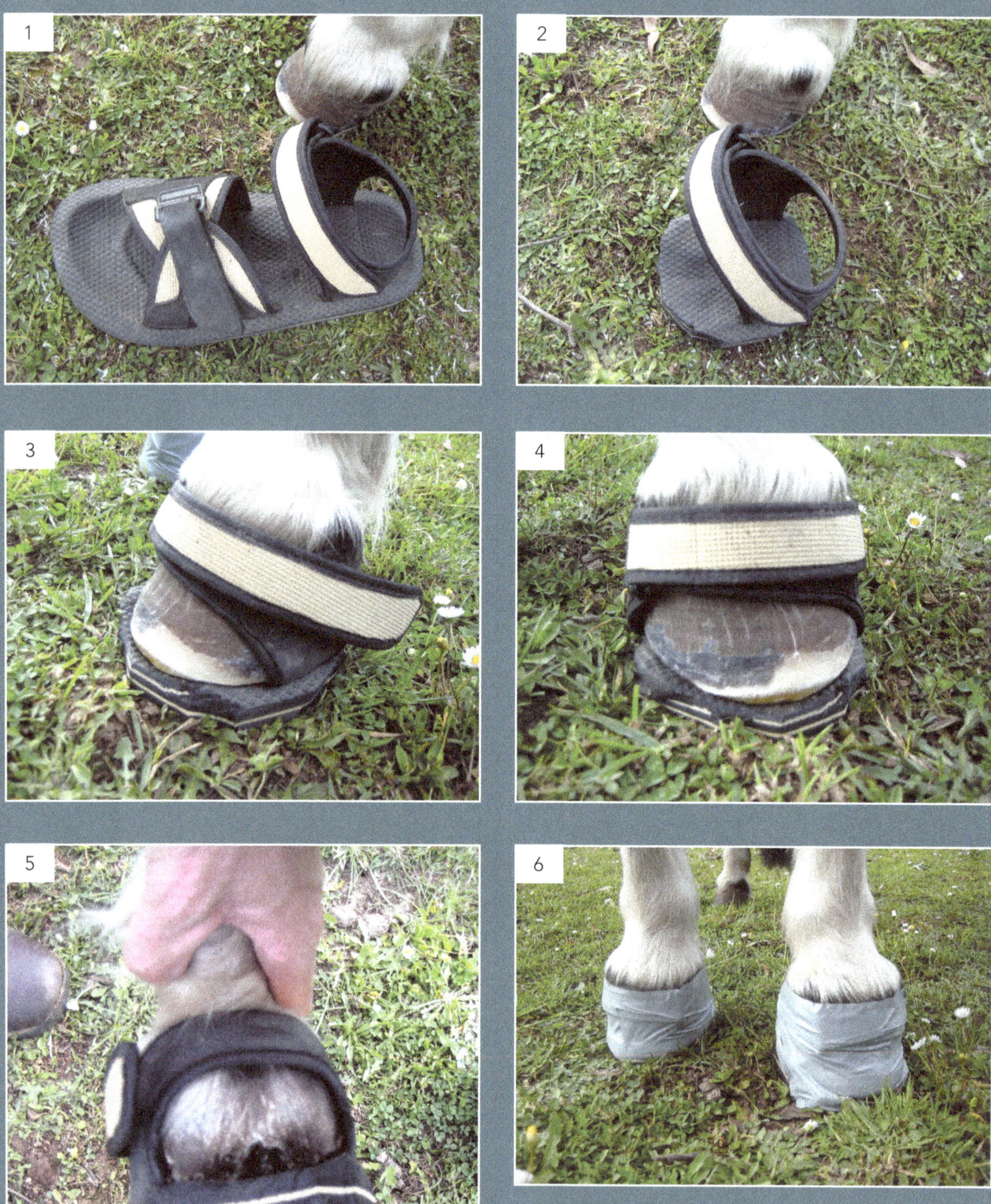

Emergency insoles made out of old foam sandals
(concept and photos: Cynthia Cooper)

EMERGENCY INSOLES

Emergency insoles can be easily made out of XPS insulation boards (polyurethane foam) that are sold at the hardware (DIY) store:

1. Place the horse, with correctly trimmed hooves on a 2 cm (3/4") thick XPS foam board.
2. Cut the foam board around the impression the hoof has made. This is the first layer of the insole.
3. Remove the part of the foam insole where the coffin bone presses against the sole. If necessary this location can be established with hoof testers.
4. The remaining foam board provides support to the back of the hoof and collateral grooves. Tape this part under the sole with duct tape.
5. Cut a second insole out of the foam board. Attach this insole with duct tape underneath the hoof as a second layer of protection.

On the opposite page you can see how a quick emergency solution can easily be realised with old foam sandals.

SUPPORTIVE CARE

Supportive care is intended to alleviate or treat clinical signs and treatment-related side effects. In the context of laminitis, this means we are predominantly talking about horses that are so severely injured that they cannot stand for long periods of time, or are unable to even stand at all. The intensity of this care should not be underestimated; you may wish to consult with your veterinarian about whether your horse would not better off in a veterinary clinic. Let's have a look at the steps you can take if you do choose to provide supportive care for your horse yourself.

LYING DOWN FOR TOO LONG

Both respiratory and circulatory problems may develop in horses that lie down for a prolonged period of time. One common circulatory-related complication is painful pressure sores (decubitus). Sores might appear at the joints (hip, shoulder, hock, knee, fetlock) and at the head. Every 2 to 3 hours you will need to help the horse change their position. Try to keep the horse in the sternal position as much as possible. If you rug the horse, for their safety use only a spandex horse blanket that is fastened with Velcro. Metal or hard plastic closures can injure the horse. This also applies to the edges and closures of hoof boots.

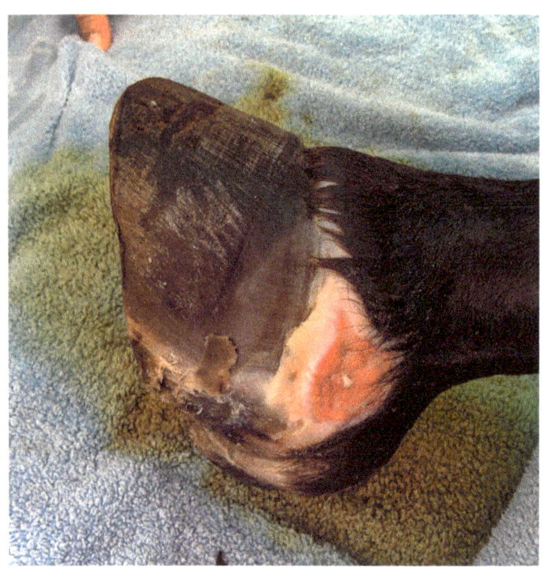

Decubitus
(photo: Wesley De Candt)

HYGIENE

Apply a thick layer of bedding. Ideally the horse will lie on 30 centimetres of straw or sawdust with a top layer of peat moss. Keep the bedding clean, removing dirt, urine and manure immediately after defecation. Clean the genitals and surrounding skin with lukewarm water and soft soap after urination. Fluff up the bedding a few times a day. If, despite these precautions, there are still pressure sores, clean them with Betadine and apply an oily, non-perfumed skin ointment.

If your horse is wearing hoof boots for an extended period of time, use hoof socks, bandages or tape to protect the coronary band, bulb groove and hoof balls. Socks, bandages or tape should be changed and the heel bulbs checked on a daily basis for any areas of rubbing.

Install an anti-insect lamp to prevent your horse from being attacked by flies and, if necessary, provide a fly mask. Keep his eyes clean; dust particles or sawdust can get into his eyes because of the prolonged recumbency.

A recumbent horse cannot easily lose his heat, so make sure that the ambient temperature is low, especially if it has a fever. If the horse sweats less, the risk of developing pressure sores is lower. Fresh air is also important because dust particles can make breathing more difficult. So, ventilate well.

SAFETY

A horse that cannot get up or reposition itself can easily injure itself. Often it tries to change position by 'clawing' with only the front or hind legs. This might result in the horse becoming cast. Attention should be paid if the horse manages to stand up too, as it may fall due to a disturbed sense of balance, due to stiff muscles after lying down for too long or because his feet are too painful. Also, think of your own safety and that of the veterinarian and hoof care provider. A falling horse can be dangerous. Make sure that the place where your horse is located is large enough and clear of any objects that could injure it. Cover concrete or brick walls with wood, insulation boards or tarpaulin.

Regularly check that your horse is still safe and comfortable. Consider installing an observation camera. Some horses react differently in the presence of people than when they feel they are unwatched. In the latter case, they may show different or more pain reactions. In case of an impending coronary band separation or prolapse, some horses nibble their hooves. You will also want to make sure you observe the early signs of a colic caused by lying down for too long.

NUTRITION AND HYDRATION

It is imperative that the horse is offered high quality hay or soaked beet pulp, a salt lick and fresh drinking water. With a horse that does not stand up, stay seated until it has drunk, after which you should remove the bucket. If he does not want to drink in your presence, retreat and come back later to take the bucket away. You do not want it to be hurt by an empty bucket. Repeat this at least every two hours.

PHYSICAL AND MENTAL WELL-BEING

Pay attention to whether there are changes in physiological characteristics or your horse's behaviour. Important physiological indicators of a worsening condition include: strong pulse with an increased frequency, muscle tremors, excessive sweating, signs of dehydration, dilated pupils, excessive blood flow to the eye mucosa, widened nostrils, ears stiffly turned backwards, increased respiratory rate, increase in body temperature. Behavioural indicators of concern may include irritability, anxiety, being withdrawn, tired sighing or groaning. Communicate notable changes to any of these physiological, behavioural or pain-related indicators directly to your veterinarian. In particular, changes in the pulse and respiratory rate are important.

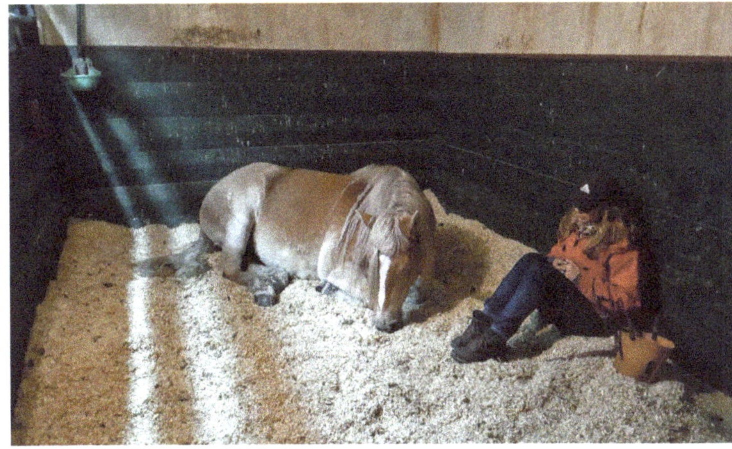

A safe place for the sick horse
(photo: Laura Vos)

Spend time with your ill horse. A prey animal that feels it can no longer flee if needed feels particularly vulnerable. Be there with your horse and provide it with reassurance and encouragement. Social interaction – also with the owner – is of great importance for the mental and emotional well-being of a horse and whoever feels better heals better. Even if this were not true, your own motivation and perseverance in the fight against laminitis will be bolstered.

TRIMMING A LAMINITIC HOOF

Many horse owners are quite capable of maintaining the healthy hooves of their own horse after following at least one hoof trimming course. When you have questions or the slightest doubt occurs about your trimming skills, get in touch with a professional hoof care provider. To have the hooves checked at least twice a year by a professional is a good idea anyway. If your horse has laminitis it is certainly highly recommended to have it trimmed by a professional hoof care provider. The experience with laminitis a professional has and all related knowledge will be indispensable, especially in the first stage of the healing process.

> To think trimming alone will cure laminitis is a mistake. By now you will probably understand that laminitis is not just a hoof problem. You will have to broaden your perspective and act on more levels in order to help the horse effectively.

PREPARATION

It goes without saying that you should be present when the hoof care provider is there. They can explain important things to you and will need to ask you questions about your horse and his illness. They will explain how you can help maintain the hooves in between his trims. You can ask them your questions before and after they trim the horse. Do not do this during trimming.

In any case, make sure that you are well prepared so that your hoof care provider can work safely and with full attention to the hooves. A clean, level surface is important. It is important that the trimming is done in a place that your horse knows and where it feels safe. Put it there some time before your hoof care provider arrives.

If your horse cannot stand still properly due to the pain or other causes, consider giving it a mild painkiller. Trimming a laminitic hoof requires more time and more attention to detail than is the case with a healthy hoof. A horse that is restlessly moving back and forth does not make work any easier. If it is too painful for your horse to lift one front leg, a hoof boot on the other front leg can help. A gardening knee mat, a piece of insulation board or a bit of straw to stand on can also make a difference.

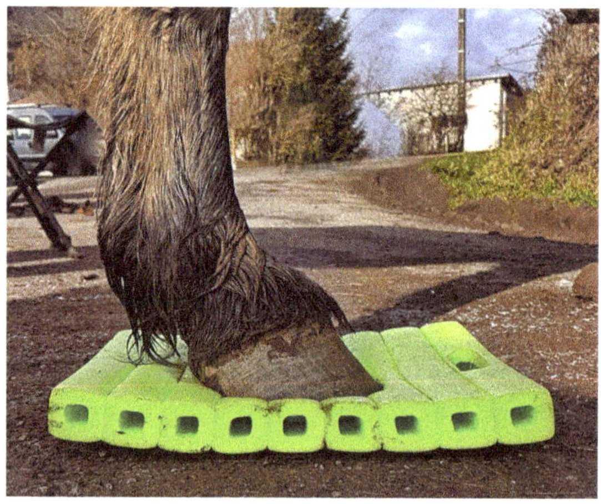

Support with a knee mat

If the horse is not able to stand on three legs at all, it is possible to build a construction to support the horse. Make sure this construction is strong enough. Some hoof care providers can bring a mobile crush or chute. They are possibly even for rent.

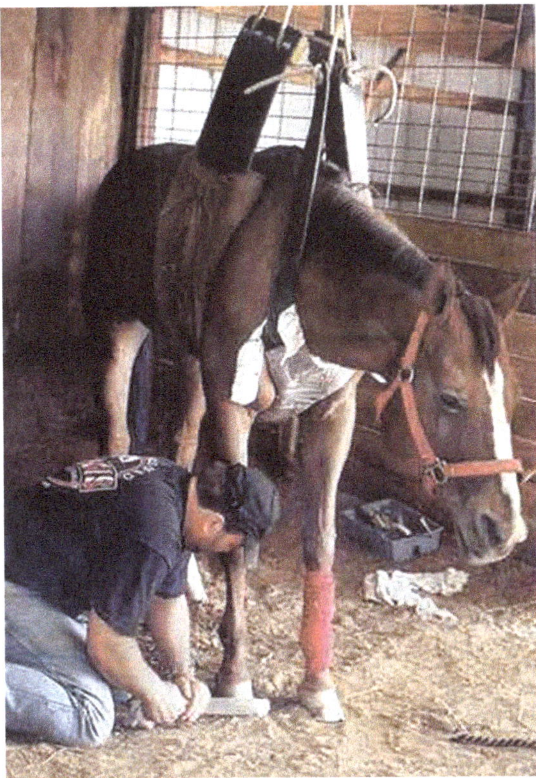

Support construction
(photo: Gretschen Fathauer)

Make sure to give the hooves that do not show signs of laminitis a very accurate trim as well. They might need hoof boots and insoles when they are at risk of traumatic laminitis because of the extra load they carry.

TRIM

The trim is noninvasive. This means that, as long as this is possible, sensitive living tissue is not being cut, touched or exposed. It contributes to the welfare of the horse and minimises the risk of complications.

The hind hooves are trimmed first for the simple reason they are usually less affected by laminitis. While the front hooves are being trimmed the horse will be able to carry its weight better on the trimmed hind feet.

A laminitic hoof is trimmed in the following steps:

- Pulling the shoes
- Cleaning and checking the sole
- Removing excess bar
- Trimming the hoof wall and white line
- Lowering the heels
- Lowering the hoof wall
- Removing the lamellar wedge
- Rounding off the wall's edge
- Trimming and debridement of the white line, lamellar wedge and frog
- Removing flares

Of course not all steps will be relevant or in the exact order.

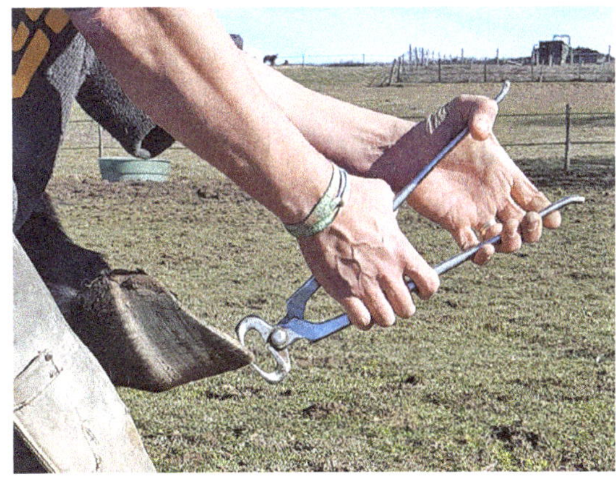

Pulling the shoes

In case the horse is shod, the shoes are pulled first. This is done with care. The nails are removed one by one rather than pulling of the shoe with shoe pullers. This protects the painful lamellar connection between hoof wall and coffin bone, and avoids damage to the hoof wall.

Cleaning and checking the sole

The sole is cleaned and checked for signs of disease and abscesses underneath. Normal sole tissue remains untouched because all healthy sole provides valuable cushioning.

Removing excess bar

The bars are trimmed the same way as in regular hoof maintenance, to avoid bruising of the underlying tissue and to allow hoof mechanism.

Trimming the hoof wall and white line

To be able to work with accuracy the hoof wall and white line are trimmed.

Lowering the heels

Low heels facilitate the typical laminitic stance. The horse adopts this posture to contribute to the healing process. It takes weight off the toe area, relieves pressure on the coronary band and decreases the pressure from the tip of the coffin bone onto the sole. It also promotes hoof mechanism and therefore circulation. Lowering the heels promotes heel first landing, which protects the sensitive toe.

Drastic lowering of the heels is not recommended in the acute phase. It suddenly increases the tensile force of the deep digital flexor tendon. Even though this tendon is not the cause of the coffin bone rotation, its pulling force may increase the degree of rotation. As mentioned earlier, the cause of rotation is the inability of the lamellae and extensor tendon to offer counter force. The increased pull will last until the tension of the deep digital flexor muscle has adapted and therefore the pulling forces on the tendon decrease. A good hoof care provider takes this into account and reduces the heel no more than one cm (3/8") at a time.

To test how much to reduce the heels place a piece of wood of the same height as the heel you are planning to remove, underneath the toe. If a dent occurs at the front of the coronary band or the horse shows signs of increased pain you have to proceed conservatively.

Lowering the hoof wall

The hoof care provider needs to trim the hoof wall to prevent it from touching the ground, especially at the front of the hoof. The hoof wall is shortened considerably. Some trimmers follow a slightly different approach by leaving some wall touching the ground further towards the back of the hoof.

Removing the lamellar wedge

The lamellar wedge needs to be removed at a certain point. Different hoof care methods use different criteria to determine the best moment to do this.

Rounding off the wall's edge

The edge of the hoof wall is rounded off with a rasp and file. It is important not to thin the toe region too much by making the bevel too large, especially in small breeds with small hooves, for example Shetland ponies or Falabellas.

Trimming and debridement of the white line, lamellar wedge and frog

When the stretched white line and the lamellar wedge are trimmed, pockets of bacterial and fungal disease can be pared away. All damaged, diseased and necrotic tissue is removed as well. In case of drastic tissue removal it is recommended to disinfect the hoof for at least three days with diluted (1:25) Dettol, Halamid or a similar product. Loose parts of the frog will be cut off.

Removing flares

Wall flares are removed as they generate excessive stress to the lamellar connection.

TIPS FOR HOOF CARE PROVIDERS

As a professional hoof care provider you might think this list simply describes all the best practices that you employ on a daily basis. Still, it will be useful to read it through once and check if every point applies fully to the way you work.

There is no strict protocol for treating laminitis. Stay alert and do not try to solve each case in exactly the same way.
For one horse the main focus might be on diet, while in another case the trim might be the decisive factor.

When treatment does not work sufficiently, try to find out what causes it. Remain open minded and critical about your own knowledge and competence. Laminitis is a complicated disease. Even if you do everything as well as you possibly can, the treatment could still fail.

During treatment, complications can occur. Try to be prepared for them. Make sure the horse owner is prepared as well.

Make sure you are well aware of the expectations of the horse owner. Know what options they have to help the horse. Do they have the time, space, resources, motivation? If you think a positive outcome is not possible within the existing circumstances, it might be better not to get involved.

Horse owners can be very opinionated but often lack the knowledge and expertise in regards to laminitis. This combined with a stubborn attitude can hinder the chances of a positive outcome. It is your job to educate the horse owner. On the other hand, always stay open minded to the insights and experiences of the customer. They see their horse every day, not you.

Do not give up too soon. As long as the horse and its owner have not given up, you should not either.

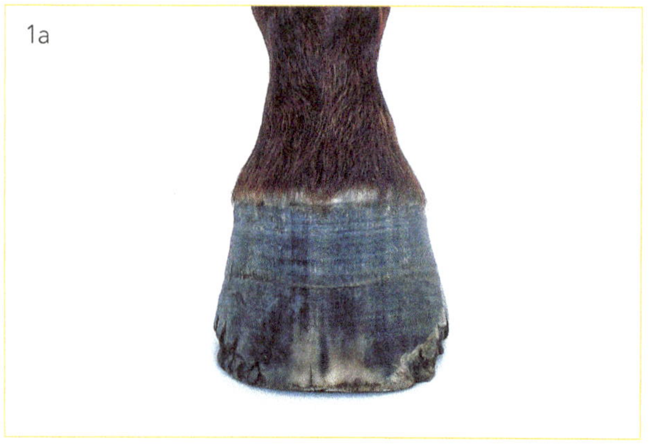

Before trim

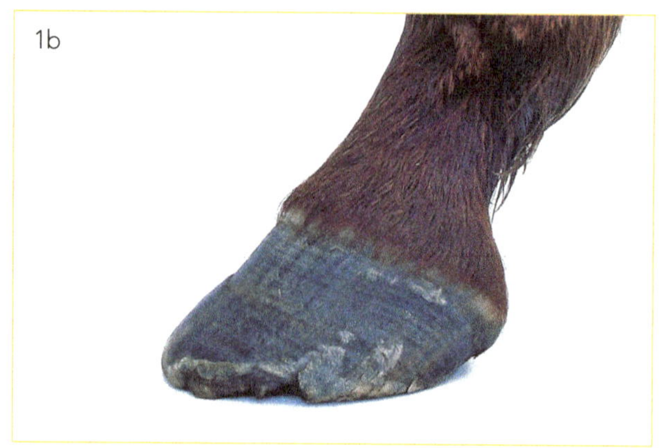

Before trim

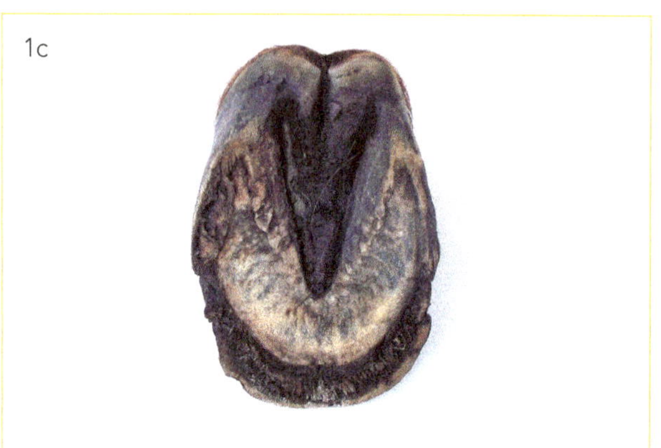

Before trim

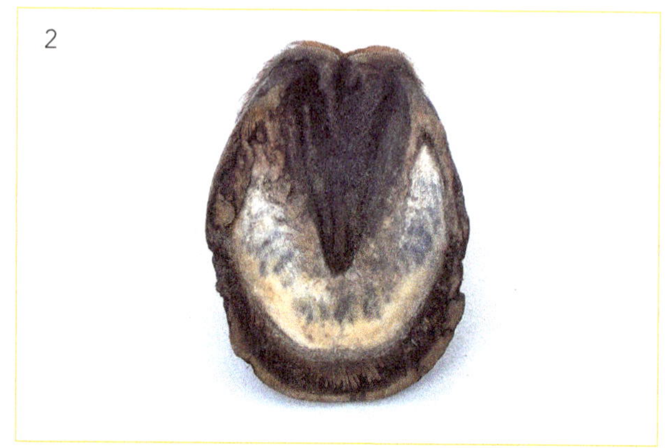

Cleaning and checking the sole

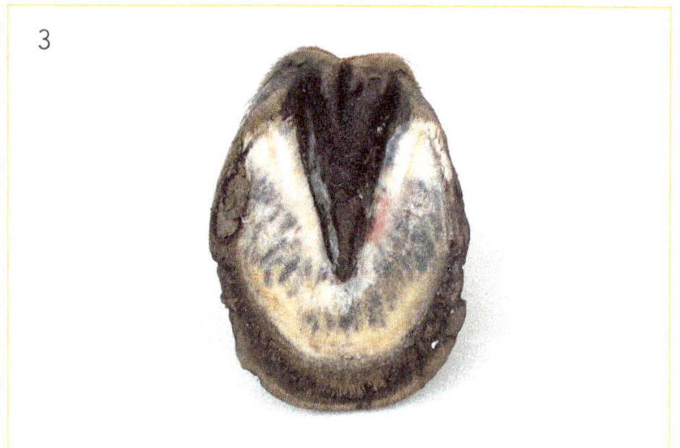

Removing excess bar and trimming the frog

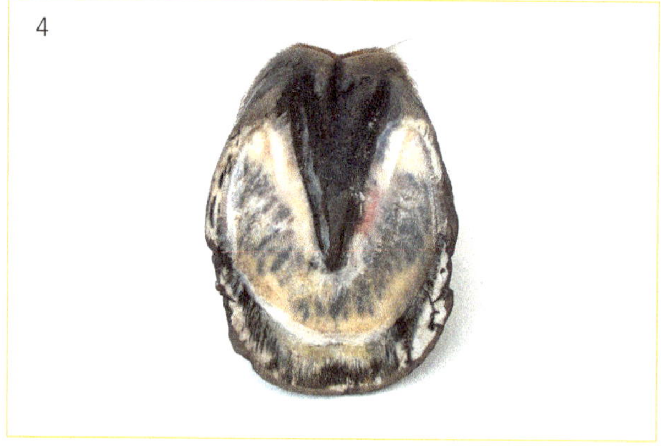

Trimming the hoof wall and white line

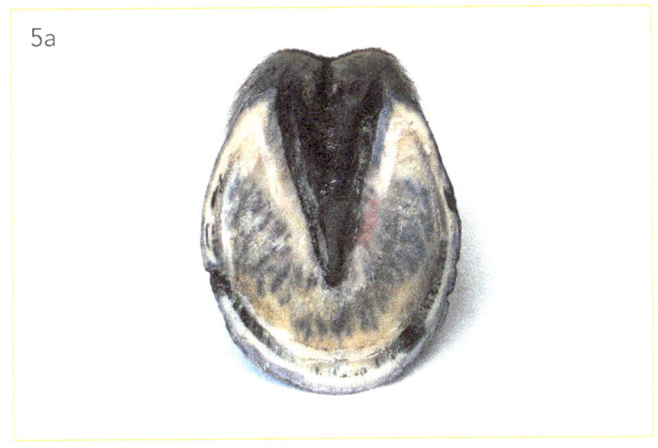

Lowering the heels and hoof wall

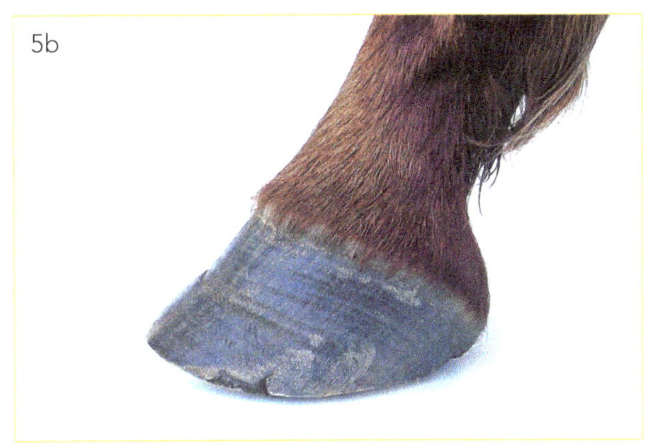

Lowering the heels and hoof wall

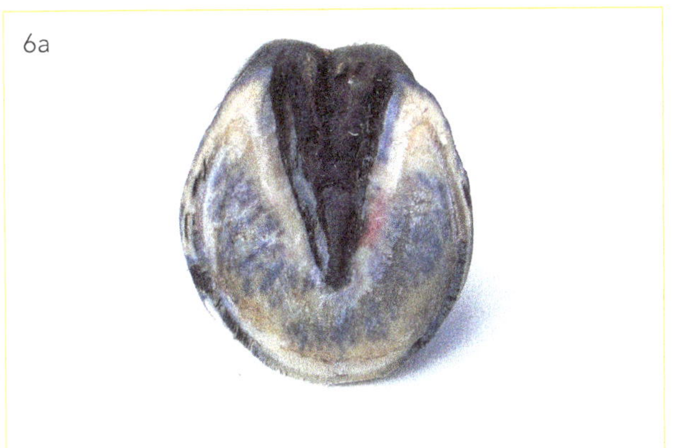

Removing the lamellar wedge

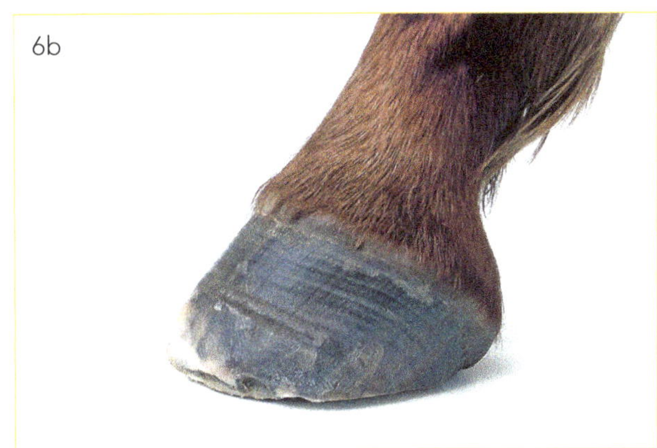

Removing the lamellar wedge

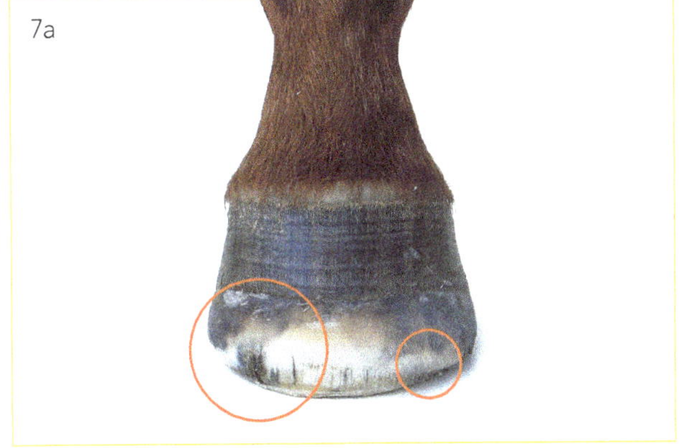

Debridement of the white line/ lamellar wedge (before)

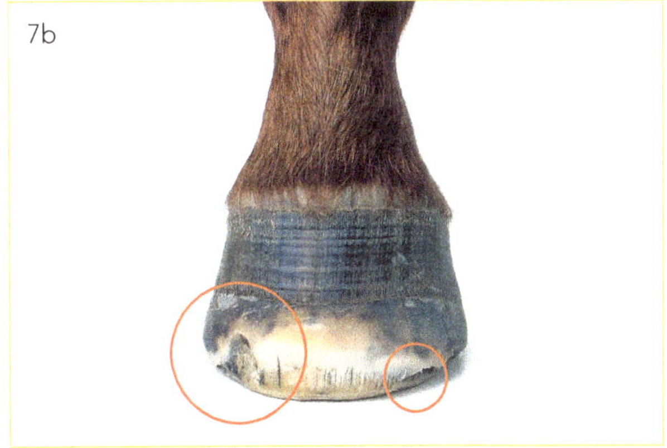

Debridement of the white line/ lamellar wedge (after)

NATURAL HEALING

After some time, sometimes in a matter of days, a laminitic ring in the hoof wall appears, growing down from the coronary band. The wall above this ring shows the correct, steeper angle and can be seen as the start of a new, connected, healthy hoof. As soon as this ring has grown down to approximately one-third of the wall, the lamellar connection is strong enough to be loaded again. This takes about four months.

The new lamellar connection between hoof wall and coffin bone rotates the coffin bone back into position, regardless of the degree of rotation.

> Based on the position of the laminitic rings it is possible to roughly gauge how long ago laminitis started. It takes about a year to produce a new hoof wall. When the location of the ring is halfway, laminitis must have begun half a year ago.

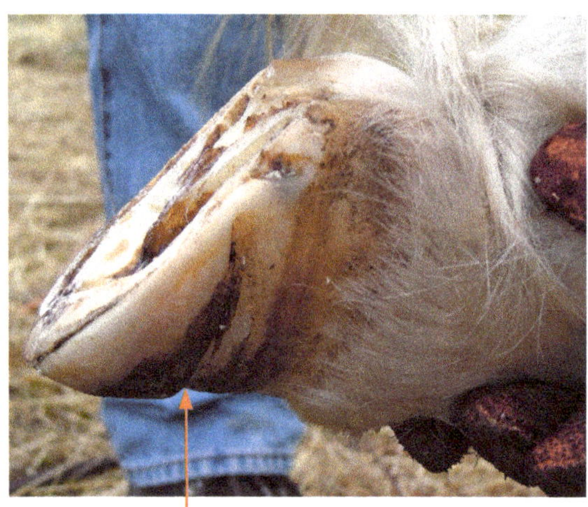

Natural healing process
Note the difference in angle between the new growth and old wall (photo: Cynthia Cooper)

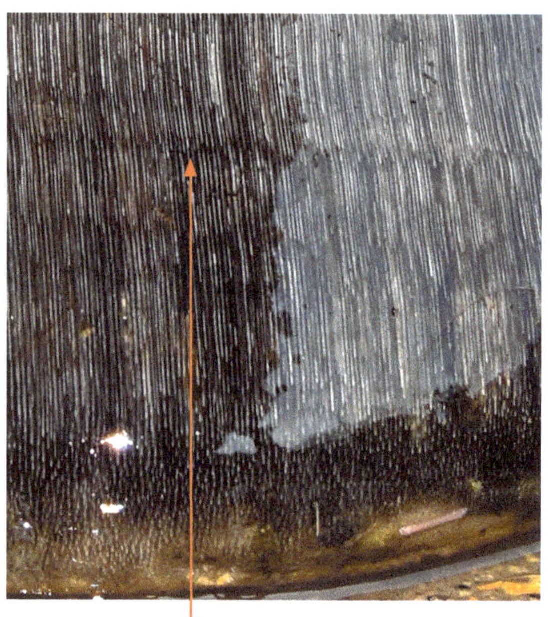

Close-up view of a laminitic ring (photo: Lacelynn Seibel)

When the coffin bone regains its suspended position, higher within the hoof capsule, the sole will recover its original concavity. After all, the sole is connected to the base of the coffin bone. The concave sole increases the resilience of the hoof, which improves the hoof mechanism. Better hoof mechanism creates better circulation. An upward spiral.

In the early stages it is recommended to have the hooves trimmed by a hoof care provider at least every three to four weeks. You can take care of interim hoof maintenance yourself but only in close consultation with the hoof care provider and after attending a good hoof care course. The costs of hoof care should never be a deciding factor in how often hooves need to be maintained.

The checklist page 237 might provide a helpful overview of the current situation of your horse. The questionnaire is designed to be filled in by the horse owner and hoof care provider together.

TREATING COMPLICATIONS

> ➤ Treating complications that can occur with laminitis falls under the heading of veterinary care and is therefore the job of the veterinarian. Do not experiment yourself if your horse needs this care. The vet can tell you what part of the care you can eventually provide yourself.

ABSCESSES

Abscesses can appear one to two months after the onset of laminitis. They may erupt at the coronary band, the white line or at the heel bulbs. They are caused by infection of accumulated blood (serum) or necrotic tissue. A rotated coffin bone increases the pressure on the sole from the inside. Also this contributes to tissue dying of. As the abscess grows, the pressure increases on surrounding tissue, and therefore pain also increases.

Some abscesses should be considered as part of the healing process. They drain the waste products of the inflammation that occurs with laminitis.

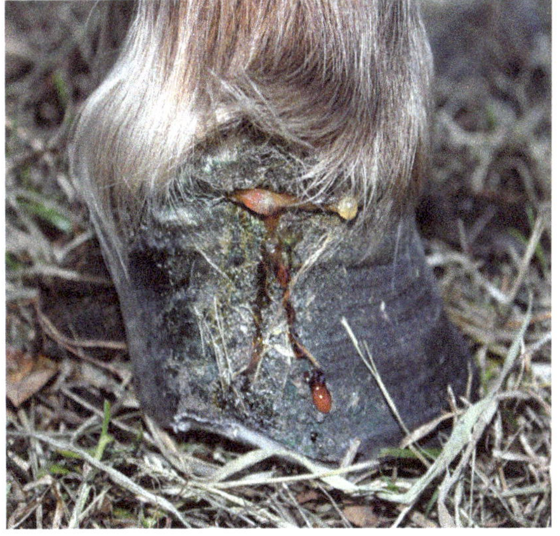

Coronary band abscess
(photo: Tanja Boeve)

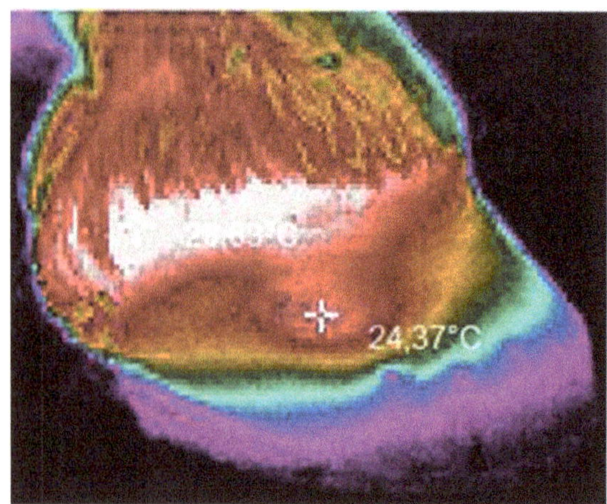

Thermographic image of a coronary band abscess
(photo: Cindy Altorf)

TREATMENT

It is absolutely true that cutting open an abscess provides instant relief. Unfortunately, outside a veterinary clinic it is nearly impossible to carry out this procedure in a sterile way. Providing sterile aftercare is very difficult as well. The probability of a new abscess or further infection is therefore unacceptably high. In most cases it is better to give the abscess time to mature. Furthermore, anti-inflammatory or antibiotic drugs should be avoided. They cause abscesses to mature too slow or not mature at all. Studies even show that horses with abscesses that were intensively treated needed more time to recover.

To accelerate the maturing process of an abscess juniper or rosemary oil can be used. Read more about this on page 152 under 'Essential oils' Soaking in lukewarm water with a natural soap or enzymatic laundry powder contributes to the maturation of abscesses as well. Making the horse walk on a hard surface could stimulate an abscess to erupt. Obviously this is only possible if the now extra sore, laminitic horse can handle it.

In case an abscess refuses to erupt action needs to be taken. In severe cases, abscesses can spread and result in infections of joints and bones (osteomyelitis). Cutting an abscess open through the sole should only be done in

ABSCESS OR LAMINITIS?

The clinical signs of an abscess can be very similar to those of laminitis. Horse owners often mistake these clinical signs for laminitis not healing properly or a relapse. Some signs to determine whether the horse has an abscess instead of laminitis:

- One to two months after the onset of laminitis your horse suddenly starts limping.
- One leg shows significantly more clinical signs (lameness, elevated pulse and body temperature) than another.
- You have taken all possible preventive and curative measures against laminitis. Nothing has changed in the circumstances and suddenly this lameness occurs including pulsations and elevated temperature.
- The horse is in even more pain than with acute laminitis.
- The lameness started not long after a trim.

exceptional cases because there the risk of complications is especially high. By using the white line, or even through the hoof wall, most persistent abscesses can be reached. Unfortunately, it has become customary for hoof care providers to take on this task. As you have read before, it is very important that this surgical procedure is performed under sterile conditions. This is a task for a veterinarian, not a hoof care provider.

Once the abscess has erupted naturally or has been opened up surgically it must be kept extremely clean. Apple cider vinegar with water (1:1) or iodine are suitable means for this. The gap in the hoof wall, created by the abscess erupting at the coronary band, will naturally grow down. Keep an eye on the hole because it can easily become a place for disease and fungus to hide. If this is the case, the hole usually becomes wider by the pressure of the proliferating fungi. Treat fungi with a fungicide. Talk to your hoof care provider about which products to use. Often treatment with white vinegar and a few drops of tea tree oil is sufficient.

In some cases, there is so much necrotic tissue to expel that abscesses rip up the whole coronary band. This looks very serious. Keeping it clean and free of disease is important. Just wait and observe how the divested part of the hoof wall grows down. Make sure the hoof care provider keeps the edge of the hoof wall off the ground with his nippers. Rasping or filing a hoof wall that has disconnected at the coronet is painful for the horse. A new hoof wall will grow behind the loose one. After several months the hoof care provider may remove the loose part.

(A)SEPTIC OSTEITIS AND OSTEOMYELITIS

Aseptic osteitis is inflammation of the bone without a bacterial infection. If there is a bacterial infection, we speak of septic osteitis. Osteomyelitis is inflammation and infection of the bone and bone marrow. Coffin bone osteitis is a common complication of chronic laminitis. In the case of septic osteitis, the bone will need to be surgically curetted and rinsed. This is not the case with the aseptic variant. After the operation, the horse will be given antibiotic drugs. Recovery can take a long time. The hole in the hoof wall along which the operation was performed will already have closed after a few weeks.

SOLE PERFORATION

The coffin bone can rotate, sink and press on the sole from the inside to such an extent that the sole is no longer able to withstand this pressure. The tip of the coffin bone pierces the sole and can be seen from the outside. Sole perforation is a painful complication that also carries a serious risk of infection.

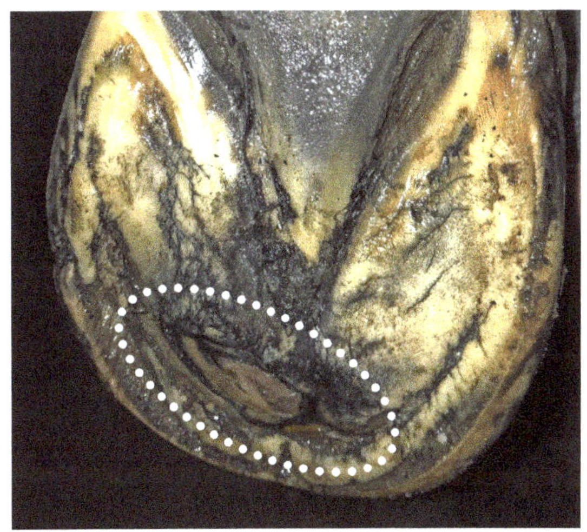

Sole perforation

Treatment

Your hoof care provider will try to optimise the position of the coffin bone as soon as possible to avoid aggravating the situation. The wound must be cleaned and maintained very thoroughly. The hoof is then bandaged. Hoof boots with insoles can also be used. Where the exposed coffin bone touches the sole of the boot, part of the insole can be cut out. The hoof boot and insoles must always be kept clean and disinfected. The horse is given antibiotic drugs.

WHITE LINE DISEASE

Also known as seedy toe, white line disease is an attack on the white line by a combination of bacteria and fungi. It is the hoof care provider's task to treat this complication. Often a significant part of the hoof wall needs to be removed. Diligent treatment with a variety of possible products obviously remains a task for the horse owner.

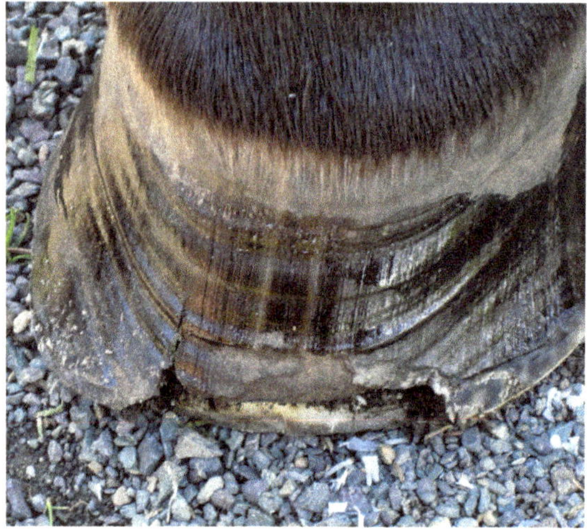

White line disease
(photo: Mike Harris)

Infection

Tissue affected by white line disease can provide access for bacteria to create an infection. This is not the same kind of infection as an abscess described above. The hoof care provider should treat the infection simultaneously with the white line disease.

Treatment

Recommended products to support the treatment of the hoof care provider vary from vinegar diluted with water up to copper sulphate, unpasteurised honey, chlorine (dioxide), Imaverol and colloidal silver. The more aggressive the product the greater the risk of dehydration and damage to healthy tissue or regenerating horn. Talk to your hoof care provider or veterinarian about which products to use.

Prevention

Prevention is more important than treatment. Try to find out why the quality of the hoof horn is so bad. In many cases this can be traced back to nutrition. Shortages of trace elements such as zinc and copper are associated with poor horn. Just like disturbances in the balance between iron, copper, zinc and manganese. The amino acids methionine and lysine are indispensable for a healthy hoof wall too.

Mechanical forces, generated by a long hoof wall, overload and stress the horn. Small cracks and other damage to the wall become easy access for fungi and bacteria. Urea and ammonia in the horse's urine and faeces attack the corneocytes (horn cells). Wet ground softens the hoof tissue, while hooves that are too dry crack more easily. The opportunistic microbes benefit directly from this. Also holes created by hoof nails are often the starting point of white line disease. Much can be gained by optimising housing, so the horses are offered dry footing and the place is easy to keep clean .

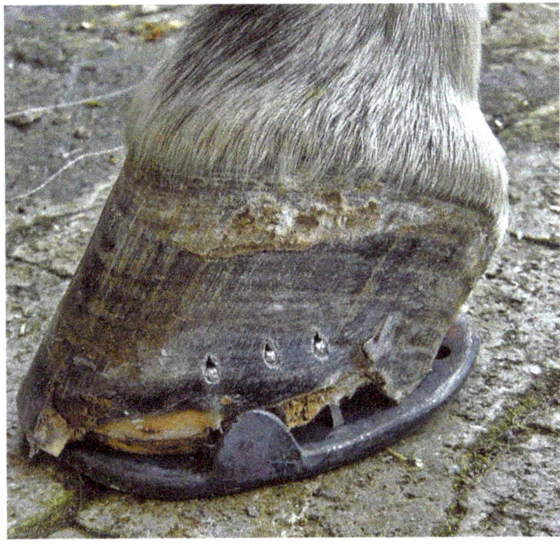

White line disease in a shod hoof
(photo: Patrick Brunner)

FROG INFECTION

A thrush-like infection of the frog could develop accompanied by a corresponding penetrating smell. Treat this complication as thrush. This means cutting away the affected tissue and treating the frog with a bactericide.

Do not use hoof tar. Tar seals the bacteria off from oxygen but these anaerobic bacteria thrive without oxygen. Furthermore tar contains carcinogens (polycyclic aromatic hydrocarbons/ PAH). Your horse is unlikely to get cancer from it, but prolonged and frequent use is definitely not recommended because of the presence of the PAH.

SEPSIS

Sepsis or blood poisoning is a possible complication of hoof abscesses. Clinical signs of sepsis include fever, weakness, confusion and lack of appetite. Call your veterinarian immediately if you think this is the case.

DETOXIFICATION

Detoxification (detox for short) is the removal of toxic substances (toxins) from the horse's body. On page 77 and beyond several types of toxins are listed. Determine if there are toxins that may be affecting your horse. Many toxins are easy to avoid by making dietary modifications, alterations in the worming and vaccinating regime and withholding or changing some types of medication. Toxins as a result of chronic kidney or liver problems, sepsis or exertional myopathies (like ER or AM) require treatment of these primary problems.

Lymphatic drainage is claimed to reduce oedema, remove necrotic tissue, affect glucose metabolism favourably, activate the parasympathetic nervous system, lower blood pressure and reduce pain. As yet no scientific research is available to confirm this.

Mycotoxin binders are available that disable toxic by-products of mould, fungi and yeasts in food.

The most efficient way to get rid of toxins is still by relying on a well-functioning liver, kidneys, urinary system and intestines. By providing movement, offering a high fibre diet to the intestines, keeping waste product levels low and of course, by making sure no new toxins are introduced.

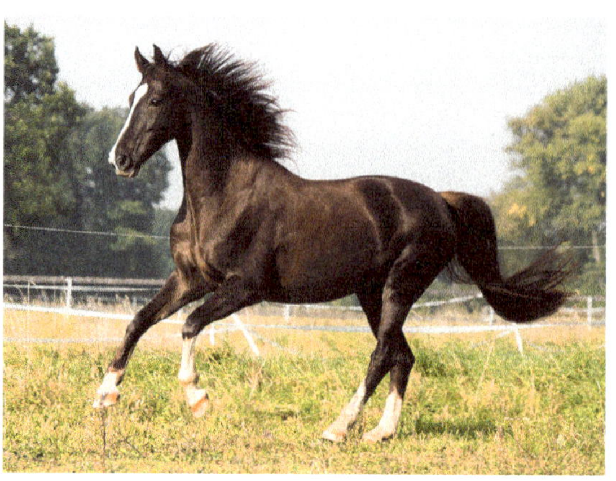

Detox by movement

WEIGHT MANAGEMENT

A fat horse is not normal and not healthy. If you don't want your horse to get laminitis, make sure it doesn't become overweight.

There are two types of fat horses:

- Overweight through excessive consumption
- Overweight due to hormonal problems

The first type has a big belly and is heavier than it should be. This horse has obesity. Dietary changes and exercise work wonders. The second type has a strange fat distribution: Fat deposits above the eyes, on the neck, shoulders, on top of the rump, above the tail and around the sheath or udder. This kind of overweight is called adiposity. Adiposity often occurs in horses with EMS. Obesity and adiposity may also occur together. For convenience, from here, we discuss both types under the term overweight.

Apart from a hereditary component in EMS, in both types of overweight an unsuitable diet and lack of exercise are to blame. This is usually caused by insufficient knowledge of the dietary needs of horses in general, often based on misinformation especially given by food manufacturers. Breeds originating from arid or cold areas have lower energy requirements and are therefore easily overfed. These ponies are 'designed' to gain weight in the abundant season (spring and summer) and loose the weight again in the lean season (autumn and winter). Domestication disturbs this system because we prevent horses from burning their excess fat. Then there are horses that do not get enough movement and exercise or not often enough.

As long as most horses are too fat it will remain the norm. Fat horses are regarded by many people as healthy or beautiful. Unfortunately there are still many owners who do not want to be different from other horse owners, change habits or deviate from tradition.

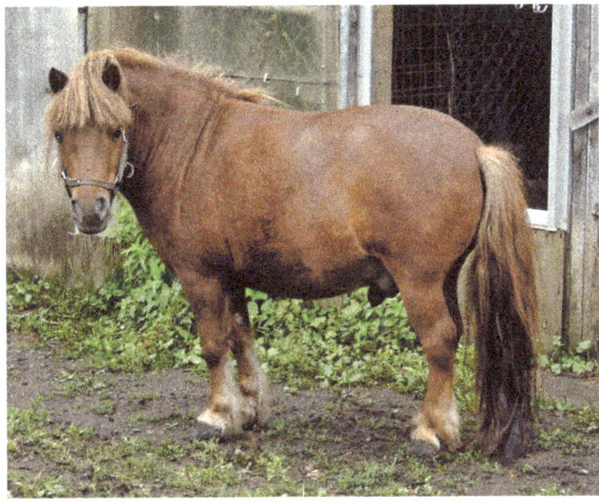

A fat horse is not normal and not healthy *(photo: Deanna Fenwick)*

WEIGHT LOSS

In the context of this chapter, weight loss is understood to mean intentional loss of fat mass. Provide nutrition with less NSC and more fibre. Restrict grazing (see page 187 under 'NSC prevention'). In case grazing restrictions are difficult to maintain it might be better to take the horse off the pasture altogether. Especially EMS and PPID horses are often better off on a hay only diet.

To determine the daily amount of hay to feed, 1.5% of the target weight is a good amount to start with in the first month. After that, the daily ration can be lowered to 1% of the target weight. An overweight horse with a 500 kg (1100 lbs) target weight is fed 7.5 kg (16.5 lbs) of hay the first month and 5 kg (11 lbs) of hay in subsequent months.

Make the horse move more. This is so important that even when you are unable to exercise your horse yourself, make sure somebody else does. Even if the horse does not lose weight, movement will certainly improve insulin sensitivity. Read also the section 'Nutrition and pasture management' on page 175 attentively.

Measure the horse and record the following weekly to keep track of progress:

- Weight (see sidebar 'Determine the horse's weight')
- CNS and BCS (see sidebars on pages 81 and 83 resp.)
- Neck size (see page 171 under 'Log')

Make sure the weight loss is gradual and not too fast. Rapid weight loss, especially in Shetland and Welsh ponies, Haflingers and donkeys can cause hyperlipidemia, which can result in vasoconstriction, another potential cause of laminitis. When too much fat is released too fast it can cause fatty degeneration and thus organ damage (steatosis). The liver is especially sensitive to this. Weight loss of up to 1% of the target weight per week is safe.

Fat horses are more prone to laminitis but have better chances of recovery once weight is brought under control. Of course this is only true in cases of laminitis caused by obesity.

DRUGS

Sometimes synthetic thyroid hormones are prescribed to achieve weight loss. Only give these drugs when exercise and diet really (!) don't achieve sufficient results. Realise that making a horse lose weight often takes just as much self-control as losing weight yourself. Drugs should never substitute discipline. On page 159 under 'Levothyroxine' more about this hormone.

DETERMINE THE HORSE'S WEIGHT

- Preferably weigh the horse on a weighbridge or use the Carroll & Huntington formula:
  - Measure the girth. Measure around the midsection, immediately behind the elbow and withers
  - Keep the measuring tape tight and wait until the horse has exhaled
  - Measure the body length. Measure from the point of the shoulder to the point of the buttock (tuber ischii)
  - The horse's weight is calculated by a formula that uses a constant which depends on the system you use, metric or imperial
  - The horse's weight in kilograms is:

    $$\frac{\text{Girth squared x body length (in centimetres)}}{11900}$$

    Example (centimetres > kilograms):

    Girth = 170 cm, body length = 210 cm

    $$\frac{(170 \times 170) \times 210}{11900} = 510 \text{ kilo}$$

  - The horse's weight in lbs is:

    $$\frac{\text{Girth squared x body length (in inches)}}{330}$$

    Example (inches > lbs):

    Girth = 67", body length = 83"

    $$\frac{(67 \times 67) \times 83}{330} = 1129 \text{ lbs}$$

- The formula has a 10% margin
- The formula for foals up to two months old:
  Metric: (chest size in centimetres minus 62.5) / 0.7
  Imperial: (chest size in inches minus 24.5) / 0.13
- Determining the weight by using a weight tape is not very accurate. On average it results in a weight that is 65 kilograms out (143 lbs). This can be either 65 kilograms too heavy or too light.

HOOF PROTECTION

Because it is difficult to watch your horse suffer from pain or because you hoof care provider thinks it is possible to accelerate the healing process using horseshoes, solutions for laminitic horses are often sought in hoof protection. Unfortunately metal or plastic shoes are not beneficial. Hoof boots however, can be very useful.

THERAPEUTIC SHOEING

Often (therapeutic) shoeing is used to treat laminitis. The range of corrective shoes for laminitic horses varies from open-toed shoes or even reversed shoes to shoes resembling an unshod natural hoof, from egg bar shoes to shoes with adjustable heel height and synthetic glue on shoes. The shoes are attached with or without all kinds of insoles and shock absorbing materials. Some shoes include frog support (heart bar shoes), or even a screw mechanism that can be used to increase or decrease the pressure on the frog.

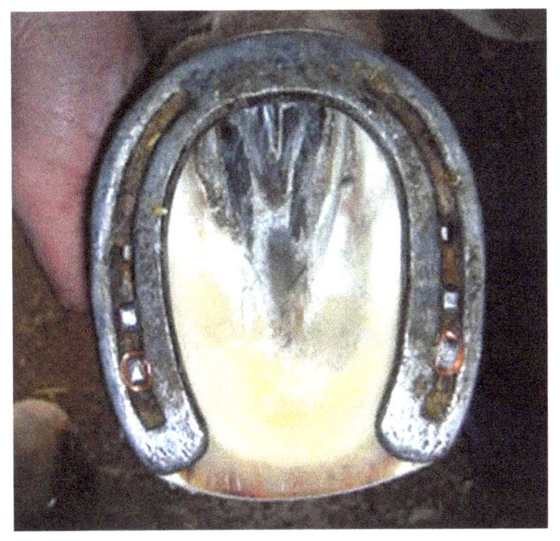

Reversed shoe
(photo: Andrew Grimm)

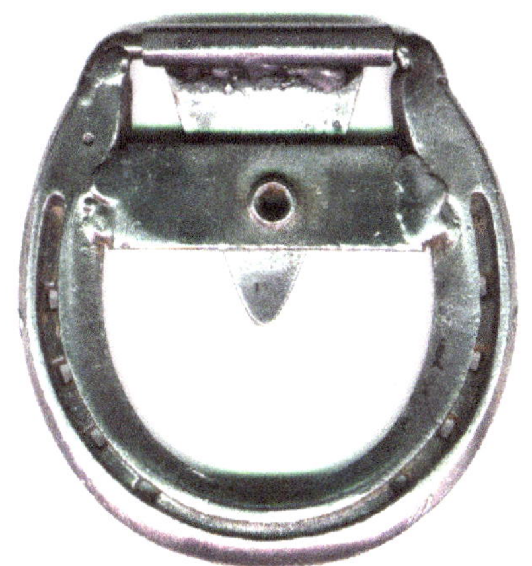

Heart bar shoe with screw mechanism
(photo: Mary Bayard Fitzpatrick)

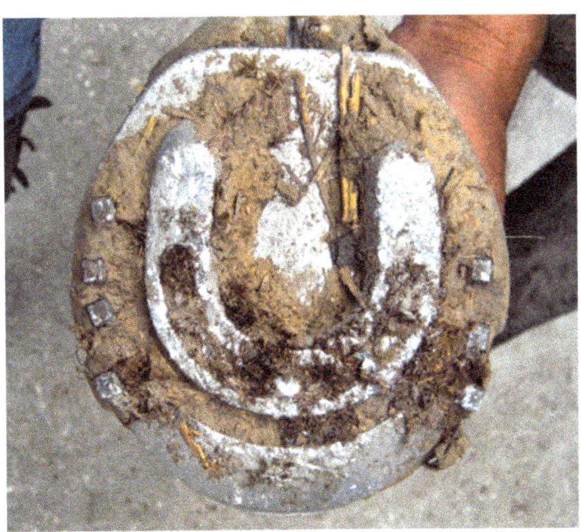

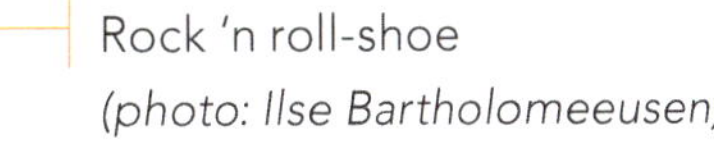

Rock 'n roll-shoe
(photo: Ilse Bartholomeeusen)

Disadvantages

Shoes have so many disadvantages that their use is strongly discouraged. Shoes decrease hoof mechanism, which results in a limited supply of oxygenated blood and removal of carbonated blood. The same applies to the supply and transport of nutrients and removal of waste products. Dead lamellar tissue and inflammation residue accumulates which can disrupt the metabolism. The frog will become more prone to infection as well.

Besides affecting the hooves, also the bones, joints and vascular system in the lower leg suffer from both the vibration and the centrifugal force caused by metal shoes. In the short term this has negative consequences for the circulation as described above. In the long term it may result in osteoarthritis and ossification of cartilage tissue. Especially for laminitic horses this can be part of the problem because the hoof cartilages are important for shock absorption. Shod hooves cannot break over properly. This may result in overloading and even ossification of the hoof cartilages.

Horseshoes are nailed, screwed or glued to the partially detached hoof wall while the hooves are trying to recover by growing a well-connected hoof wall. The shoes stress the growth of healthy lamellar tissue and the new connection keeps keeps being torn loose by the mechanical force created by the shoes. Piercing the hoof wall and white line with nails weakens the structure of the hoof wall and causes drying out of the horn tissue around the nail holes. Bacteria, microbes, and ammonia compounds from dirt and faeces penetrate into the hoof through the nail holes, increasing the risk of white line disease.

In between shoeing appointments the hoof wall cannot be maintained with a rasp or knife. The outer wall can quickly become too long and will then start pulling on the lamellar connection like a lever. The frog will receive little or no ground pressure, causing it to develop insufficiently. This leads to reduced shock absorption and a preference for toe first landing which increases the risk of overloading and traumatic laminitis.

To be able to notice improvement or worsening of sole sensitivity is important. Because the sole of a shod hoof is lifted off the ground you will not be able to judge the situation. The sole will not harden sufficiently. A solid sole will provide more protection to the coffin bone that is pushing against it from the inside. Sole flexibility reduces when hooves are shod, increasing the chance of sole bruising. Sole bruising will make horses more reluctant to walk while this is so important for the healing process.

Shoes with raised heels are used to reduce the tension of the deep digital flexor tendon, but increase the pressure on the tip of the coffin bone and the lamellar connection at the front of the hoof. In addition, the deep flexor muscle tension will adjust to the new position. This causes the forces exerted by the tendon to return to the old level quite quickly. Raising the heels is a temporary solution that unfortunately is often applied for too long. Moreover, it is not the pulling force of the tendon that causes the coffin bone to rotate, but the inability of the lamellae and extensor tendon to counter act this pull.

Shod horses cannot feel the surface they walk on. They stumble more often and occasionally slip. For laminitic horses this is very painful and may result in less movement than is beneficial.

If you still want to use shoes despite all the disadvantages mentioned above, choose plastic over metal and glue rather than nails.

It is easy to understand why horse owners are tempted to have their horse shod. The horse will seem to walk relatively pain free. However, it is the lack of proper circulation that partially numbs the leg. The horse tends to move more, longer and faster than the recovering tissue can handle. The apparent benefit of being pain free in the short term will be compensated for by a prolongation of the problem in the long term.

Transitional phase

When deshoeing it is important to realise that the discomfort of being barefoot is not caused by the removal of the shoes but the result of being shod (for years) previously. The tissues in the hoof have suffered all that time because of the compromised circulation. The sole is still sensitive. In case the horse has been shod since an early age the digital cushion and hoof cartilages might be underdeveloped. It sounds harsh, but the horse will have to get through this transitional phase. Hoof boots can offer a solution in this case. A good hoof care provider can advise you on this. They also know how to trim your horse's hooves to minimise or prevent discomfort. Now, let's have a look at hoof boots.

HOOF BOOTS

Some people believe that all horses should be able to be barefoot in all circumstances. Hoof boots are rejected by them as an option. This is regrettable and unjustified. Using boots is not a failure, but a way to get through the difficult times, speeding up recovery by reducing pain and encouraging movement. The use of hoof boots can be discontinued over time.

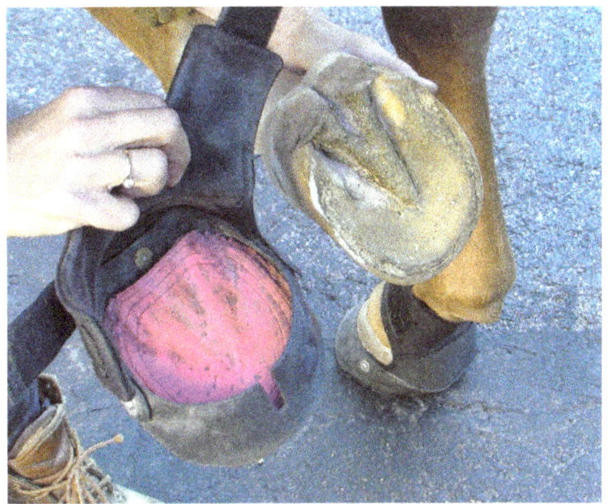

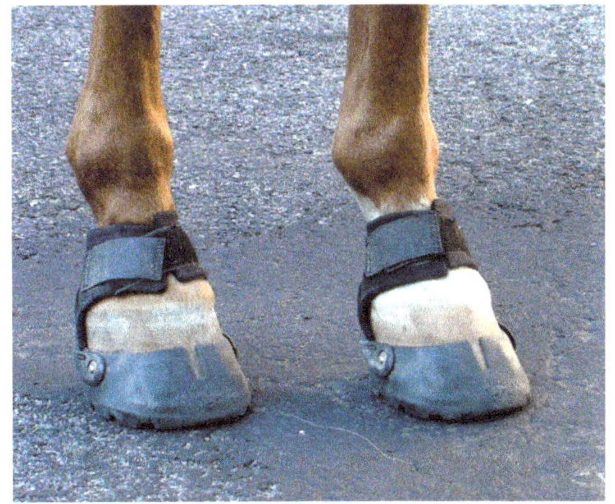

Hoof boots
(photo: Sherilyn Allen)

Advantages

Hoof boots provide extra cushioning which relieves the pain. Pain-free movement stimulates circulation and therefore a faster development of shock and vibration-absorbing tissues, such as the digital cushion and hoof cartilage. Improved blood flow also ensures a better supply of oxygenated and and removal of carbonated blood. The supply of nutrients such as enzymes increases and the removal of bodily substances like waste products improves. This contributes to a faster healing of the laminitis itself, and of that of possible complications like abscesses. Proper movement accelerates the reduction of oedema. Besides this, exercise burns energy which stimulates weight loss.

Soft insoles stimulate the frog and therefore the hoof growth (see sidebar 'Frog contact and hoof growth' on page 32). In case of a sole perforation, some material of the inner part of the insole can be removed to relieve pressure on the tip of the rotated coffin bone.

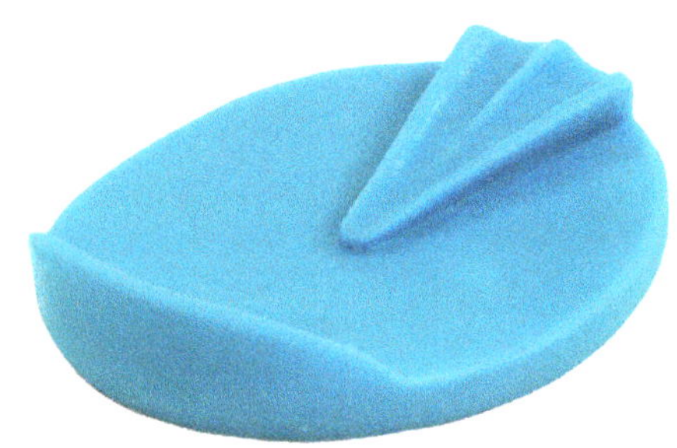

Insoles with frog support
(photo: Soft-ride)

Most disadvantages of horseshoes do not apply for hoof boots. The big advantage is that you can put them on and take them off. This makes it possible to maintain the hooves regularly. In particular, keeping the hoof wall and toe section short is essential in the healing of laminitis.

For severely deformed hooves, boots can be made to measure. The soles could be made of extra soft material for even more cushioning. Both new and second hand boots should fit as well as possible.

Disadvantages

The disadvantage is, as with horseshoes, the centrifūgal force acting on the hooves, bones, joints and capillaries. However, most movement and exercise during the recovery period of laminitis will be in walk. Some horses may suffer from rubbing or bruising of the heel bulbs or pasterns. This can be solved by using protective socks, pastern wraps or athletic tape.

To ensure hoof boots maintain the right fit and remain easy to put on and take of, regular hoof care is essential. In case of laminitis the shape of the hoof may change substantially. Hoof boots that initially were the right size might not fit anymore once the lamellar connection recovers and the white line is no longer stretched. While this is good news for the horse, it isn't for your wallet. Costs should not be an obstacle. By using secondhand boots it is possible to reduce the costs. When buying used boots make sure they are not worn asymmetrically. Check underneath and inside the boots.

We will now look at some popular brands and models. Note that this overview is not exhaustive.

Easyboot Stratus

- + Therapeutic hoof boot
- + Adaptable for specific conditions using TheraPad System
- + Moisture drains easily
- + Good air circulation
- − Adjustments require experience

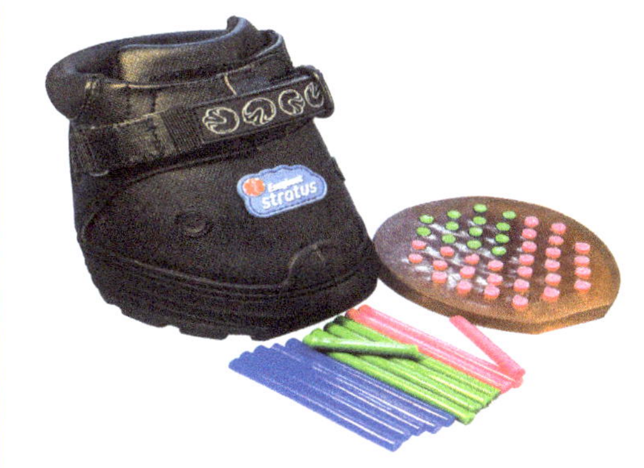

Easyboot Cloud

- + Therapeutic hoof boot specifically developed for laminitic horses
- + Soft sole
- − Not suitable for riding

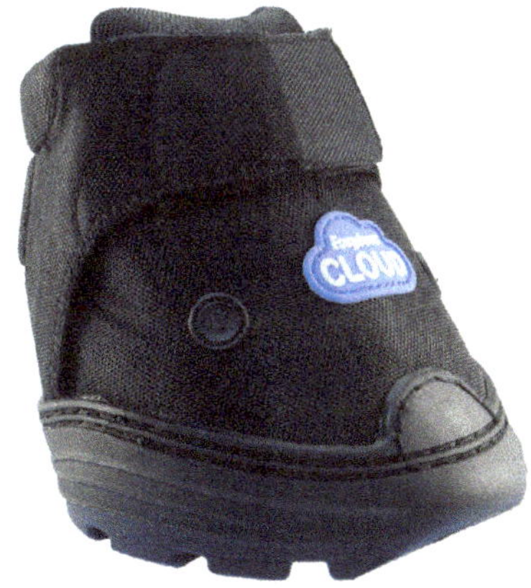

Easyboot Zip

- + Therapeutic hoof boot
- + Quick and easy solution to protect the hoof
- − Not suitable for riding

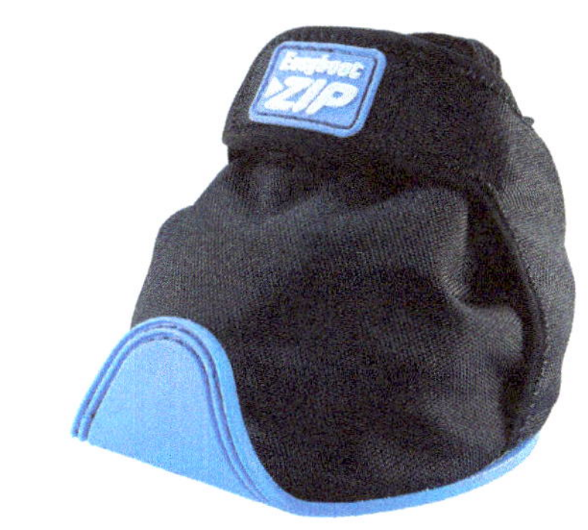

Easyboot Glove

- + Lightweight
- + Easy to put on
- + Suitable for horses with hooves which have a greater length than width
- − Difficult to take off

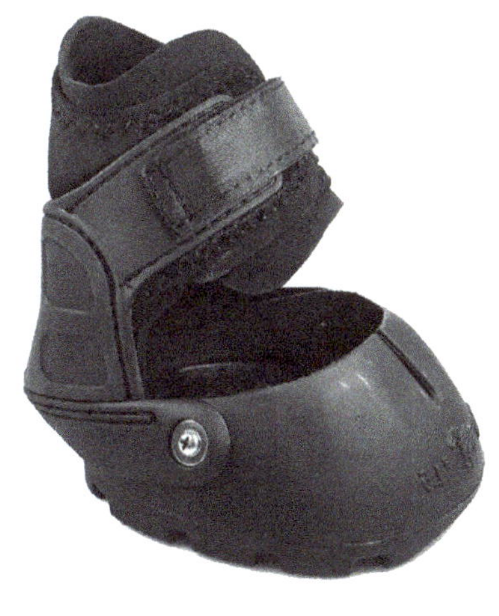

Scoot-boot

- ⊕ Lightweight
- ⊕ Easy to put on
- ⊕ Water drains easily
- ⊖ Back and closure can cause irritation

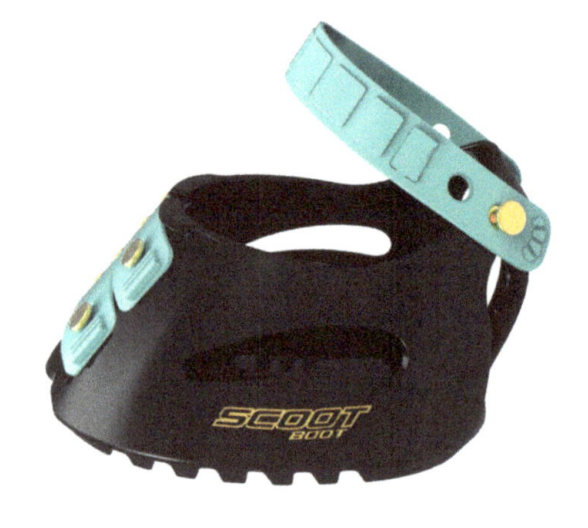

Cavallo simple

- ⊕ Easy to put on, stays well in place
- ⊕ Heel bulbs are protected
- ⊕ Suitable for horses with hooves which have a greater width than length
- ⊕ Suitable for driving
- ⊖ May cause irritation of the pastern

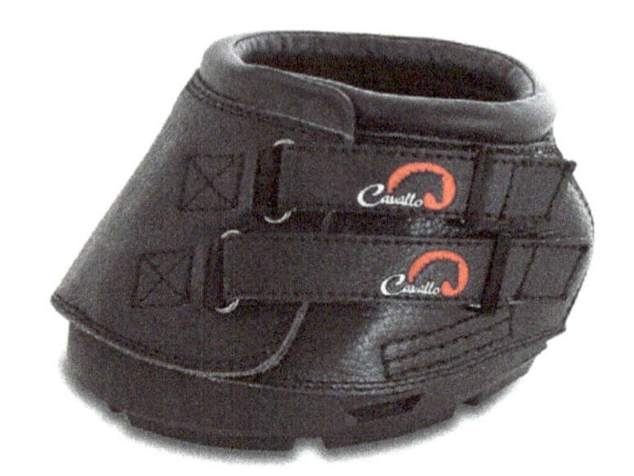

Dallmer clog

- ⊕ Easy to adjust
- ⊕ Wear resistant
- ⊕ Separate models front and hind hooves
- ⊕ Water drains easily
- ⊖ Open sole, causing peripheral loading

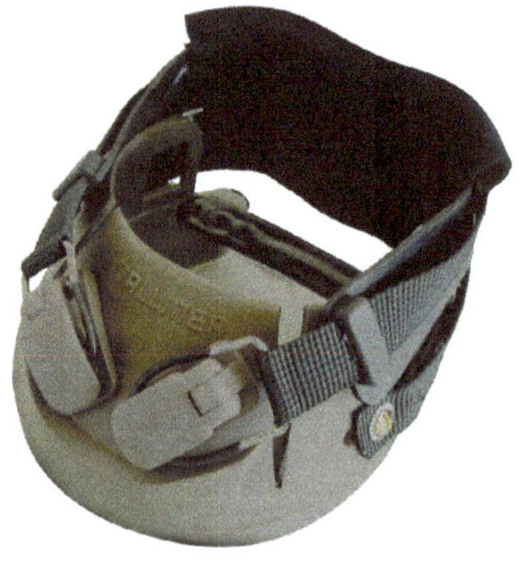

Equine fusion all terrain ultra

- ⊕ Very good shock absorption
- ⊕ Soft inside
- ⊕ Suitable for deviating hoof shapes, such as flares and lamellar wedge

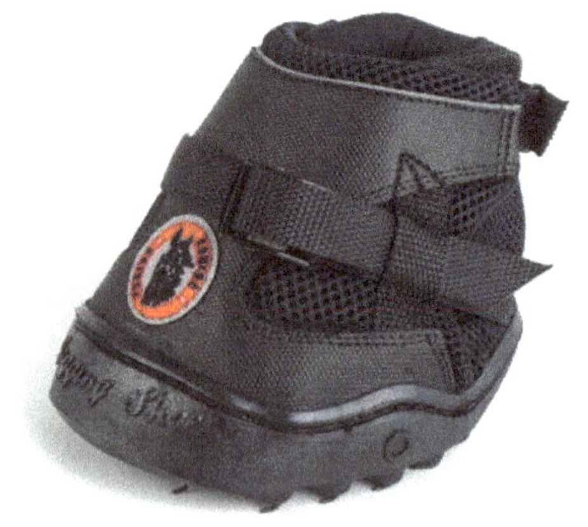

Soft ride

- ⊕ Therapeutic hoof boot
- ⊕ Extra soft insoles for optimal shock and vibration absorption
- ⊖ Not suitable for riding

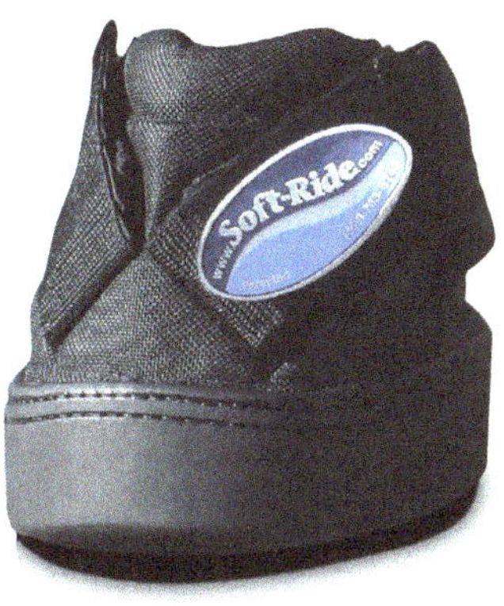

Evo boot

- ⊕ Lightweight
- ⊕ Concave sole
- ⊕ Flexible

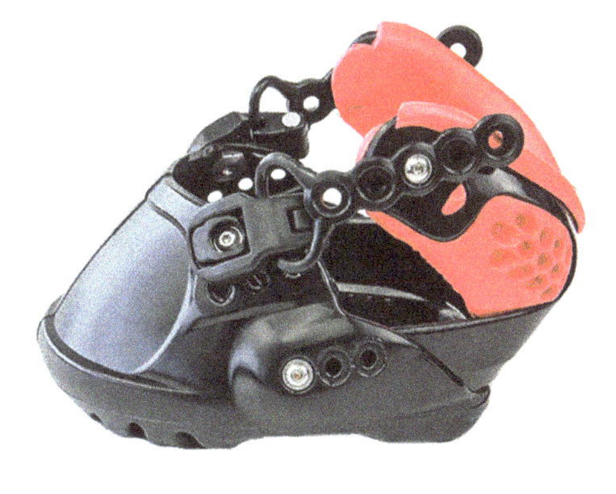

Renegade

- ⊕ Stays well in place
- ⊕ Suitable for horses with hooves which have a greater length than width
- ⊕ Water drains easily
- ⊖ Less suitable for deviating hoof shapes
- ⊖ Sole too hard and no possibility to use insoles
- ⊖ This shoe must be adapted before first use

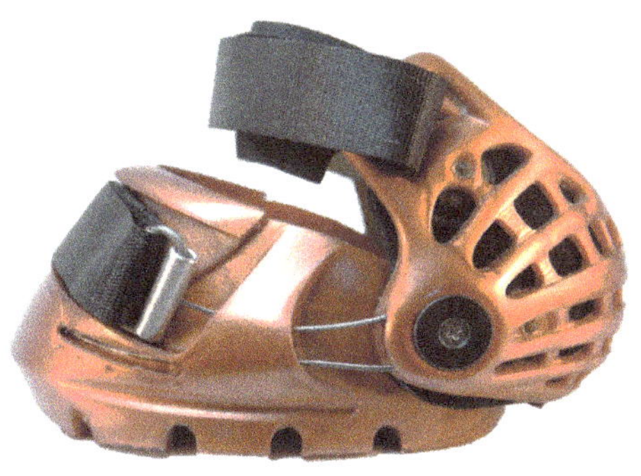

Swiss galoppers

- ⊕ Flexible, suitable for different hoof shapes
- ⊕ Good protection of heel bulbs
- ⊕ Few wear-sensitive parts
- ⊖ Sole too hard
- ⊖ Few large sizes available

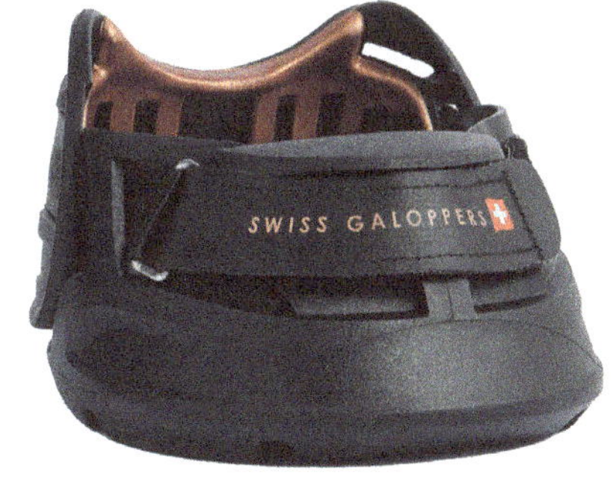

HOOF CASTING

In the acute phase, or in case of a sinker, the hoof may be casted with plaster or synthetic casting material. Sole supporting materials are included within the cast. The purpose of casting is to improve the distribution of forces on the hoof and prevent further coffin bone rotation. In some cases, casting is combined with a coronary band resection. (see page 147 under 'Coronary band resection').

Disadvantages and complications

- The cast is left on the hoof for to two up to four weeks. During this time developments of the hoof can only be observed by radiographs.
- Hoof mechanism is restricted.
- Incorrectly applied casts may constrict circulation.
- Some casting materials are not breathable, causing fungal infections.
- Risk of undetected bacterial infections.
- Nowadays the objectives of hoof casts can nearly always be achieved in other ways.

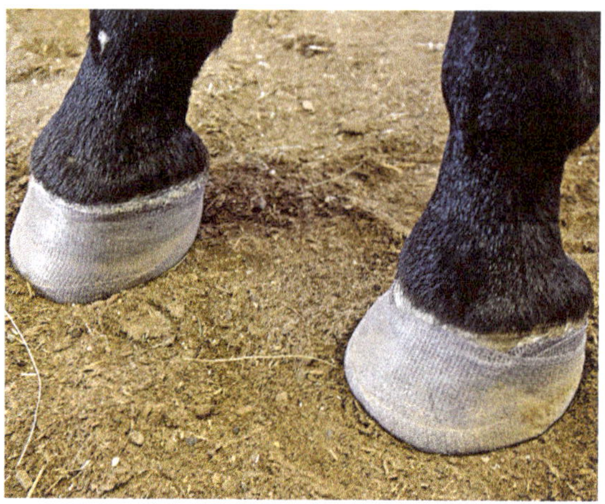

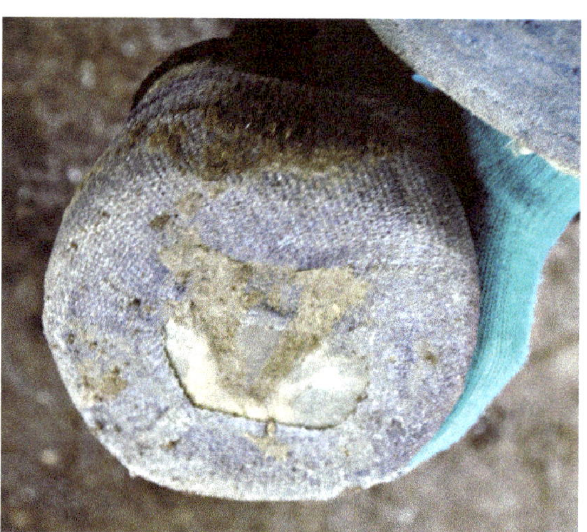

Hoof casting
(photos: Sarah Bernier)

MOVEMENT AND EXERCISE

Often, lack of sufficient movement and exercise is one of the major causes in the onset of laminitis. Lack of it also results in poor circulation and overweight. Movement is essential to successful recovery. However, if you make your laminitic horse move before he has been trimmed properly, you might make his condition worse. To be even clearer, don't let your horse move an inch before your hoof care provider has trimmed the hooves. After that, encourage every movement the horse makes, even if it means just standing up after lying down for days, but never force it to move. The weakened lamellar connection should not get damaged even further and the sole should be loaded carefully because of pressure of the rotated coffin bone against it.

Movement stimulates hoof mechanism and therefore circulation. Oxygenated blood, full of nutrients and hormones, is able to reach the hoof, while carbonated blood and waste are removed. However, a large percentage of blood does not reach the lamellar dermis as a result of shunting (see page 33). It is therefore important to find the balance between the maximum beneficial effect of movement without it causing damage to the hoof.

A laminitic horse 'knows' intuitively how much and what kind of movement (gait, speed, distance) it needs to aid the healing process. Stabling deprives the horse of this opportunity. Box rest is not a solution, but one of the causes.

Give the horse space to move in an environment where food risks are minimal (grass, acorns, beechnuts, apples, et cetera). Only give access to grazing when risks can be managed. Food risks and grazing are discussed extensively on page 175 under 'Nutrition and pasture management'.

You can start encouraging your horse to move from Obel 1, or when the horse starts to move noticeably better after one minute of walking with hoof boots and insoles, by:

- Hand walking
- Groundwork or games
- Offering social interaction with other horses (see page 197 under 'Social interaction')
- Creating several locations with hay, water and salt licks at a fair distance from each other
- Fencing off a track in the meadow or sand school with electric fencing (see page 195 under 'Paddock paradise')

> ➤ Make sure the footing is either flat and hard, or sandy. Irregularities will overload the sensitive soles too much. Sand that is too deep or heavy will also generate too much pressure on the sole.

To ride your horse in the acute phase is not a good idea. The extra weight will burden the hooves too much. Maintaining balance is harder for the horse because of its painful feet. Jumping, obviously, is out of the question.

You could start riding again from Obel 0, but only if the horse's soles are at least 1 cm (3/8") thick (ask your hoof care provider). Still, the use of hoof boots with insoles is recommended. Start with short distances, in a calm to moderate pace, and make sure not to overload the horse. Let the horse decide where to place its feet. Pay attention to signs of pain or fatigue and respect them immediately. The same applies for lunging and movement in a horse walker. The movement on a circle stresses the inner structures of the hoof too much. Movement in a horse walker becomes strained quite quickly.

Increase movement duration and intensity slowly and gradually over time. Not only owners, but also some horses want to go too fast too soon. When exercise causes deterioration, you have to slow down immediately.

SURGERY

For completeness, or even as a warning, the surgical procedures that are sometimes used are described in this book. Obviously there are situations where this type of intervention might be useful or necessary. Please discuss the options with your veterinarian and try to get an objective idea of the most negative outcome as possible. Ask for a second opinion from another veterinarian. Finally, it might be good to reflect on the reasons for surgery. Is it for the welfare of the horse or your own benefit? The adjustment of your own expectations will always be less invasive than surgery.

TENOTOMY AND DESMOTOMY

Tenotomy, the division of the deep digital flexor tendon and desmotomy, the cutting of the check ligament, are procedures that aim to eliminate the rotation of the coffin bone. The purpose of this type of surgery is to remove the tensile force of the deep digital flexor tendon on the coffin bone.

This surgical intervention is often undertaken despite the fact this tensile force is not the problem. The rotation of the coffin bone is caused by the inability of the lamellae, along with the extensor tendon, to offer counter force. In other words, it is the detachment of the hoof wall rather than the rotation of the coffin bone that is the problem. Usually this method is applied in a very late stage of laminitis, and mostly just to prolong the life of the horse, a goal that is hardly ever attained by it.

Disadvantages and complications

To counteract the changed forces on the hoof, therapeutic shoeing is often applied, combined with aggressive trimming to force the coffin bone parallel to the ground. This can have serious drawbacks.

Swelling, pain, inflammation, osteomyelitis, connective tissue tumours, osteoarthritis, joint deformities and permanent tendon contraction may occur as complications. Long and intensive aftercare is required.

HOOF WALL RESECTION

A hoof wall resection is the partial or complete removal of the hoof wall. In case of laminitis, a part of the dorsal hoof wall is resected. In the chronic phase, this is done with the objective of:

- Removal of necrotic tissue
- Treatment of abscesses
- Removal of pressure.
  - The same result can be achieved by drilling small holes in the hoof wall, which can be closed again after fluid and blood serum have drained.

DISADVANTAGES AND COMPLICATIONS

The hoof's quarters can be affected by the increased pressure if they are not trimmed properly. This can result in the aggravation of preexisting white line separation. Without adequate aftercare complications can occur like inflammation, abscesses and excessive growth of granulation tissue (proud flesh).

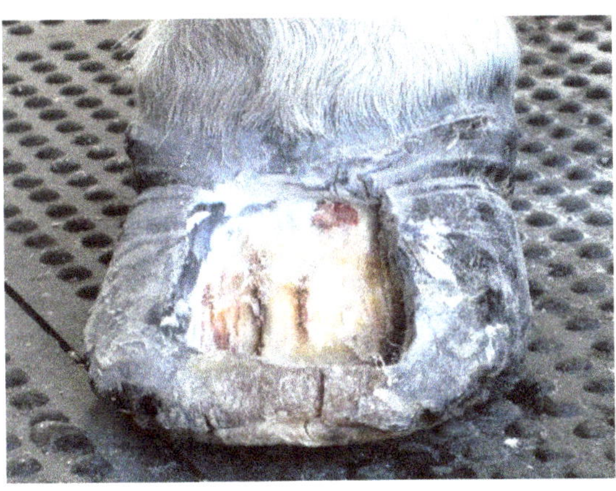

Partial hoof wall resection
(photo: Simon Constable)

CORONARY BAND RESECTION

A coronary band resection is the removal of a small portion of the hoof wall just below the coronet with the objective of:

- Stimulation of proper wall growth in the toe region
- Removal of the pressure exerted by the hoof wall that is constricting the circulation
- Removal of pressure on the coronary dermis

DISADVANTAGES AND COMPLICATIONS

This procedure weakens the hoof wall increasing the risk of further coffin bone rotation. A coronary band resection has the same potential complications as a hoof wall resection. The edges of the created groove may constrict the circulation and cause swelling. A coronary band prolapse is one of the potential undesirable side effects.

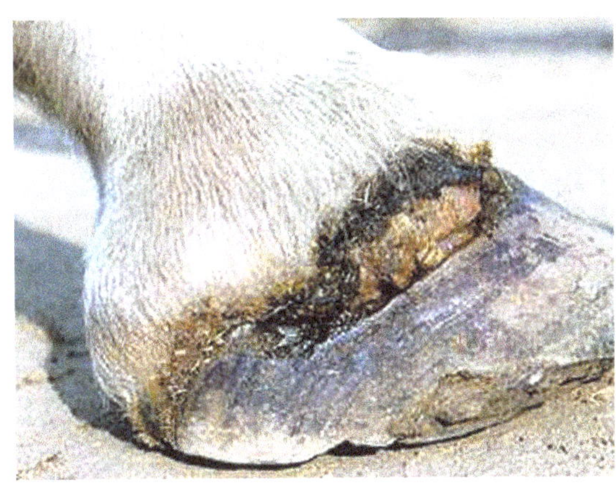

Coronary band prolapse as a result of a coronary resection
(photo: Gretschen Fathauer)

STEM CELL TRANSPLANT

Epidermal cells are constantly being renewed. This process, called epidermal regeneration, also takes place in the hoof. It is part of normal growth and repair of the hoof wall. The germinal layer of the epidermis contains stem cells, that generate the specific cells required for epidermal renewal. The protein P63 is involved in the maintenance of the stem cells. In chronic laminitic horses the activity of P63 seems to differ from that in healthy horses. As a result, the stem cells produce insufficient horn cells, weakening the lamellar connection. Transplantation of stem cells of the horse's own body could provide a solution.

Disadvantages

Stem cell transplant is very expensive and specialised surgery. You may wonder if this kind of treatment isn't a bit too complicated for the type of illness laminitis actually is. In the future this treatment might offer a solution in very rare cases of laminitis, when all other solutions fail.

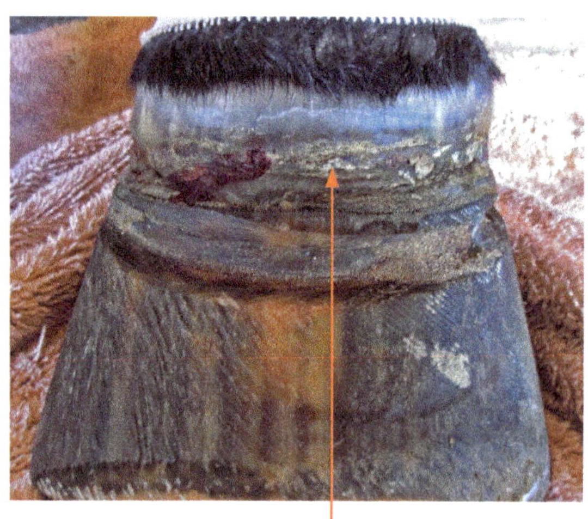

New wall growth after stem cell treatment *(photo: Rood & Riddle stem cell laboratory)*

BLOODLETTING

Bloodletting (phlebotomy), is an ancient treatment that nowadays occasionally is used again. By draining blood an attempt is made to lower the blood pressure. The idea behind this is twofold. Firstly, a lower blood pressure slightly reduces the flow of MMPs. Secondly, the lowering of blood pressure helps to prevent blood serum leaking from the capillaries which slightly decreases the risk of oedema formation between the hoof wall and the coffin bone. The pulsations in the hoof reduce which eases the pain. However, soon after treatment the blood pressure will recover, although usually not completely up to previous levels. With regard to oedema formation bloodletting remains just a symptomatic measure. Also the decreased supply of MMPs is a short-lived effect.

A second aim is to reduce the viscosity of the blood. After bloodletting the body tries to restore the blood volume as quickly as possible. To make this happen, fluid is drawn from tissues and added to the blood. The idea behind it is blood that flows more easily will provide better circulation. This brings the bloodletting treatment in line with the circulation and trauma theories. Again, the viscosity of the blood will quickly return to its previous level.

Disadvantages and complications

The rapid changes in blood volume and fluid balance have adverse effects on mineral concentrations in the body. Besides, bloodletting potentially has the following complications:

- Bruising
- Microthromboses
- Vascular infections
- Nerve or tissue damage by keeping the tourniquet on for too long

MAGGOT THERAPY

Maggot therapy is an unusual bio-surgical treatment that is still in the experimental stage. Although chances are very small your horse will ever undergo this treatment, it has been added to this book nonetheless.

Until the invention of antibiotics in the nineteen thirties, the use of maggots was fairly common in human medicine. Infected or necrotic tissue is removed very effectively by the sterile maggots of the flesh fly. The bacteria in the tissue are digested by the maggots. Healthy or healing tissue is left untouched.

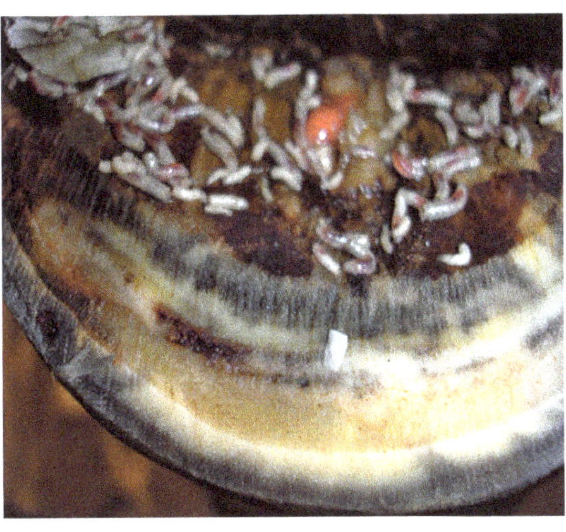

Maggot therapy
(photo: Scott Morrison)

The presence of maggots changes the acidity of the surrounding tissue causing bacterial multiplication to slow down. Maggots also secrete allantoin, a substance that is able to stimulate tissue to create new cells. A second substance they release is ammonia, that has a disinfecting effect. Besides this, maggots produce enzymes that have an anti-inflammatory effect, soften necrotic tissue, stimulate the production of capillaries and delay the clumping of blood platelets. This last feature causes the wound to stay open longer, ensuring the maggots to continue their good work. Lastly, there is the movement the maggots make. The constant wriggling stimulates the tissue and causes the body to more rapidly generate granulation tissue. The only known side effect is the result of this movement of the maggots. The horse can become irritated by it and start scraping or striking the hoof, for instance against the stable wall.

Every three days, the maggots are replaced by fresh ones. They are held in place with special oxygen and moisture-permeable bandages, that are changed daily. Another method is casting the hoof and creating an opening through which the wound can be reached.

When maggots are needed to work on the sole, the horse is shod with a hospital plate. That way, the maggots are not crushed by the horse's weight. It may be that this treatment is worse than the disease. Given the experimental nature of the therapy, other treatment is probably possible without maggots and therefore without the need to shoe the horse.

Maggots don't need anything but oxygen and their buffet of infected and necrotic tissue. Especially in places with poor circulation they can do good work. On page 47 under 'Shape and condition of the coffin bone' you read that dead tissue is, among others, caused by pinched blood vessels.

The most commonly used form of maggot therapy with regards to laminitis is when the coffin bone is infected (osteomyelitis). An opening in the hoof wall needs to be made to get the maggots in the designated place. Also in cases with severe sole perforation, with complicating infections and chronic sole abscesses, this therapy seems to deliver beneficial results.

LEECH THERAPY

Leech therapy is a second type of bio-surgery. Medicinal leeches have been used against many diseases for thousands of years. Leech saliva contains substances that have anticoagulant, antibiotic, analgesic and anti-inflammatory properties. Some of these substances are actually extracted from leeches for medicinal purposes. Complementary medicine has shown a renewed interest in leech therapy which can be applied as an alternative to chemical or phytotherapeutic drugs with the characteristics listed above. Also, the alleged benefits mentioned about bloodletting are pursued while using leeches.

DISADVANTAGES AND COMPLICATIONS

Leech therapy potentially has the following disadvantages and complications:

- The bite is painful, causes itching and possible allergic reactions.
- Anemia
- Pathogens can be transmitted including a bacterium that lives in the leech's intestines. This may cause a severe infection.
- Fever
- After the leeches have been removed, the wound remains open and bleed for quite some time because of the coagulation-inhibiting agent hirudin, secreted by the leech. When the wound finally closes, scar tissue may form.

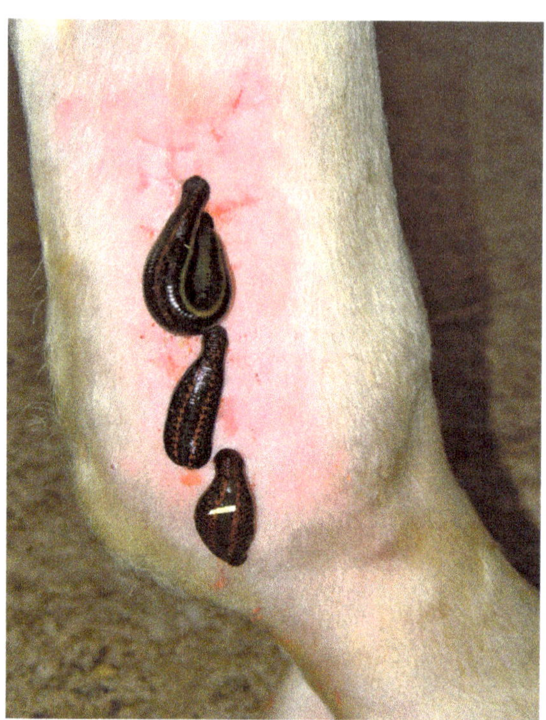

Leech therapy
(photo: Kathmann Vital)

All in all, this treatment has quite a few disadvantages, while modern alternatives are available that do not have these complications. Of course, the treatment might have a positive effect because of its action and the substances involved, but you may wonder if the end justifies the means.

COMPLEMENTARY THERAPIES

You now know that you have to focus on eliminating the primary and facilitating causes of laminitis and treat its complications. Later in this book you will read how improving your horse's living conditions can contribute to a speedy recovery. Besides these lifestyle changes, a wide range of complementary and alternative therapies is available. Complementary therapies to reduce inflammation, pain or oedema, improve circulation or bring the body back into balance include homeopathy, aroma and flower therapy, magnetic and electrotherapy. Reiki, craniosacral therapy, bio-resonance, healing gemstones and spiritual healing are also said to be beneficial, supporting the process or even curing laminitis completely.

It is beyond the scope of this book to discuss all these possibilities or to assess their therapeutic value on a scientific basis. If you feel comfortable with this form of treatment, you should consider using them in the healing process or prevention of laminitis. Just make sure they don't interfere with the treatment as described in this book. Also watch out for the pitfall of having 'two captains on one ship'. Different care providers giving conflicting advice will certainly not accelerate the healing of your horse.

Try not to lose sight of the facts. An acupuncturist can help to reduce your horse's oedema. There is even scientific evidence that acupuncture can have a positive effect on glucose metabolism. But if your horse is severely insulin resistant you will really have to change diet and exercise as well.

On the next pages some of the therapies that have shown to be effective as complementary therapy will be discussed. There is no evidence, other than anecdotal, that one of these therapies alone can cure laminitis.

ACUPUNCTURE, ACUPRESSURE, SHIATSU

Acupuncture, acupressure and shiatsu could enhance the beneficial effects of (conventional) treatment and limit side effects. This is partly because these therapies help to relieve pain by releasing endorphins in the blood. They are able to improve circulation and reduce oedema as well. Earlier in this book you have read that the augmented supply of MMPs is a possible cause of laminitis. To have your horse treated with acupuncture to promote circulation during the developmental or acute phase is therefore not recommended.

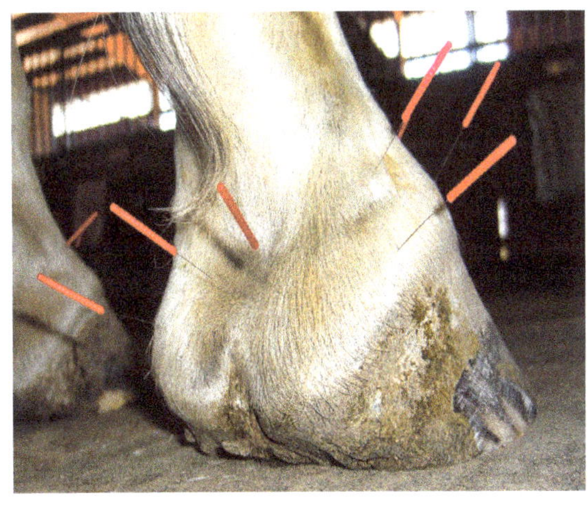

Acupuncture
(photo: Lisa Lancaster)

> Studies in humans have shown that the increased production of endorphins is independent of where the acupuncture needle was inserted on the body. Treatment on the meridians did not yield a better result. The researchers stated that the increased production is a response to the pain caused by the needle.

MASSAGE

The laminitic stance often causes muscle aches. Massaging can provide relief. Feel if you can discover hard, tense muscles. Muscles in chest, back and hind can be especially sore.

First, rub the muscles to warm them up, using both hands, then start the actual massage. Simply kneading the muscles helps well. Drumming loosely with your fists on the buttocks is also a simple massage technique. Be careful not to drum on joints or other sensitive areas.

Chronic tension in the shoulder muscles will eventually increase tension on the deep digital flexor tendon. A simple treatment to loosen the muscles and connective tissue: lift the front leg and gently pull it forward. Support the leg below the knee and hoof. You might need some practice, but if done in the right way, you will notice that the horse will start to extend the foreleg by itself. Hold the hoof in line with the shoulder, and close to the ground. Stretch the leg that way for about four times. Then gently put the leg back onto the ground. You can stretch both front legs daily.

A severely laminitic horse will not be happy with this exercise. He is not comfortable standing on three legs and it adds even more stress to the tendon. If your horse indicates that the massage feels unpleasant you have to stop immediately. Try the same massage again, but even more gently. If your horse still thinks a massage is not a great idea, then stop completely. You can also ask help from a physiotherapist or horse masseur.

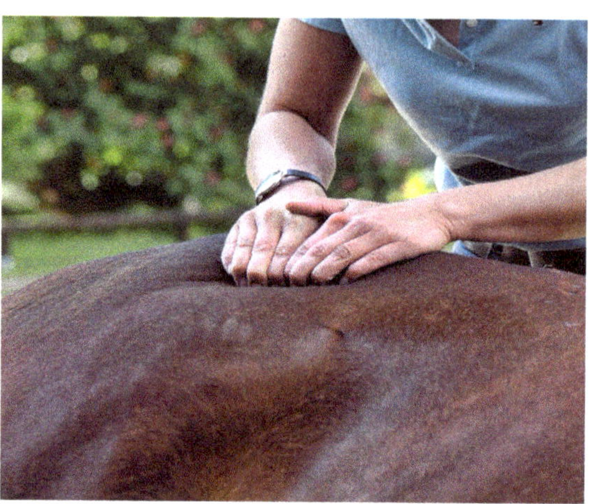

Massage
(photo: Wide open pets)

ESSENTIAL OILS

Rosemary and juniper oil can be used to stimulate blood flow. As previously mentioned, increasing circulation is not beneficial in the first two stages of laminitis, however in the chronic phase the hooves do benefit from it.

- Only use pure essential oils.
- Mix ten drops of rosemary oil with five drops of juniper oil and 100 ml. (3 oz) jojoba oil.

- Firmly massage the entire leg with this oil on a daily basis, rubbing the oil all the way down to the coronary band. The hoof itself should not be treated.
- In case the coronary band becomes irritated, you can increase the quantity of jojoba oil to 150 or 200 ml (5 to 7 oz).

PHYTOTHERAPY

Herbs are not necessarily more innocent than chemical drugs. Whether the antibiotic active ingredient is extracted from a plant or prepared in a laboratory does not alter the fact that you are administering antibiotics. Always consult a phytotherapist (herbal therapist) before using therapeutic herbs.

Some frequently used herbal therapies:

- Buckwheat, nettle, yarrow, hawthorn and cleavers stimulate blood flow to the hooves.
- Rosehip (dog rose) contains a lot of vitamin H (B8, biotin).
- Thistle, gentian, laurel and hazel leaves enhance the production of red blood cells.
- Dandelion contains vitamin A, B1-2-3-5-6-9, C, E, H, P, phosphorus, potassium, manganese, magnesium and zinc.
  In addition, it is said to have a detoxifying effect on the liver and kidneys. As mentioned earlier, dandelion contains relatively high quantities of NSC (ca. 27%) including the fructans inulin and oligofructose.
- Cinnamon and fenugreek may have a positive influence on sugar metabolism.
  We'll discuss why it is better not to give them later in this chapter.
- Blond psyllium has a positive effect on both insulin and blood sugar levels.

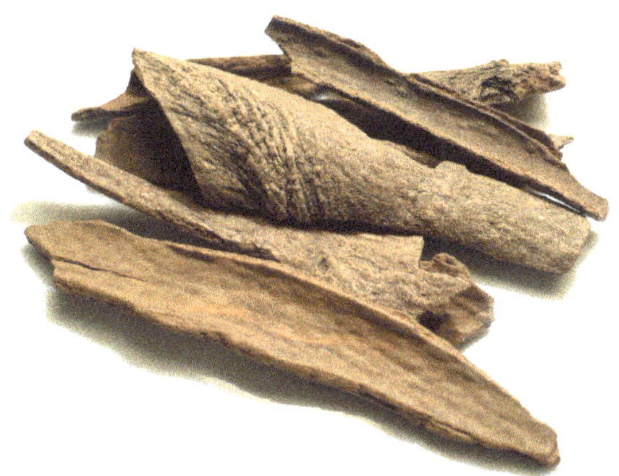

Cinnamon

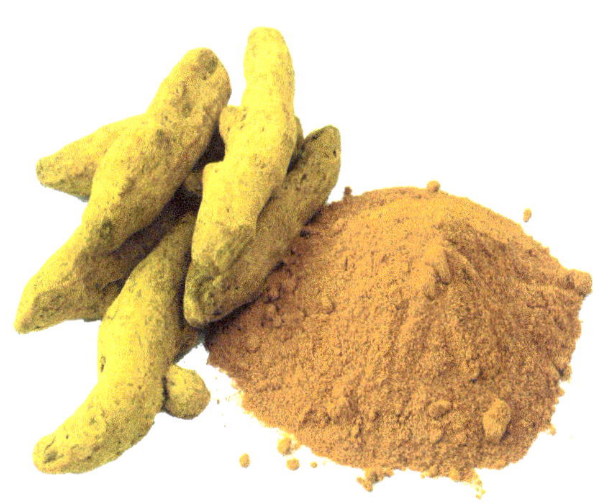

Turmeric

- Turmeric (curcuma) can be used for its anti-inflammatory properties and is known to be a strong antioxidant. Scientific sources contradict each other about the supposed beneficial influences turmeric has on lowering glucose and insulin levels.

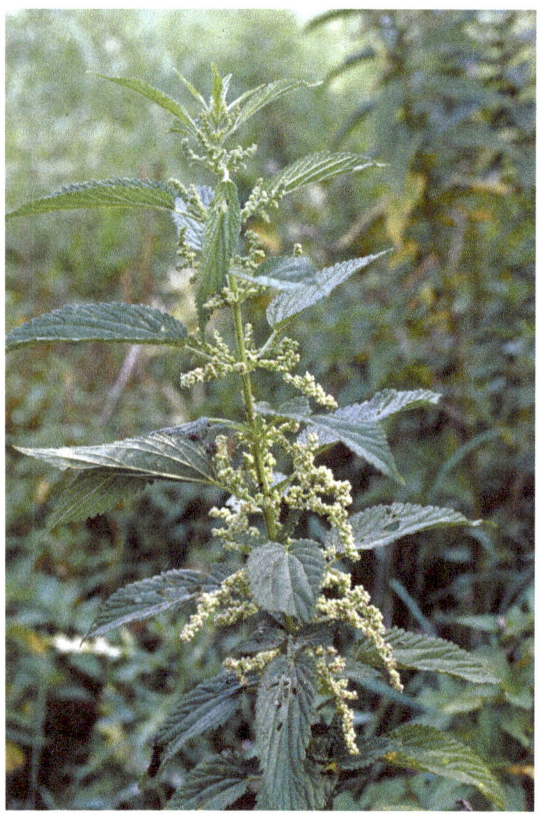

Nettle
(photo: Theodore Webster)

- Nettle stimulates circulation and contains a lot of silica.
- Beet pulp without molasses stimulates the excretion of ammonia and therefore relieves the liver. It contains very little NSC and makes a good (temporary) substitute for grass.

As mentioned before, giving pain relief is usually not recommended. What you can do is offer the horse willow branches. Almond willow is especially high in salicin, a natural analgesic. The horse can gnaw at the bark when he needs it. Salicin is bad for the stomach, so do not give too much of it.

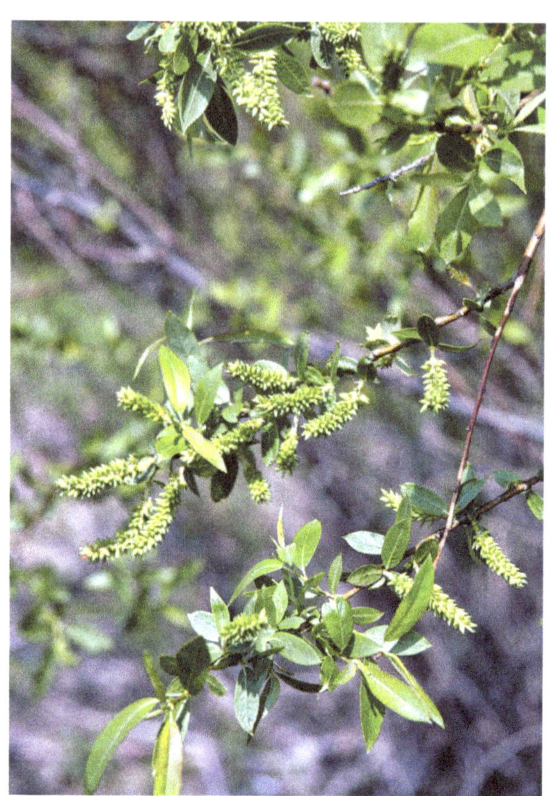

Almond willow contains salicin
(photo: Robert Vidéki)

SUPPLEMENTS, HORMONES AND REMEDIES

To support the healing process or prevent reoccurrence of laminitis it is sometimes useful to give supplements, hormones or remedies (amongst which mainly drugs). The range of available products is so large that it is impossible to cover them all. On the following pages several commonly used products and substances will be discussed, as well as two relatively new drugs. Scientific evidence is available for some. For others, like magnesium, only anecdotal evidence exists. Be aware that all (pharmaceutical) manufacturers are confident that their product makes a real difference in the treatment or prevention of laminitis. However, not all drugs have been proven effective by thorough research and testing.

> A manufacturer may place a broad spectrum vitamin and mineral supplement onto the market with the addition of some herbs that are known to have some positive effect on laminitis. Even when the name of the product contains something with 'lamina' or 'hoof' it is not guaranteed this product actually works.

SUPPLEMENTS

All sorts of supplements are being prescribed and sold. The usefulness and necessity of these substances is sometimes quite doubtful. For some supplements it is not even known whether they have the opposite effect. Most substances the horse needs he ingests through food, salt lick or by producing them in his own body. Supplements that stimulate the quality and quantity of hoof growth, are not important in the early stages of laminitis.

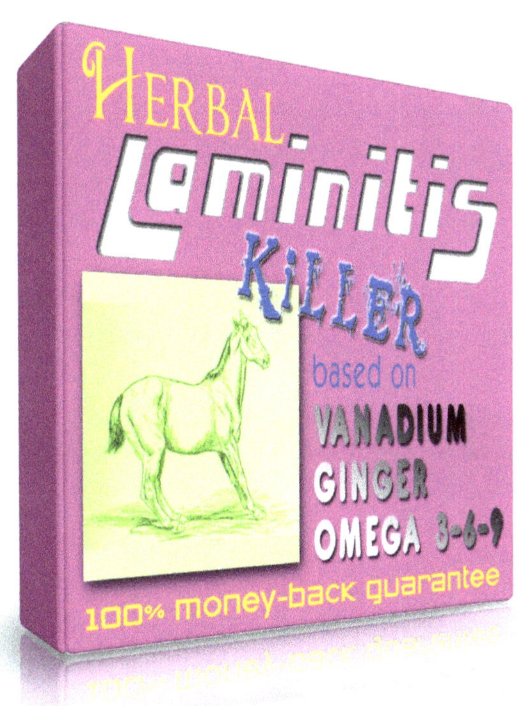

Miracle cure?

An excess of certain vitamins or minerals can be just as harmful as a deficiency. Do not supplement anything until it is clear the horse is actually lacking it, for instance by having a blood test or hair analysis done. Bio-resonance is said to be able to detect deficiencies as well, although there is no scientific evidence for this. Neither has it been scientifically proven that it is not possible to detect deficiencies by using that method.

Supplements include:

- Vitamins and minerals
- Fatty acids
- Hoof growth promoters

VITAMINS AND MINERALS

CHROMIUM, MAGNESIUM AND VANADIUM

The minerals chromium, magnesium and vanadium seem to have a beneficial effect on insulin resistance in horses. This is because they increase the sensitivity of the muscle cells to insulin.

The effect of magnesium may be adversely affected by an excess of potassium in the soil (see sidebar 'Potassium' on page 193). Fertiliser or incorrect soil acidity levels can also influence magnesium levels negatively. Too much calcium or phosphorus interferes with the absorption of magnesium.

SIDE EFFECTS

Normally, magnesium does not burden the kidneys, but his does not apply to horses with kidney problems. Too much magnesium may, combined with a high acidity in the intestines, cause intestinal stones (enteroliths). Diarrhoea is listed as a side effect.

HERBAL SUPPLEMENTS

Herbal supplements can be cinnamon, fenugreek, black cohosh and chastetree berry. But because these plants are so called phytoestrogens their use is not advisable. The effect they have is similar to oestrogen (see page 94). Black cohosh may even be toxic and can cause liver problems. A safe plant variety is dandelion. It contains relatively high levels of magnesium, omega-3 fatty acids and vitamin A. Unfortunately, it also contains relatively high NSC (27%) including quite a bit of starch. Vitamin D (sunlight) may have a beneficial effect as well.

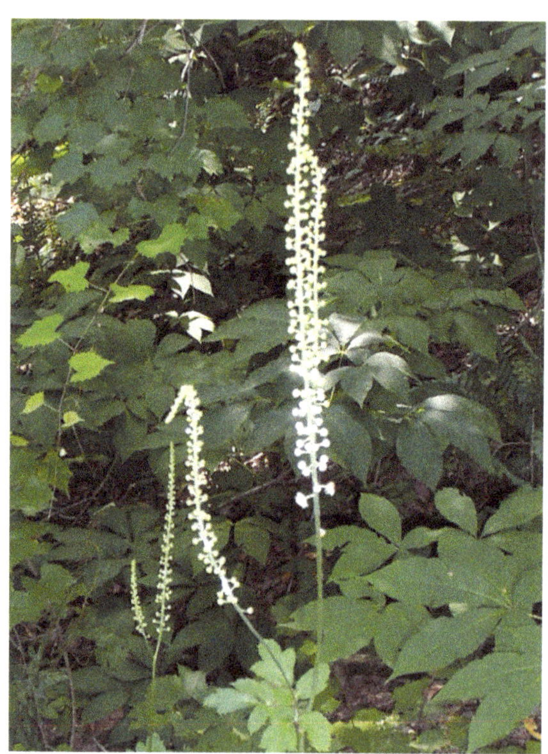

Black cohosh
(photo: David Stephens)

MAGNESIUM COMPOUNDS

Organic magnesium compounds like magnesium chelate and citrate, are absorbed most effectively by the horse's body.

The inorganic magnesium oxide is used by many horse owners, however the uptake of magnesium from this compound is low. According to some estimates, the absorption is nearly four times lower than most other compounds. Besides, magnesium oxide has a laxative effect.

The use of magnesium sulphate (Epsom salts) is not recommended. It contains little magnesium, is also poorly absorbed and irritates the intestines.

Magnesium aspartate and magnesium glutamate are neurotoxic and can cause damage to the brains and nervous system when used long term.

Magnesium deficiency

A structural magnesium deficiency in the horse's body cannot be determined based on a blood test. Of course, the magnesium content of the blood can be measured but this is primarily an indicator of the amount of magnesium in the food the horse ate shortly before the blood was drawn. A muscle biopsy may provide more accurate information about the magnesium reserves in the body.

Horses do not get a structural magnesium deficiency easily just by a low intake of the mineral. In scientific research, attempts were made to cause magnesium deficiency in young, growing horses. It was remarkable how long magnesium had to be withheld from the diet before a deficiency occurred. The reason appears to be, in particular excessive intake of calcium interferes with the absorption of magnesium. High levels of calcium in the body can even make kidneys excrete magnesium.

Manganese

Lack of manganese could play a role in the development of insulin resistance and bone demineralisation as well. Make sure only to supplement manganese if there actually is a proven manganese deficiency.

The vitamins and minerals mentioned above are not a miracle cure. In cases where insulin resistance is not the cause of laminitis they will have little or no effect.

Vitamin E and selenium

A vitamin E deficiency may occur in a laminitic horse as a result of the inflammation in the lamellae. When horses are deficient they will become more prone to other deficiencies as well. If you decide to add vitamin E, preferably supplement this combined with selenium.

> ➤ Make sure not to overdose selenium as it may result in chronic selenium poisoning. One of the possible complications of selenium poisoning is laminitis.

Only supplement vitamin E when a deficiency has been determined by a veterinarian. Have at least two different blood tests done because the concentrations of vitamin E tend to fluctuate.

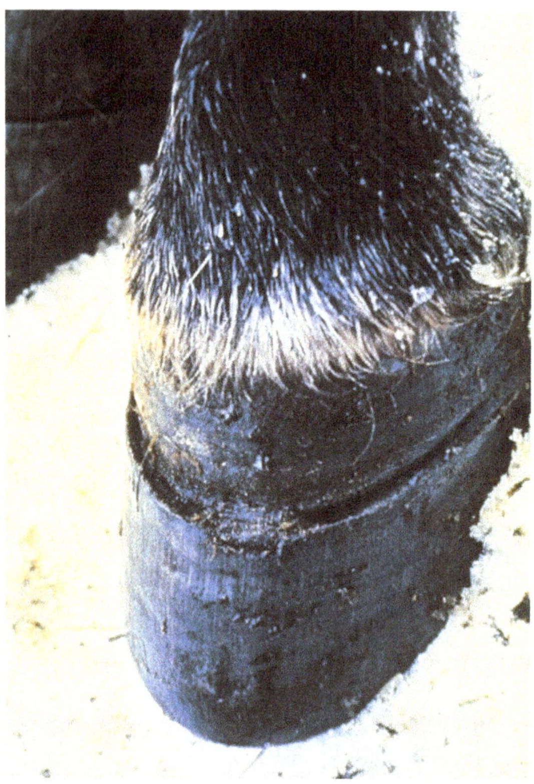

A sharp horizontal edge in the hoof indicates selenium poisoning *(photo: N.A. Irlbeck)*

Fatty acids

Omega-3 fatty acids have anti-inflammatory properties. They also seem to reduce vasoconstriction and have a positive influence on blood pressure. Horses that get enough omega-3 are less affected by high blood pressure. High blood pressure could contribute to the increased supply of both TIMPs as MMPs and their triggers as described on page 59 under 'Enzyme theory'. According to this theory, vasoconstriction is not a problem in the developmental phase. In that regard omega-3 can therefore have both a desired and undesired effect. Omega-3 reduces the production of the cartilage-degrading enzyme ADAMTS-4. Lastly omega-3 reduces microthromboses.

The horse gets omega-3 from green grass. In the winter or if the horse enjoys grazing control measures, flax seed is a good source

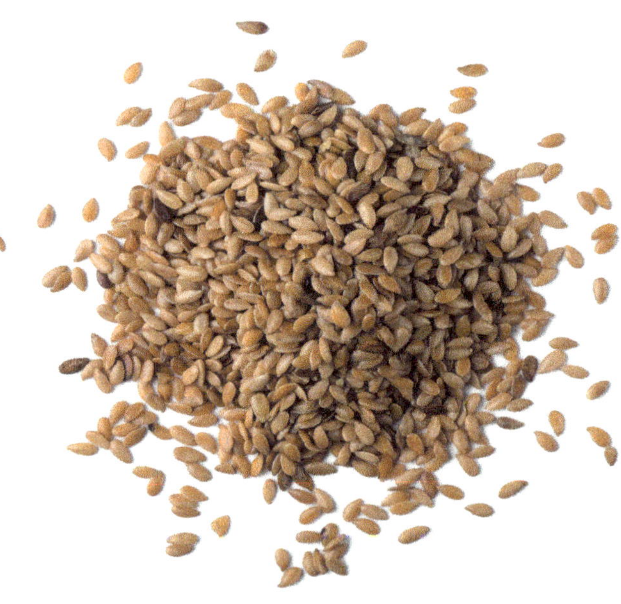

Flax seed is a source of omega-3

Hoof growth promoters

There are some substances that may have a positive effect on hoof growth. These are:

- Methionine, a sulphur-rich amino acid that influences the density of the horn tissue
- Lysine, an amino acid that contributes to the formation of collagen, cartilage and other connective tissue
- Sulphur, to prevent disturbances in the production of keratin
- Zinc, that affects the hardness of horn tissue
- Vitamin H (B8/biotin), also sulphurous, influences the hoof growth

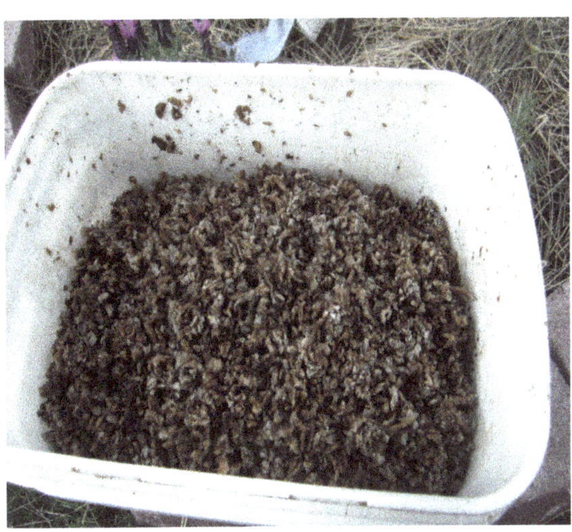

Beet pulp contains methionine
(photo: Haiku farm)

It is true that for the healing of laminitis a whole new hoof wall needs to grow. When primary causes are eliminated and nutrition has been optimised the horse usually is provided with all that is needed for healthy hoof growth. Besides, it is questionable whether hoof growth needs acceleration. If the hoof is growing at a healthy pace, patience is more important than supplements like the ones mentioned above.

HORMONES

In some cases, veterinarians may prescribe synthetic hormones to intervene in the endocrine system of the horse. These include:

- Thyroid hormones
- Dopamine-agonists and serotonin-antagonists

Thyroid hormones

As described in chapter "Theories and causes", for a long time the clinical signs of laminitis were attributed to a reduced thyroid function. The increased production of endogenous glucocorticoids (natural corticosteroids, secreted by the adrenal gland) disturbs the pituitary gland function which in return negatively influences the thyroid gland. But there is nothing wrong with the thyroid itself. Prescribing synthetic thyroid hormones on the assumption that the thyroid is not working properly is completely pointless.

Levothyroxine

Levothyroxine (also: T4-hormone, L-thyroxine, or Thyro-L) is a synthetic thyroid hormone that, when given in high doses, increases thyroid action. This speeds up the metabolism with weight loss as a result. For that reason it is ironically called 'diet in a jar'. Studies show it increases insulin sensitivity. Undoubtedly changes in diet and exercise are by far preferable to combat overweight. Still, in some cases this drug could be useful. A laminitic horse that absolutely needs to lose weight but is unable to move because of the pain could benefit from this drug in the mean time. Of course also the diet needs to be adjusted during treatment with levothyroxine. Keep in mind that the drug increases the appetite. Great vigilance is advised with horses grazing on pasture.

Once the horse is able to move again, the use of levothyroxine needs to be gradually reduced. Take four weeks to wean the horse of the drug by slowly lowering the dose. During this phase or after the discontinuation of the drug, weight gain can be expected because of the slowing down of the metabolism.

> ➤ Only administer Levothyroxine under supervision of a veterinarian who has experience with this drug. And only, as mentioned before, when exercise and diet really don't work. Realise that making your horse lose weight often takes just as much self-discipline as loosing weight yourself. Medication should never substitute discipline.

Dopamine-agonists and serotonin-antagonists

These drugs are given to PPID and EMS horses to respectively activate the dopamine receptors and de-activate the serotonin receptors. That way veterinarians try to limit ACTH production. Dopamine-agonists are sometimes administered combined with synthetic enzyme inhibiting drugs, which will slow down the breakdown of dopamine. Clinical signs will reduce but these drugs do not solve the real problem. In the long term, they can cause liver damage.

Pergolide

Pergolide is commercialised under the brand name Prascend. It has been the only dopamine agonist to be prescribed for veterinary use since October 2012. The use of Permax and Celance - drugs prescribed in human medicine for Parkinson's disease - has since been banned.

In many cases, the dosage can be lowered after 'starting' this drug. During the seasonal rise in ACTH (see page 89), it is recommended to increase the dose. From December, the horse can then be given its normal dosage again.

Bromocriptine

The use of Parlodel (active substance bromocriptine) is not recommended because of the side effects. Also, it is not absorbed as efficiently as Prascend when administered orally.

Cyproheptadine

Cyproheptadine is a serotonin-antagonist and anti-histamine which may be prescribed when the maximum dose of pergolide is not sufficient to suppress clinical signs. It is sold under the brand name Periactin.

CURATIVE REMEDIES

These include not only problem solving remedies as well as remedies that suppress or conceal clinical signs.

Curative remedies include:

- Antibiotic drugs
- Analgesic and anti-inflammatory drugs
- Nerve blocking drugs
- Antihypertensive drugs
- Anticoagulant drugs
- Vasodilator drugs
- Antidiabetic drugs
- Antihistamine drugs
- Enzyme inhibiting drugs
- Antioxidants
- Botulin toxin

> ➤ All remedies have potential side effects. In laminitic horses side effects often aggravate the disease.

ANTIBIOTIC DRUGS

Antibiotics are often prescribed to reduce inflammation. One of the clinical signs of laminitis is sterile inflammation (an infection without bacteria being involved). The use of antibiotics is therefore completely pointless. Furthermore antibiotics kill the good bacteria in the horse's body as well. In case of a sole perforation, accompanied by infection, often antibiotic treatment is necessary.

ANALGESIC AND ANTI-INFLAMMATORY DRUGS

Most analgesic drugs are also anti-inflammatory. These are so-called NSAIDs (non-steroidal anti-inflammatory drugs). Often prescribed drugs are phenylbutazone ('bute' or equipalazone) flunixin (banamine) and ketoprofen. They are referred to as non-selective NSAIDs.

Analgesic drugs mask the pain and inflammation and make the horse moves more or differently than is beneficial. The lamellar connection has already been compromised and will continue to get damaged by overloading, especially when the hooves are not trimmed correctly.

Possible complications of (excessive) use of NSAIDs:

- Stomach ulcers
- Colitis
- Liver problems
- Kidney problems
- Fluid retention
- Oedema
- Blood clotting problems

Stomach ulcers are partially preventable with stomach lining protecting drugs. A 'new generation' of selective NSAIDs is now available: Suxibuzone and Firocoxib. These drugs cause less side effects including fewer stomach problems. Selective NSAIDs may cause adverse reactions to the heart.

The problems of NSAIDs mentioned above, the masking of inflammation and pain and therefore the risk of overloading, are also valid for the selective NSAIDs. The same applies to herbal remedies including devil's claw and No-Bute.

> Don't give products containing devil's claw to pregnant mares. It could cause a miscarriage.

> Often sugar is added to these products to increase palatability. A laminitic horse should not be given any sugar. Take this into account.

Fentanyl patches, known from human medicine, are also starting to be used on horses. These patches affect the central nervous system by slowly releasing the strong painkiller fentanyl. Fentanyl belongs to the opiates, just like morphine. Little is known about the side effects. One disadvantage is that the dosage of patches cannot be adjusted. The active substance accumulates in the subcutaneous fat tissue and will still be active for some time after the removal of the patch. Another disadvantage is that the ambient temperature influences the effect of this drug.

Positive effects

Opposite the listed disadvantages, pain relief can also have positive effects. Too much pain stimulates the production of the hormones epinephrine, norepinephrine and dopamine, the so-called catecholamines. These hormones cause blood sugar levels to increase and blood vessels to constrict. Take this into account in your decision to provide pain relief or not.

> When dealing with laminitis the often difficult choice needs to be made whether or not to use pain relief. In making this decision the balance needs to be found between what is 'humane' and what is beneficial for the horse. The analgesic effect should certainly not be overstated. Analgesic drugs are not 'good' or 'bad' by definition. The basic principle should be: Don't use analgesic drugs, unless withholding them impedes healing.

Nerve blocking drugs

These drugs block the nerves' ability to transmit pain signals. Whereas the analgesic effect of NSAIDs should not be overestimated, the effect of nerve blockers should certainly not be underestimated. A horse that has been given nerve blockers is not able to feel any pain. The chance of damaging the fragile hoof tissues is large. A veterinarian will have to come up with a very good reason to justify the use of nerve blocking drugs.

GASTROINTESTINAL PROBLEMS AND NON-SELECTIVE NSAIDS AND ASPIRIN

COX (Cyclo-oxygenases) are enzymes involved in inflammation. Some NSAIDs may inhibit COX. Two types of COX can be distinguished: COX-1 and COX-2. Non-selective NSAIDs and aspirin do not distinguish between these two types.

COX-1 has not only a positive influence on inflammation, but is important for the normal function of the gastrointestinal tract as well. The intestines become disturbed by the enzyme inhibitory action of the non-selective NSAIDs. Fighting inflammation affects unintentionally, the natural activity of COX-1.

Antihypertensive drugs

Blood pressure plays a small role in the enzyme theory. Lowering the blood pressure during the acute or developmental phase could possibly slow down the process somewhat. The effect is probably fairly small as well. In the circulation theory, decreased blood pressure is said to help prevent blood serum leaking from the capillaries. The risk of oedema formation between the hoof wall and coffin bone may be lowered. However the increased pressure in the capillaries is not a cause, just one of the many consequences of laminitis. Antihypertensives are therefore used to relieve clinical signs. Garlic has blood pressure reducing properties as well and is often given as an alternative. Be aware that garlic is not good for the kidneys.

> Research has shown that garlic is toxic to horses. At a daily dose of 0.2 grams freeze-dried garlic per kilogram of body weight (0.3 ounces per 100 lbs body weight), the horse can already develop some type of anemia. For a 600 kilo horse, this is 120 grams (1323 lbs/4 ounces, resp.). This is the equivalent of about 350 grams (12.3 ounces) of fresh garlic. If your pasture is not overgrown with wild garlic, the chances of your horse taking in such amounts are negligible.

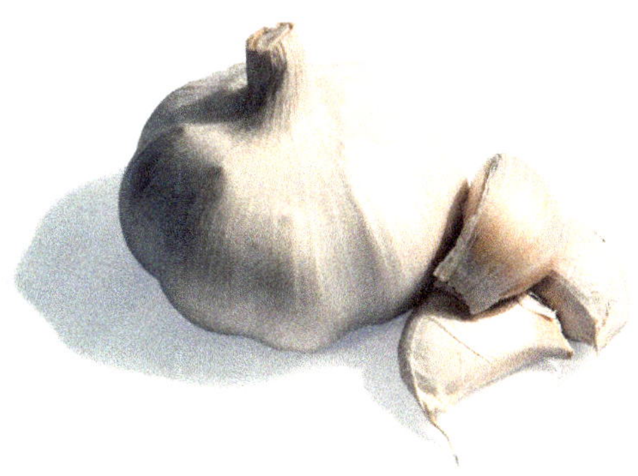

Anticoagulant drugs

As mentioned before, anticoagulants are often erroneously called blood thinners. By inhibiting the clotting properties of blood, superficial wounds will indeed continue to bleed longer. This gave reason to believe these drugs make the blood thinner. However this is not the case. The thickness of the blood is not the problem. Researchers do not agree with each other on this point. From Obel 3 anticoagulants like heparin could be prescribed to prevent or dissolve microthromboses.

Aspirin

Aspirin is prescribed as an anticoagulant too. It has an inhibitory effect on the binding of blood platelets. This effect is short lived as aspirin is broken down in the horse's body fairly quickly. When in addition to aspirin NSAIDs are administered as well, the anticoagulant effect decreases even more.

Activation of thrombocytes and the subsequent formation of microthromboses does not take place at all in endocrinopathic laminitis. It is not yet known whether coagulation problems play a role in traumatic laminitis. Only in SIRS-related laminitis would the use of aspirin as a coagulation inhibitor be justifiable. It should be noted that the activation of thrombocytes in this form of laminitis is a result of the inflammation in the lamellar tissue and not a cause. Fighting the inflammation with a more effective anti-inflammatory than aspirin should be enough. Aspirin has the weak-est anti-inflammatory and analgesic effect of any horse NSAID.

Garlic has antihypertensive properties
(photo: Dominic Morel)

The sharp edge of the hoof bone can, in the event of a coffin bone rotation, damage the blood vessels in the solar dermis. If the horse is given aspirin, the anti-coagulation effect can cause bruising.

Other anticoagulant drugs

The effects of the activation of thrombocytes can also be limited with DMSO, phenylbutazone ('bute' or Equipalazone), flunixin (Banamine) and ketoprofen (Dinalgen).

Vasodilator drugs

Pentoxifylline is prescribed in order to dilate blood vessels, to prevent blood cells from clumping together and to reduce blood clotting. Its effectiveness is minimal.

Acepromazine ('ace') is a sedative that has a vasodilator and blood pressure decreasing effect. It is not known if this effect extends to the lamellae. If it is so, then only after injection into a vein (intravenously) but not after oral administration or injection into a muscle (intramuscular). PPID horses that are administered pergolide should certainly not be given Acepromazine. Pergolide is a dopamine-*agonist*, while Acepromazine is a dopamine-*antagonist*.

The amino acid arginine has a vasodilator effect which is used for instance in cases of so called winter laminitis (see page 92 under 'Winter laminitis').

Antidiabetic drugs

Drugs that are used in the treatment of diabetes type 2 in humans that also have an effect on insulin-resistant horses are metformin and pioglitazone.

Metformin

Metformin inhibits the formation of glucose from proteins and fats in the liver. Additionally, it promotes glucose uptake by muscle cells.
It is assumed that it inhibits the absorption of glucose in the small intestine as well. Because of these effects blood sugar levels are more regulated which has a positive effect on the body's insulin sensitivity.

Disadvantages

One disadvantage is that only a limited quantity of the active ingredient actually reaches the horse's liver when administered orally. When given over a longer period of time, the efficacy decreases even further. Not enough is known about the exact effect of the increased supply of sugar to the caecum and large intestine when less sugar is absorbed by the small intestine. Acidification might occur with consequences as described on page 69 under 'Bacteria in the digestive system'.

> The same as for Levothyroxine applies to metformin: use this drug only after changes in diet and exercise regime have proven to be insufficient to get insulin resistance under control. Horses that cannot be exercised enough because of the pain could benefit from this drug initially. Once movement is possible again, horses have to be weaned of gradually. Discuss the use of this drug with your veterinarian in case you think the horse would benefit from it.

Pioglitazone

Pioglitazone is another insulin sensitivity enhancing drug that is tested for the use in horses. Test results still leave many unanswered questions. Besides, this drug appears to be carcinogenic.

Antihistamine drugs

Endogenous histamine plays a role in inflammation and injury. It has a strong vasodilator effect. Antihistamines are sometimes used in an attempt to constrict blood vessels in order to decrease the supply of both TIMPS as MMPs as well as their triggers.

Histamine also appears to play a part in the production of ACTH. With the administration of antihistamines an indirect attempt is made to reduce this hormone in PPID horses. Cyproheptadine (see page 160) is such an antihistamine drug.

Enzyme inhibiting drugs

In chapter 'Theories and causes' you can read how an imbalance between the protein degrading enzymes MMP-2, MMP-9, ADAMTS-4 and their endogenous enzyme inhibitors (TIMPs) can contribute to the progress of laminitis during the acute phase of the disease.

Administration of exogenous (synthetic) enzyme inhibitors could reduce the activity of MMPs and ADAMTS – significantly slowing this progress or even stopping it altogether. Enzyme inhibiting drugs used for this purpose – although as yet experimentally - are Marimastat and Batimastat.

Intravenous administration

Unfortunately the active ingredients in these drugs break down rapidly when administered intravenously. In addition it appears to be difficult to get them to reach the appropriate location in the hoof. It should be added that this applies to many other drugs targeting the lamellar tissue. In addition, these drugs can cause many and serious side effects when administered this way.

Basement membrane

The basal cells that are responsible for the lamellar attachment are located at the avascular epidermal side of the basement membrane. Oxygen, nutrients and hormones reach these cells by means of diffusion through the basement membrane, from the capillaries of the dermal lamellae. This same process of diffusion applies to the active ingredients of the enzyme inhibiting drugs described here.

Shunting

The circulation in the capillaries is, however, influenced to a significant extent by the action of arteriovenous anastomoses (shunts) in the hoof. These direct connections between arteries and veins can open or close, through which they control the blood supply to the hoof. This mechanism, called shunting, makes it difficult to predict if, and to which extent, the active agents of the drug will achieve proximity to the basal cells.

Intraosseous administration

The blood supply to the dermal lamellae is established, for the most part, through blood vessels that come from the coffin bone. It seems more effective, therefore, to inject the drug directly into the marrow of the coffin bone. This must be done with the animal under sedation and a regional nerve blockade in place. A disadvantage is that each leg has to be treated separately.

Regional limb perfusion

In this procedure, the blood supply of the leg is temporarily isolated from the rest of the body using a tourniquet. Then (with sedation and a nerve blockade) the drug is injected into the blood vessels. Subsequently, the drug circulates for approximately 45 minutes in the lower leg. The treatment is repeated a few times, at 6-hour intervals. Because the drug doesn't reach vital body parts a relatively high dose can be used. In the case of Marimastat and Batimastat, regional limb perfusion appears to be much more effective than intravenous administration. The risk of systemic side effects is lower. As with intraosseous administration, each leg must be treated separately. There is also a risk of complications, such as vascular inflammation (vasculitis), inflammation of subcutaneous tissue (cellulitis), limb swelling, or haematoma formation. Nerve or tissue damage may also result if the tourniquet is kept on for too long.

Antioxidants

Free radicals are molecular by-products of normal metabolism, inflammation, drugs, residual pesticides in foods, strenuous exercise, stress, obesity and adiposity that could cause all kinds of negative effects. Free radicals are suspected to weaken blood vessels and cause damage to enzymes. Conclusive scientific evidence for the application of antioxidants to counteract the damage of free radicals has yet to be found.

Many of the commonly used antioxidants would also be beneficial in other areas, like circulation, blood pressure, detoxification of the liver and improvement of fat contents of the blood.

Well-known antioxidants are:

- Dimethyl sulphoxide (DMSO)
- Dimethyl glycine (DMG)
- Vitamin E and selenium (among other effective with iron excess)
- Vitamin C (produced by the horse itself)
- Methylsulphonyl-methane (MSM), containing sulphur
- Coenzyme Q10
- Superoxide dismutase (SOD)
- Zinc
- Copper
- Sulphur

Botulin toxin

Botulin toxin (mainly known under the brand name Botox) is injected into the deep digital flexor muscle to partly paralyse it. As a result, the deep digital flexor tendon's pulling force at the front of the hoof is lowered to facilitate the healing process. This treatment is still in an experimental phase.

PREVENTIVE REMEDIES

Preventive remedies are especially useful in the acute phase of laminitis. Especially horses that are prone to laminitis, can sometimes be guarded from a new episode of illness by administering some of these.

Preventive remedies include:

- Antibiotic drugs
- Probiotics
- Oils
- Intestinal cleansing remedies
- Buffer solution

> Obviously you cannot have full confidence in these remedies. It cannot be emphasised enough that the focus has to remain on discovering and removing the root causes of laminitis.

Antibiotic drugs

In the acute phase, antibiotics can be orally administered to reduce the excessive presence of streptococci and lactic acid bacilli in the large intestine. A popular product is Founder Guard. This is a so called virginiamycin. This type of antibiotic has been used in life stock farming for 30 years and bacteria have started to become resistant to it. Founder Guard is not available in every country but it can be ordered online.

Probiotics

Probiotics are live bacteria and yeasts that can be given to restore the acidity and bacterial balance in the intestines. Whether these microorganisms actually reach the intestines, and are not killed in the stomach before they actually arrive there, remains a question.

Bacteria that are used as probiotics are mannan-oligosaccharides, brewer's yeast and lactic acid bacilli.

Oils

In case of excessive grain consumption, it is important to prevent colic by inserting paraffin or vegetable oils. Besides a laxative effect it also blocks the absorption of toxins through the intestinal wall.

> Administering other laxatives in the acute phase is not recommended. Many horses in this stage already suffer from dehydration.

Intestinal cleansing remedies

Activated carbon and Fuller's earth have a strong purifying effect on the intestines. Do not experiment yourself with for instance Norit. It is important that the horse receives the proper dosage.

Hippo-ex-laminitis is a product that claims to restore intestinal balance and support the liver by detoxification.

Buffer solution

The acidity of the intestines can be decreased by inserting a buffer solution, or acidity regulator by means of a cannula or surgically, through the abdominal wall. By intervention of the acidity in an early stage, an attempt is made to prevent a chain of events from happening. This treatment is still in an experimental stage but so far has not been successful in preventing the onset of laminitis. However it has proven to be a method that significantly delays the process which gives the owner and care providers more time for further treatment.

Oral administration of a buffer solution such as sodium bicarbonate in cold water can, in an emergency like excessive grain intake, help to prevent the pH level of the intestines to decrease too extremely. The cold water slows down the fermentation process a bit as well.

However, it is not certain whether sodium bicarbonate reaches the colon before it is absorbed. Another form of sodium bicarbonate exists that is known to pass through the stomach and small intestine intact. Equishure is such a product. Not in all countries this product is for sale but it can be ordered online. Administration via a nasogastric tube has been proven to increase the efficacy.

EUTHANASIA

No horse has ever died of laminitis. It is the severity and the duration of the disease and the complications, in combination with the lack of hope of recovery that make it necessary, at a certain moment, to ask ourselves whether it is still ethically acceptable to let the horse live.

Horses cannot represent their own interests. The responsibility to decide whether or not to euthanise a horse will therefore always be yours, as owner. You know your horse like no other; you are familiar with its history and recognise abnormalities in his behavioural characteristics. So, you are the first in line to assess the quality of your horse's life. Although the final decision lies with you, in most cases the veterinarian is best able to make well-informed judgments about the balance between prognosis and well-being of the horse. They can see the situation of your horse in a broader perspective and compare it with other horses they have had in their practice.

A good veterinarian makes an objective assessment in which they will once again look extensively at the nature and severity of the causes, the lameness and the complications. They will critically evaluate the treatment methods that have been attempted and their outcomes. The success of pain management is very important in this. This ideal veterinarian consults with the other practitioners who treat your horse, such as the hoof care provider. Ideally, they are honest enough to also see to what extent you are able to provide the necessary care. If it is – for whatever reason – not possible to adequately help your horse, then it is not fair to let it suffer. It is up to you to decide what the outcome will be in that case.

The good veterinarian described here only makes statements about the interests and well-being of your horse. What the consequences for your career as a show jumper will be, now that your horse will be less usable for sports, is not their expertise. Moreover, there is no emotional connection biasing the outcomes of their objective assessment; something that can hardly ever said of the owner of the horse.

It is a difficult decision to make, and one that often takes the owner more time than the veterinarian considers desirable for the horse's interest. Fortunately, they know that this is part of their work. They will give you the time to think about their advice. During this process, you should not hesitate to ask them again, if necessary, to expand on their recommendation. Ask the opinion of a second veterinarian if necessary. If you are convinced of a veterinarian's recommendation to euthanise but you really cannot let go of your horse, terminal or palliative care may still be an option. Whether this is in the interest of your horse is uncertain.

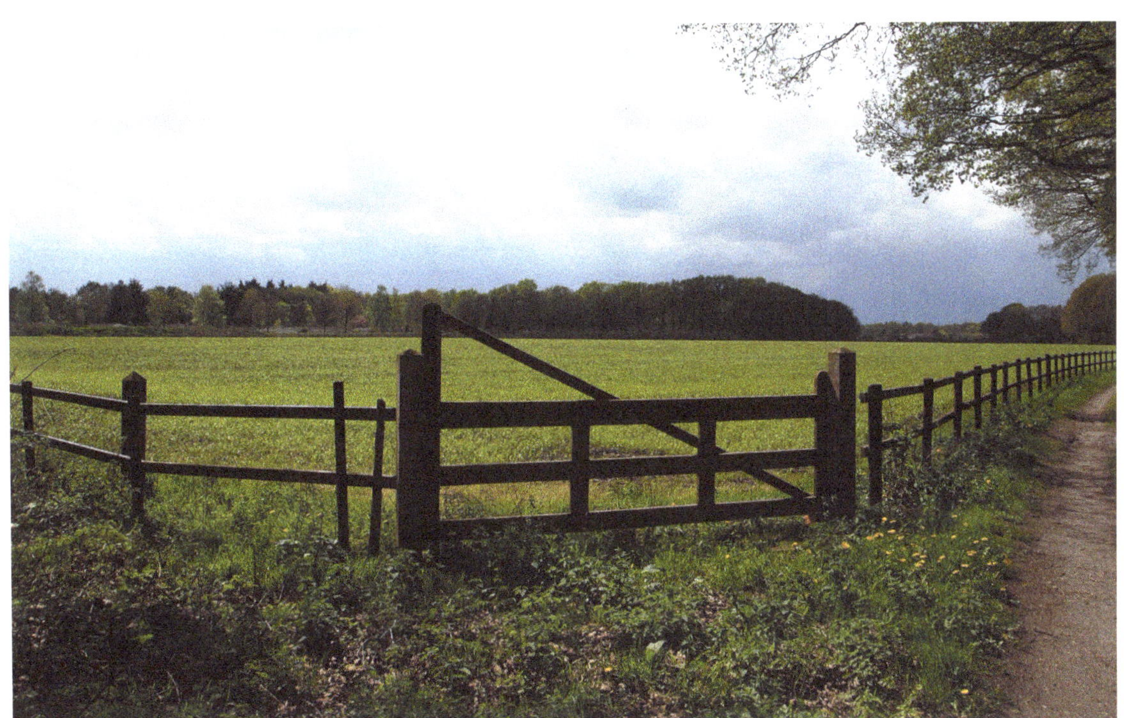

PREVENTION

Chances are real, you are reading this book because your horse has laminitis. For that reason, a large part of the book is dedicated to treatment. Prevention is equally important, also to prevent laminitis from reoccurring.

Unfortunately, prevention is not always possible. Earlier in this book you have read that laminitis is in a sense not a disease, but a manifestation of problems elsewhere in the horse's body. It is a complex clinical sign of one or more conditions.

The chapter 'Theories and causes' explains which ailments and problems can cause laminitis. Recognising all these factors and then keeping them under constant and complete control is a hopeless task. Some conditions can also be incurable. Sooner or later this will lead to such an increased risk of laminitis that a small push is enough to start the misery. If, despite all precautions and good care, your horse has become laminitic, then you should focus on preventing aggravation and the occurrence of complications. The somewhat pessimistic message is that it is better to let go of the idea that laminitis can always be prevented. This does not alter the fact that the aim must be to limit the risk as much as possible.

Practically all instructions in this chapter and the following chapter on nutrition, exercise, housing and social interaction can be regarded as preventive measures.

HORSES AT RISK

Prevention begins with determining whether your horse belongs to a risk group. In that case, all the following information deserves extra attention.

Risk groups:

- Welsh, Exmoor, Shetland and New Forest ponies, cobs, Appaloosas and Icelandic horses
- Older horses, as they might have been exposed to risk factors longer than younger horses and often have had laminitis before
- Certain bloodlines within other breeds
- Large draught horses
- Obese horses, with insulin resistance, EMS or PPID
- Horses suffering from another disease, an acute infection or chronic inflammation somewhere else in the body
- Mares that recently had a foal
- All horses whose natural needs are insufficiently met, in terms of housing, movement, nutrition and hoof care

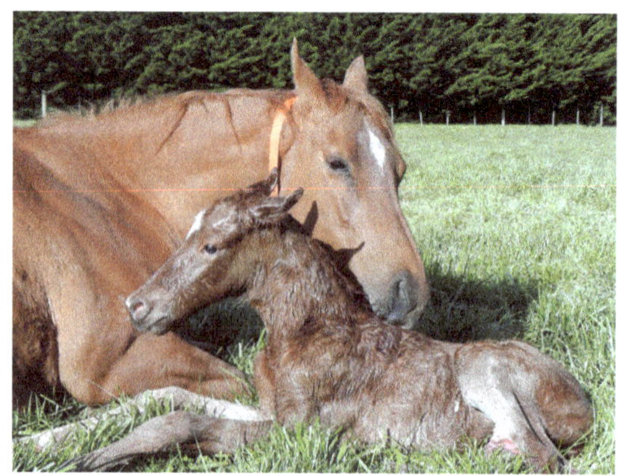

Mares are at risk of laminitis after foaling *(photo: Haiku farm)*

PREVENTIVE MEASURES

Regardless whether your horse belongs to a risk group, the following are useful preventive measures:

- Create living conditions for your horse that are as natural as possible.
- Feed your horse a diet low in NSC
- Keep an eye on the weight and fat distribution of your horse. A cresty neck score (see page 81) higher than three, combined with a body condition score higher than six results in a 75% chance of laminitis.
- Supplement magnesium if your insulin resistant horse responds well to it.
- Provide sufficient, good quality exercise.
- Keep your horse barefoot.
- Avoid toxins.
- Prevent traumatic laminitis by avoiding overloading.
- Do not breed with horses from risk groups that have suffered from laminitis more than once or for 'inexplicable' reasons.

RISK OF REOCCURRENCE

Look after horses that have had laminitis before extra carefully. They are at greater risk of having it again because of the following possible reasons:

- The damaged or recovering lamellae are more susceptible to the laminitis causing factors.
- They will experience pain in the hoof quicker due to tissue and nerve damage. Pain causes increased blood sugar levels and vasoconstriction.
- A compacted sole provides less protection so the horse will experience more pain.
- Not all primary or facilitative causes have completely been eliminated.

LOG

Does the horse get laminitis repeatedly, despite all the efforts, one aspect might still remain overlooked by you, the owner and the veterinarian. In that case, having kept a log can prove to be of great importance. Include at least the following information:

- Neck size. Measure the neck in the middle (between poll and withers) with a tape measure. The neck must be relaxed while the head is up.
- Weight (see sidebar 'Determine the horse's weight' on page 136)
- CNS (page 81)
- BCS (page 83)
- Photos
- Obel score (page 38)
- Administered drugs, supplements and the like

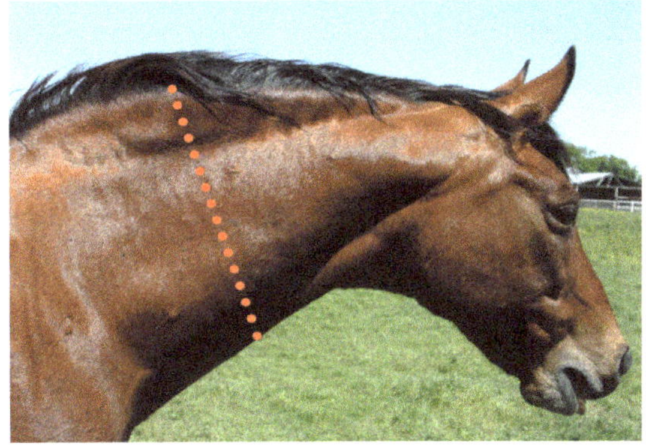

Neck size
(photo: Mark DePaolo)

Write down as well:

- Diet changes
- Remarkable weather conditions
- Changes in living circumstances
- Pasture hours
- Quantity of exercise
- Vaccinations, drugs, worm treatment (date, type, dosage)
- Notable changes in attitude and behaviour of your horse

Over time you might discover patterns that can help to find hidden causes. Don't look for more than one cause at the time but concentrate on one aspect. Is that is not the problem, then focus on the next. Record your quest in the log as well.

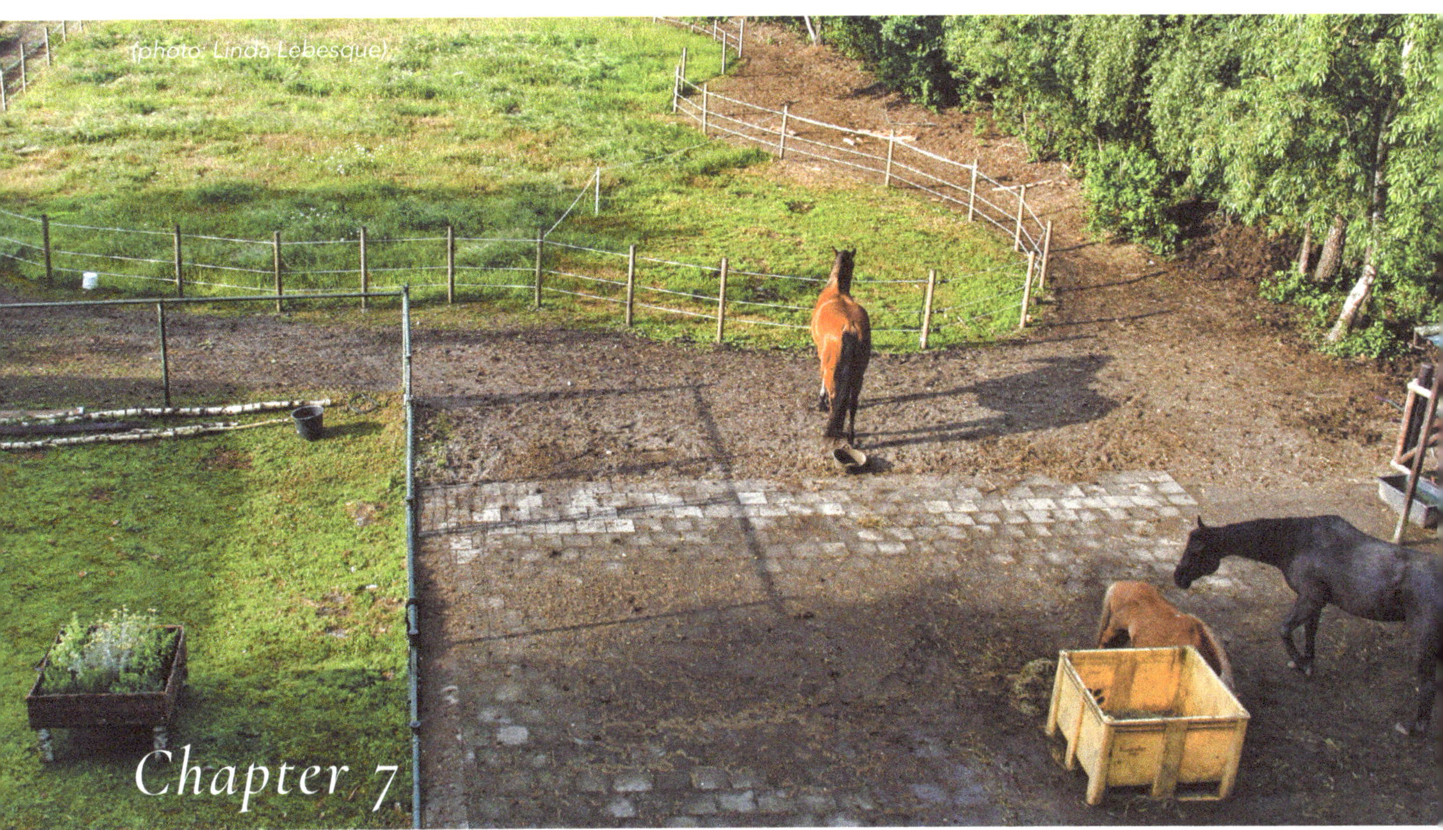
(photo: Linda Lebesque)

Chapter 7

LIVING CONDITIONS

DOMESTICATION OF THE HORSE IS A VIOLATION OF THE ESSENCE OF ITS BEING. ANYONE WHO HAS EVER OBSERVED A HERD OF WILD HORSES IN THEIR NATURAL ENVIRONMENT KNOWS HOW MUCH WE FALL SHORT IN THE WAY WE KEEP OUR HORSES, DESPITE ALL OUR GOOD INTENTIONS. A HORSE IS A SOCIAL ANIMAL THAT NEEDS SPACE AND MORE SOCIAL INTERACTION THAN IS USUALLY PROVIDED BY US. A WILD HORSE HAS FREE CHOICE OF FOOD. WE DEPRIVE THEM OF THAT CHOICE. A HORSE CAN GO WHEREVER AND WHENEVER IT WANTS. BUT NOT WITH US. WHEN IT COMES TO LIVING CONDITIONS THERE IS ALWAYS ROOM FOR IMPROVEMENT.

This chapter, along with the previous sections on trimming and movement, is perhaps the most important part of this book. If the living conditions of a domestic horse were similar to that of a wild horse, vast improvements in his health would be quickly noticeable. It would benefit from good blood circulation in its hooves, gain a healthy metabolism and find a good balance between stress and relaxation. Do not underestimate the self-healing ability of the horse. A horse that lives in optimal conditions is stronger, has a better immune system and a greater zest for life. It will therefore respond better to treatment and heal faster. Simply put, the more naturally horses are kept, the greater their chance of recovery.

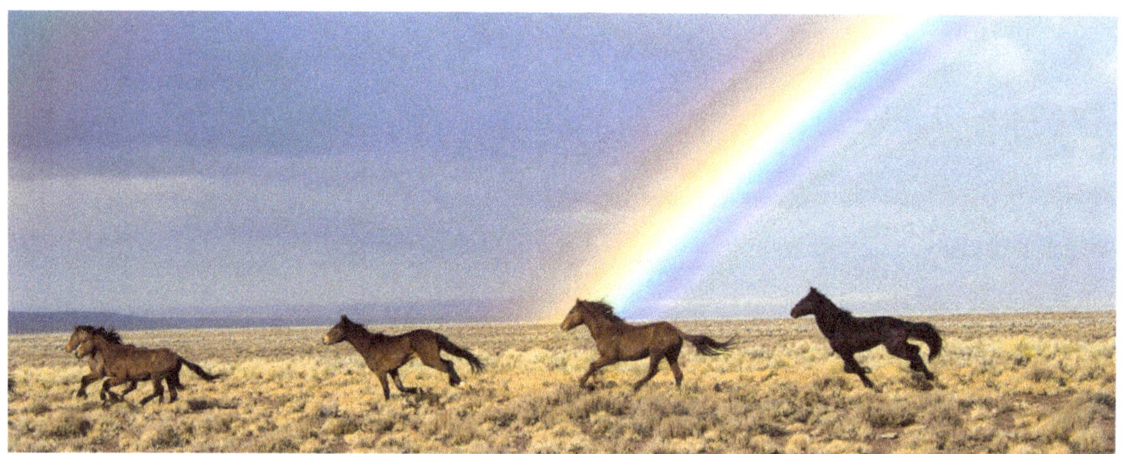

DIRECTION INSTEAD OF GOAL

Unfortunately we cannot offer our horse such living conditions. Deciding to keep a horse means limiting the freedom and options of the horse by definition. We ride them, have limited space, time and resources available and are never completely able to comprehend the horse's essence.

What we can do is try to accommodate the horse's needs as much as possible by changing their living conditions. The first and easiest thing we can do is to stop thinking of the required changes as an absolute goal. As long as the ultimate goal remains unattainable, we might conclude that it is impossible to achieve and therefore stop making an effort. We will remain satisfied with how we always kept our horses thinking 'It can't be that bad'.

When you approach improving your horse's living conditions as a direction, every little step will be a change for the better. This will be motivating and make you more inclined to persevere and keep your eyes open for new opportunities. For example, when you aim to give your horse more space, a few hours in a paddock in the morning, instead of being stabled for 23 hours a day is an improvement. Your direction will be to provide even more space and movement but for now you can be happy with the improvement. The next step is to find out how to proceed. Obviously, permanent paddock access would be the next step. Before you know it, your horse will be out on many acres of land in a naturally composed herd all year round. Or maybe even better than that.

By using your imagination and cooperating with other horse owners, much can be accomplished. Even when you are not able to completely perfect your horse's living conditions there will be progress as long as you do what you can and remain critical.

When you are truly unable to give your horse what you feel he needs, not even with all the creative solutions you can come up with, it could be better to find your horse another owner or caretaker, temporarily or permanently.

Fortunately, this is hardly ever necessary. In this chapter we will show you different ways to improve the way you keep your horse, manage your pasture, provide social interaction and, most importantly, how to feed your horse.

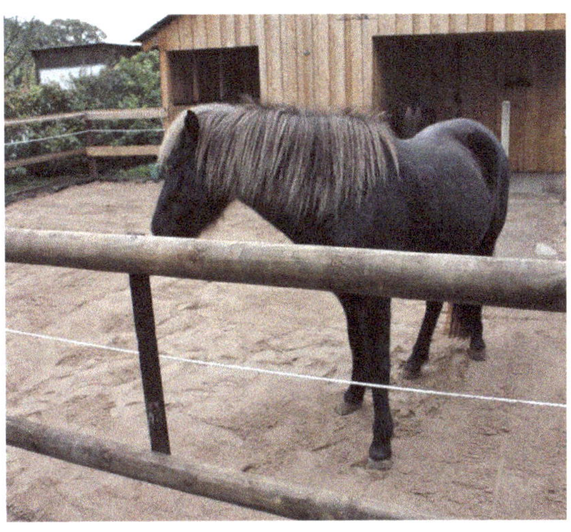

Permanent access to the paddock: a step in the right direction *(photo: Novus)*

NUTRITION AND PASTURE MANAGEMENT

Several books and web sites are available on the subject of healthy and natural horse nutrition. The information on the next pages is limited to the nutritional aspects related to laminitis.

It is very useful to analyse all aspects of the way you feed your horse. The more natural the feeding regime, the healthier and stronger the horse will become.

DIGESTIVE PROCESS

The most important part of the horse's digestive process takes place in the hind gut: the large intestine and caecum. Raw cellulose fibre and hemicellulose (two types of so called structural carbohydrates) are digested here by various types of bacteria and protozoa.

Cellulose, consisting of a long chain of carbohydrate units, is broken down into glucose by the bacteria. This glucose is fermented by the bacteria into volatile fatty acids. These fatty acids are important for the horse's digestive system. In the liver of the horse, fatty acids are converted back into glucose.

When the horse's diet contains insufficient cellulose, part of the bacteria population will die of starvation. This decline in numbers of fibre digesting microbes hinders the digestion of a new supply of cellulose.

Non-structural carbohydrates are digested in an earlier stage of the digestive process, in the small intestine. As described on page 69 under 'Bacteria in the digestive system', the horse can only process these 'fast' carbohydrates at a limited rate.

Just to repeat:

- The small intestine is not able to process large quantities of NSC.
- Undigested NSC enter the large intestine.
- Bacteria in the large intestine will then multiply rapidly to ensure the sugars and starch will still be digested.
- Excessive amounts of lactic acid are released during this process, causing the pH level of the hind gut to drop.
- Cellulose processing microbes will die in this very acidic environment.
- Fructans are only partly digested in the small intestine. They are mainly digested in the large colon.

Not only hard feeds, molasses, grass, fruit, roots and cereals are high in NSC. Certain herbs like dandelions, couch grass, stork's bill and red clover are also known for their high quantities of fructans. In addition, the fructan in dandelions has a low degree of polymerisation.

The high NSC content of dandelions allows them to survive drought. Since horses like to eat them, this may contribute to the high numbers of laminitis during drought periods.

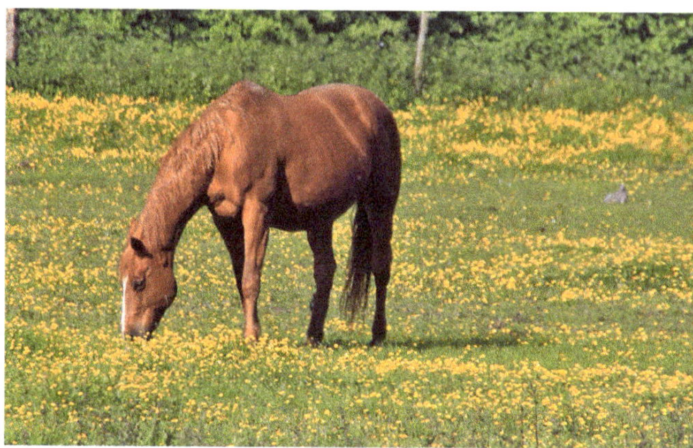

Dandelions are high in fructan

Even dead grass may contain NSC levels that are still too high. Meadow fescue for example is a type of grass that retains nutrients very well. The green colour of grass is caused by the protein chlorophyll and is no indication of NSC content.

Besides grass, wild horses eat herbs, bark, leaves, roots and even fruit and nuts. The composition of their diet depends on availability at a certain place and time of the year. A common misconception is that all food types horses are able to eat are essential in their diet. For example, it is true some horses eat berries and nuts, but it does not mean they cannot live without berries or nuts. The main part of their diet is fairly unvaried: cellulose-rich plants.

> Horses with unlimited opportunities to choose their own food have access to plants containing substances with antibiotic, analgesic or blood cleansing properties. On page 153 under 'Phytotherapy' you can read about the use of plants for these purposes.

This relatively monotonous diet however does provide the horse with sufficient vitamins, minerals and amino acids. The majority of vitamins horses need, vitamins B1, B6 and B12, C and K, are produced by bacteria living in the large intestine.

The horse relies heavily on a balanced intestinal flora and steady pH level in the intestines. Rapidly digestible NSC, as well as medications, worming and other factors, can disrupt both the microbial balance and the acidity level.

UNNATURAL DIET AND FEEDING PATTERNS

Domesticated horses are often fed an unnatural diet in an unnatural way. A few examples:

Blood sugar levels

The metabolism is not able to deal with spikes in blood sugar levels. Spikes are caused by rationing food, or feeding in portions. Horses are often given servings that are too large to eat at one time and are not fed often enough each day. The horse's system registers the variation in blood sugar levels as being hungry. This results in adjustment of the metabolic rate. Sugars are stored as fat. The horse will become fat.

NSC

Nearly all commercial feeds are cereal-based, contain molasses, or both. The NSC from these foods are a real problem. In the long term they may contribute to colic, AM (atypical myoglobinuria, Monday disease) and obesity. In the short term, it disturbs the intestinal flora and acidity of the hind gut, as described in the previous section. The link between these types of feed and laminitis is obvious.

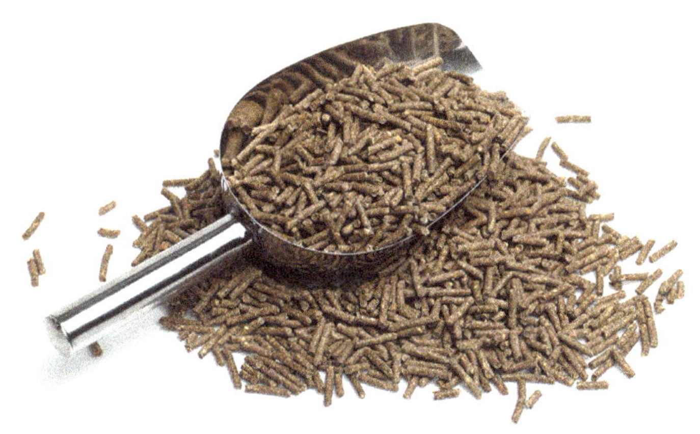

Hard feeds are unnatural

Overeating

Horses overeat out of boredom or because they are not getting what they need. A familiar problem is horses chewing wood in their stable when the cellulose content in their diet is insufficient.

Iron

Surface or bore water may contain too much iron. Iron is a free radical when absorbed in excessive quantities.

Excess iron hinders absorption of copper and zinc by binding to these minerals and complicating the uptake through the intestinal wall. Copper and zinc are important for the horse. Copper is needed for hooves and tendons as well as being an antioxidant. Zinc affects the hardness of the horn. Iron overload is associated with tying up as well.

> Do not worry when water has a rusty brown colour. Iron is less harmful when it has already oxidised.

Nutritional needs

The horse's digestive system is unable to deal with sudden changes in diet. Changes often occur when a horse is sold to a new owner, is moved to new or recently fertilised pasture, or when horses are turned out on pasture after being stabled over winter

> An abrupt transition from unlimited grazing to being hard fed, is not uncommon for many domestic horses. Especially in the first four days after this switch-over, big changes take place in the acidity level of the hind gut and therefore the amount of lactic acid bacilli and streptococci.

Poor food quality

Examples of poor quality foods:

- Old or mouldy hay
- Hay containing gravel, sand or other dirt
- Harmful bacteria in silage

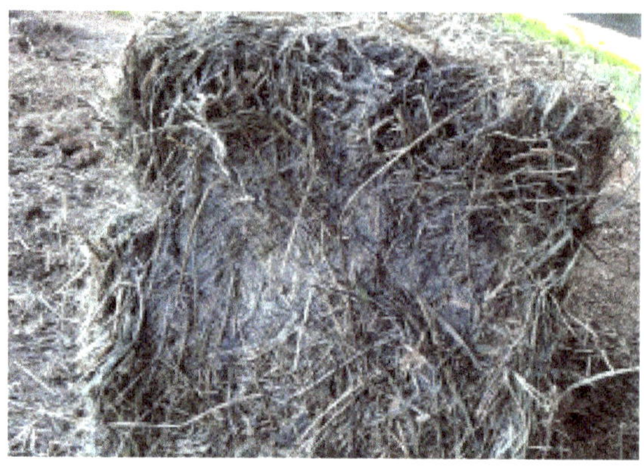

Mouldy hay
(photo: Kate Light)

POSSIBLE IMPROVEMENTS

Below are some suggestions for improving your horse's the diet. Emphasis is on optimal digestion and recovery or reduction of the risk of laminitis.

General

Avoid abrupt dietary changes. In case you need to switch to other foods, make the transition as gradual as possible. That way the intestinal flora is given the chance to adapt. In case your horse is given strenuous exercise, choose calorie sources with slow digestible crude fibre such as pectin, cellulose and hemicellulose, for example soybean meal, beet pulp and alfalfa hay. Of course, laminitic horses should not be heavily exercised until they have fully recovered.

> Some laminitic horses do not respond well to alfalfa. They probably convert proteins into sugar extremely effectively. Alfalfa contains a lot of proteins.

Horses need a constant supply of roughage to satisfy their need for dietary fibre. When fibre is insufficiently available horses will not stop grazing. In more serious cases, they will gnaw on fence posts or other available timber.

> High in fibre does not necessarily mean low in NSC.

Drinking water

Make sure fresh drinking water is always available and keep it free from:

- Algae
- Dead leaves
- Dead insects
- Manure and urine
- Rust from water pipes or troughs

It is possible to have your horse's drinking water analysed. Surface water may contain too much nitrite, nitrate, ammonia compounds, iron and salt. In that case it might be better to provide rain or tap water. Bear in mind that tap water may contain fluoride.

Besides testing for minerals, water can also be tested for heavy metals and harmful bacteria.

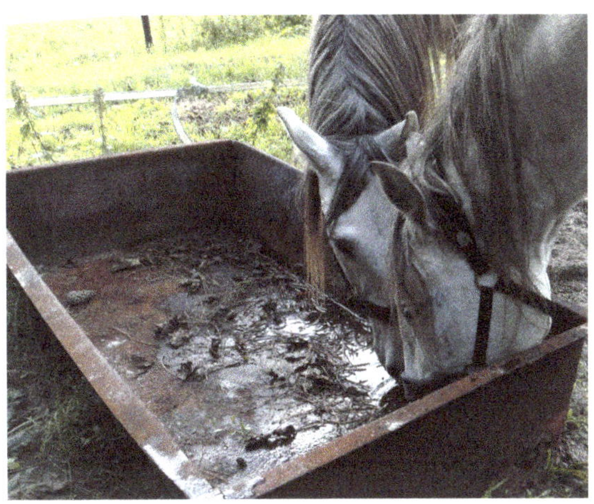

Corrosion in the pasture trough *(photo: Sabine Baron)*

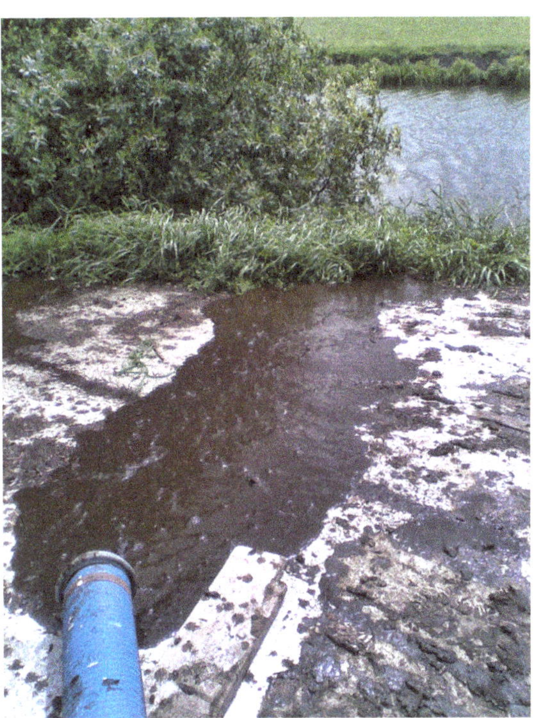

Contamination of surface water

Bore water

Shallow wells (up to 20 meters/65 feet deep) have an especially high risk of a variety of contaminants. Be extra vigilant when the well is located nearby a manure pit. Deeper wells often contain high levels of iron, sodium, fluoride, chloride and ammonium.

Rainwater

Even the quality of rainwater needs to be monitored. Zinc roofing sheets, gutters and downspouts increase the zinc content of drinking water too much. Even old zinc drinking troughs may be a source of this pollution.

Surface water

Water from streams, ditches, rivers and other types of surface water is often contaminated by manure, fertilisers, pesticides or the illegal dumping of chemicals. Also toxic algae and salmonella are often found in surface water. It is the least preferable drinking water for your horse.

Hay

Preferably choose lucerne (alfalfa) hay, grass seed hay or hay from a third or second cut. These types of hay are usually called horse hay. In the respective sidebars on page 182 the drawbacks of grass seed hay and late cuts are discussed.

Hay should originate from sensibly fertilised land, cut at a time when NSC levels are low. A good idea is to discuss this with a farmer in advance, to decide the best moment to cut and harvest the hay. Have the hay analysed for ESC, starch and fructan levels at an agricultural research laboratory. Hay with less than 10% ESC in the dry matter is relatively safe for laminitic horses.

Lucerne hay is a good choice. It contains about half the NSC percentage and is rich in magnesium. It does contain high quantities of protein which is not recommended for some horses. Grass seed hay however has a very low protein content. By feeding these two types of hay combined, the protein levels can be adjusted. Choose lucerne hay with fewer leaves and many stems.

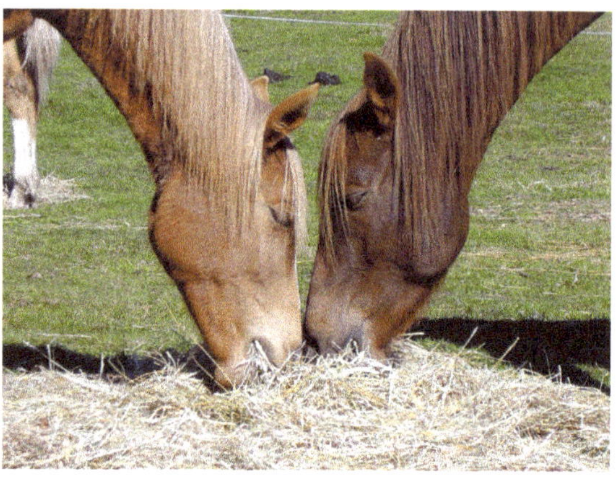

High fibre roughage
(photo: Cynthia Cooper)

Some horse owners feed old hay assuming it contains less NSC. This is not the case. Last year's hay only contains less vitamins, so it is not recommended as forage.

In some areas it is possible to buy 'natural' hay from nature reserves. Usually, the soil in these areas has not been fertilised for a long time. The nutritional content, NSC, minerals and trace elements are usually unknown and can vary per bale. The hay may also contain undesirable or toxic plants.

NSC AND FORAGE ANALYSIS

NSC content:

- Soybean meal 6%
- Lucerne hay 11%
- Wheat straw 12%
- Beet pulp 12%
- Bermuda hay 14%
- Grass seed hay 14%
- Oat hay 22%
- Wheat bran 31%
- Oats 54%
- Barley 62%
- Molasses 62%
- Corn (maize) 73%

These are average values. For some foods in this list the extremes are close to the average. Wheat straw and sugar beet pulp however, can contain up to 17% NSC under certain circumstances. Wheat bran at 30% is not an appropriate type of feed, not even as a treat, as it can reach levels of 40% NSC or even more.

Other types of feed containing NSC:

- Cereals, pellets and other types of cubes, mixes or concentrates (unless explicitly and truthfully stated differently on the packaging)
- Bread
- Carrots
- Apples and other fruits (blackberry bushes!)
- Clover and vetch.

Feeds containing high levels of NSC are definitely not suitable for horses prone to laminitis, especially horses that are in the acute phase. Don't give them half a handful of grain or a small apple because they are so sad.

To administer drugs most beet pulp can be used safely. Although some brands of beet pulp can contain up to 17% NSC, which is too high. Contact your supplier to determine which pulp is safe to use. WSC in beet pulp can be lowered even more by soaking (see sidebar 'Soaking hay' on page 117).

A positive trend in modern forage analysis (hay and grass) is the specification of NSC content. A 14% NSC content can both consist of 10% ESC and starch and 4% fructans as well as the other way round. ESC and starch are mainly digested in the small intestine by enzymes and have a much greater impact on blood sugar and insulin levels than fructans that are digested by microorganisms in the hind gut. Two batches of hay with the same overall NSC content can therefore have a different effect on an insulin-resistant horse. A good forage analysis differentiates between ESC, starch and fructans. This way a choice can be made for hay with the lowest ESC and starch content.

Please note: Some types of starch are digested in the large intestine and therefore have less influence on blood sugar levels. Most forage analysis do not distinguish between different types of starch.

GRASS SEED HAY

Grass seed hay is by-product that is left over from the cultivation of grass for seed. Grass that is mowed when the seed is fully formed is also called grass seed hay. Most of the NSC is in the seed that goes to the seed trade. The long stalks of hay that remain consist mainly of crude fibre (structural carbohydrates) and, dried into hay, form good low-energy roughage for laminitic horses or horses that need to lose weight. In addition, horses have to chew on this roughage longer. This ensures increased saliva production, which benefits digestion. The structural carbohydrates also make the intestines to work harder.

The most commonly cultivated grasses are English and Italian rye grass, red fescue and tall fescue. Sometimes Kentucky blue grass or timothy grass are used. Timothy grass and red fescue naturally contain less NSC than these other grass types. Of course, this also applies to the hay of these grasses. With a little luck, your forage company can supply you with this hay.

Yet there are also disadvantages to feeding grass seed hay. It contains less vitamins, minerals, trace elements and protein than regular hay. This problem can be resolved by supplementing the shortages. A bigger problem is a symbiotic fungus (endophyte) the grass seed grass has been deliberately contaminated with in order to make the plant stronger and protect it against insect damage. Unfortunately, this fungus releases a mycotoxin that is associated with laminitis. It can cause or aggravate inflammatory reactions. It also has a vasoconstrictor effect. This can reduce blood flow in the lamellae and increase blood pressure inside the hoof. It is impossible to determine whether grass seed hay is contaminated with endophytes with the naked eye. Therefore, it is advisable to ask the hay supplier for a document that explicitly states that the hay does not contain endophytes. A third disadvantage of grass seed hay is that most often it will have been sprayed to prevent diseases in the seed, just before harvest. Fertilizers are often used lavishly and cultivation takes place on soil that was exhausted by monoculture. Not exactly the ideal conditions for 'healthy' hay. The fact that this hay comes from only one grass species does not benefit the horse either.

CUTS

The first cut contains the entire plant, including flower heads and seeds. The plant has completed the entire growth cycle and is very nutritious because of the storage of nutrients in the seed. A first cut is likely to have been made under conditions that cause high NSC levels.

Once the plant has regrown it can be cut a second time. The plant will be smaller than at the first cut. Flowering or seed formation stage has not always been reached. The second cut is lower in yield and nutritional value. The same applies to a third cut. Usually there is less crude fibre in the second and third cuts and the grass has almost always been over-fertilised.

RESEEDING PASTURE

Remove the old grass completely. Have the soil tested and ask for fertilisation recommendations. Repeat every five years. Sow a special horse pasture mix with grass types containing low NSC levels. Give the grass on the newly sown pasture time to strengthen before allowing horses access to it. Wait at least six months or until hay has been cut twice. Sowing additional seed to patch up bare spots works best with rye grass, which is unfortunately high in NSC.

Pasture

Consider reseeding pasture with a special horse pasture mix (see sidebar).

Horses that are kept on unfertilised pasture all year round, with extra roughage provided in winter, are able to adapt to the gradual change in nutritional value of the grass.

> ➤ As mentioned earlier, all growth factors of grass should be in place. When pasture is poor or remains unfertilised the risk of high NSC levels increase.

Silage, haylage and straw

Silage

Grass that has been conserved by fermentation is called silage. The grass is wrapped in plastic when the moisture content still exceeds 70%. Silage has a high protein content. The protein is partly broken down to ammonia, which burdens the liver and kidneys. It also disrupts the bacterial culture (intestinal flora) of the hind gut. In case you do choose to feed silage, use the same selection criteria as for hay:

- Coarse and stemmy
- Second or third cut
- Low in NSC
- High dry matter content
- Low in protein

Given the characteristics of silage the last two points will be difficult to guarantee.

The fermentation process converts a large portion of ESC and fructans. Further reduction of these WSC is not only unnecessary but also unwise. Chances are a secondary fermentation process will set in. This could lead to an increase of harmful bacteria. When silage is made the old-fashioned way, grass is stored in a pit, in several layers on top of each other. This is called a 'lasagna pit'. The different cuts of hay compensate for various nutritional values. Having silage analysed for NSC content is highly advisable. However, other types of roughage remain preferable over silage.

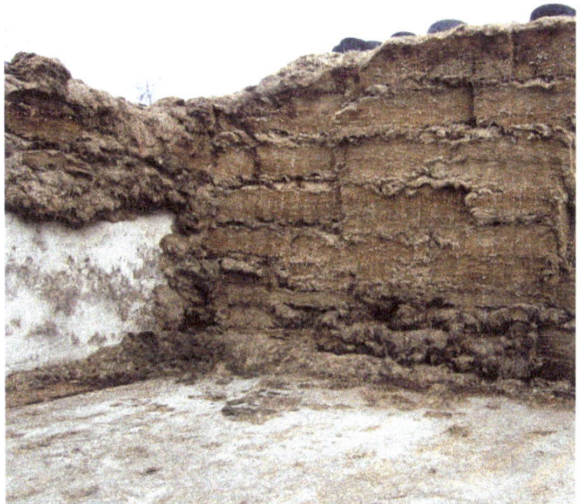

Silage lasagna pit

Haylage

Haylage is baled in plastic when the moisture content of the grass is between 40% and 60%. Haylage therefor contains a higher dry matter percentage than silage. The grass has been given the opportunity to grow taller and which makes the protein content of haylage lower than of silage.

When making haylage, fermentation occurs like in the process of making silage, although to a lesser extent. The fermentation reduces the ESC and fructan levels compared to those in hay. Of course, for choosing haylage the same criteria apply as for selecting hay.

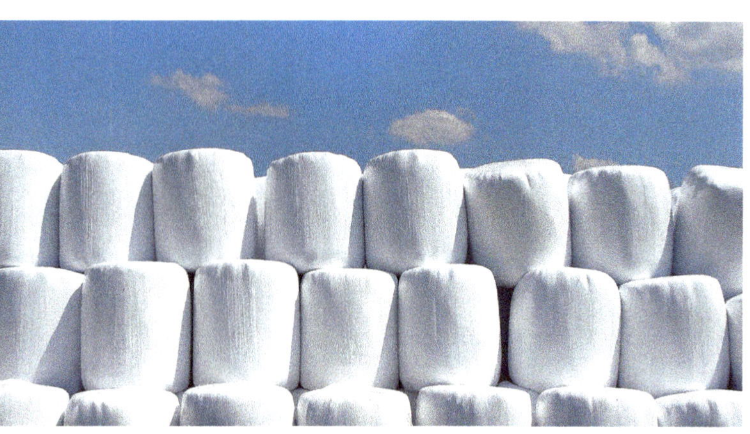

Haylage

> Silage and haylage may harbour a bacterium called Clostridium botulinum. This bacterium lives on the carcasses of small field animals and is dangerous for horses because it secretes a toxin that causes botulism. Especially in a high-protein and low-oxygen environment, such as silage or haylage, the bacterium thrives. Be sure to check for the presence of these animal carcasses.

Straw

During digestion of large amounts of straw ammonia compounds are released that burden the liver and kidneys.

Additional feeds

A healthy horse that has access to good grass, roughage, a salt lick and fresh, clean drinking water has no need for additional food. A sick horse may benefit from certain plants which may or may not grow in its pasture. If you want to start using plants or herbs to improve the health of your horse, consult a herbal practitioner for sound advice. On page 153 under 'Phytotherapy' you can read a few things about herbs.

> However much your horse loves apples, carrots, cereal, sugar cubes, vitamin biscuits and other treats: he does not need them. When your horse is prone to laminitis these little extras are especially bad for him.

Food rewards

If you want to give your horse a food reward, or just give it a little extra, the following treats are 'safe' for them:

- Celery
- Lettuce
- Cabbage leaf
- Cucumber, zucchini, pumpkin, watermelon
- Sunflower and pumpkin seeds
- Peanuts with shell
- Pea pods

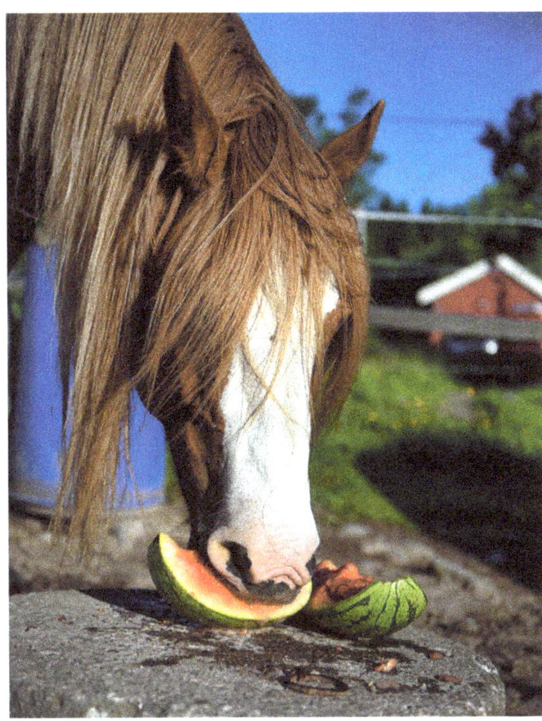

Watermelon is a safe treat
(photo: Alfaromeogirl)

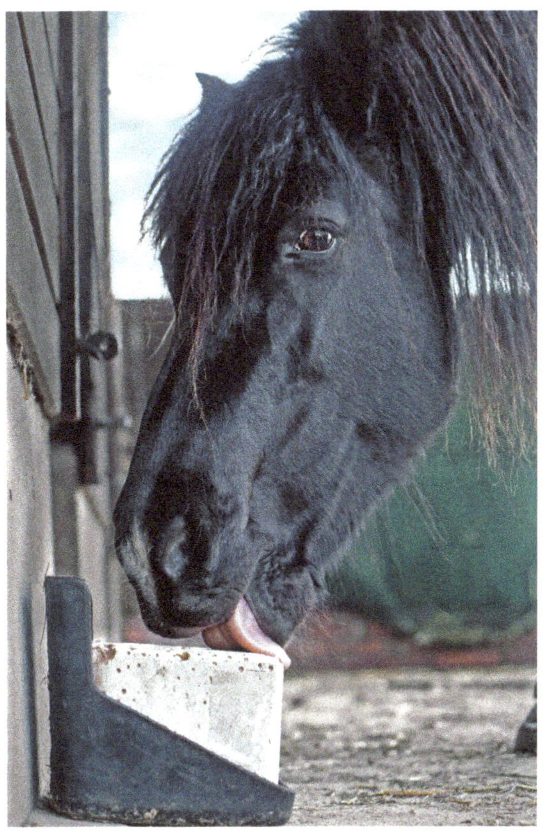

Salt lick
(photo: Karin Schouwenburg)

Salt lick

Sodium is a mineral that is often lacking in the horse's environment. Provide a good salt lick with added minerals and trace elements. For laminitic horses a low calcium lick is preferable. Too much calcium hinders the absorption of magnesium, and especially laminitic horses benefit from magnesium (see page 156 under 'Vitamins and minerals').

Himalayan salt licks contain too little zinc, copper and manganese. Its main feature is probably being flown all over the world by plane. Apple flavoured licks or licks containing molasses are best left in the store. Horses should use the lick to ingest salt and minerals, not because they like the taste of it.

Supplements

Generally, dietary supplements are not needed. All necessary vitamins, including vitamin H (B8, biotin) can be either extracted from a balanced diet or produced in the horse's hindgut (see page 155 under 'Supplements').

Losing weight

Better late than never, it is always worthwhile to try your very best to make obese horses lose weight. Be sure to do this gradually and not too drastically (see page 135 under 'Weight loss').

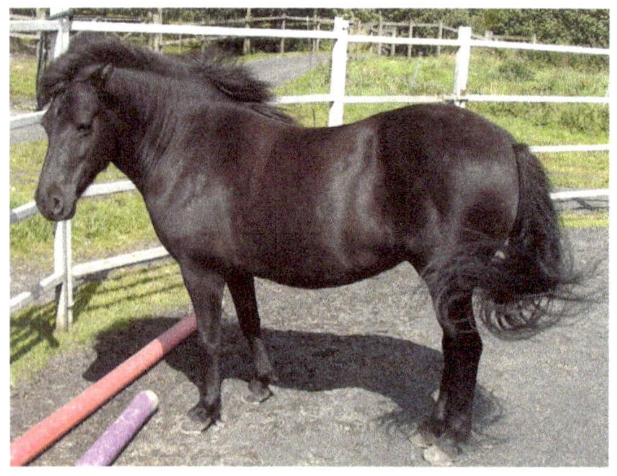

An obese horse should lose weight
(photo: Janice Hutchinson)

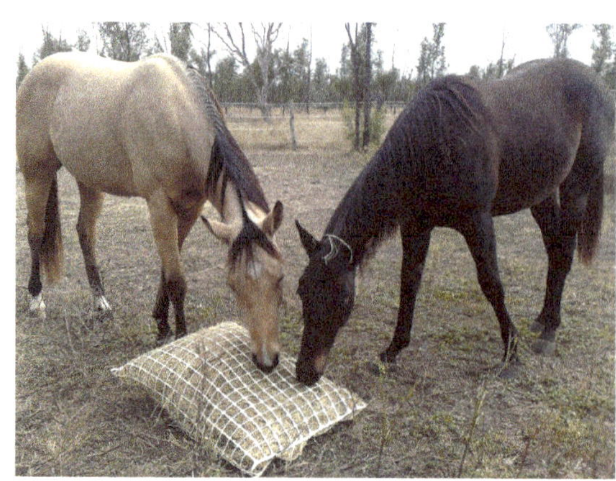

Hay pillow
(photo: Tracy Dunn)

Feeding practice

Sometimes there is room for improvement in the way food is offered to horses. Slow feeders decrease forage intake speed. They are easy to make by covering a hay box with concrete mesh or netting. Make sure the slow feeder is safe and horses cannot get stuck. With a little creativity, a hay pillow can be made quite easily as well.

Horses should eat and drink at ground level. Do not mount hay racks, mangers, salt licks or drinking troughs onto the paddock fence or stable wall. However, eating at ground level puts more pressure on the front of the feet. Therefore severely laminitic horses can benefit from being offered food at chest height for the time being. Never feed hay on sandy ground.

Place hay feeders, water and salt lick as far apart as possible. This will keep the horse moving. Although, as long as the horse is still reluctant to move because of the pain it is obviously better to offer food he can reach without much effort.

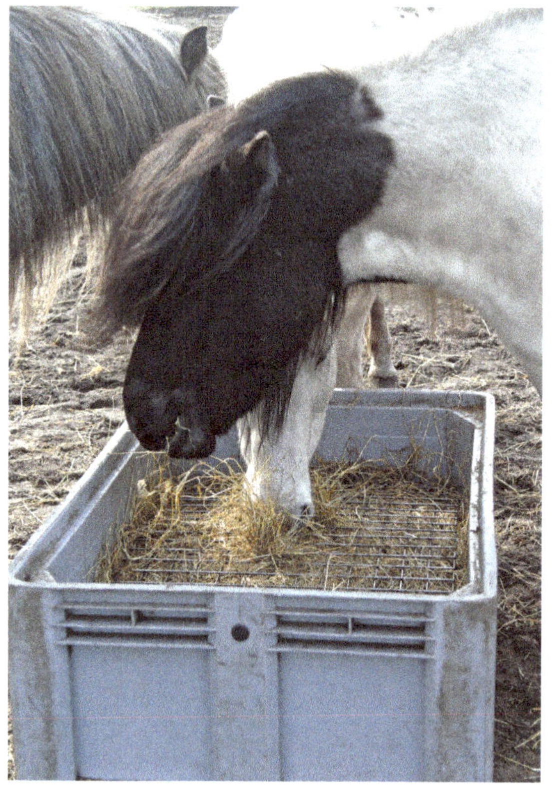

Slow feeder
(photo: Marja van Run)

NSC PREVENTION

In the next sections several ways to minimise the intake of NSC are suggested.

> To have your horse on pasture 24/7 and still keep NSC intake low will always be a difficult task. A paddock paradise with less grass will be easier to manage and has a closer resemblance to natural living conditions. More on the paddock paradise system later in this book.

GENERAL

The NSC content of grass (and herbs and weeds) fluctuates continuously. Natural, climatic and environmental factors can cause a threefold increase. These external factors play a much larger role than the genetic predisposition of certain grass types. It is sensible to feed hay to horses on pasture that is at risk of high NSC.

Rapidly growing grass contains fewer NSC. The NSC are used by the grass in order to grow. At night, NSC content in grass gradually decreases. In the absence of light, no photosynthesis takes place so no new NSC are produced. The plant continues to convert sugars into growth. Offering horses access to pasture at night only, is an option.

Mount a weatherproof sign to the pasture fence that explains why you do not appreciate people feeding your horse without your permission. Include your telephone number so that well-meaning passers-by can ask you for more information if they wish. The chance that this will happen is nil, but it shows how much you want the message to get across.

GRAZING MUZZLE

Grass leaf tips contain lower NSC levels. A grazing muzzle helps prevent the horse from grazing the grass lower down. Grazing speed decreases and food enters the digestive tract more slowly and steadily. The horse can stay out on pasture longer and therefore will get more exercise.

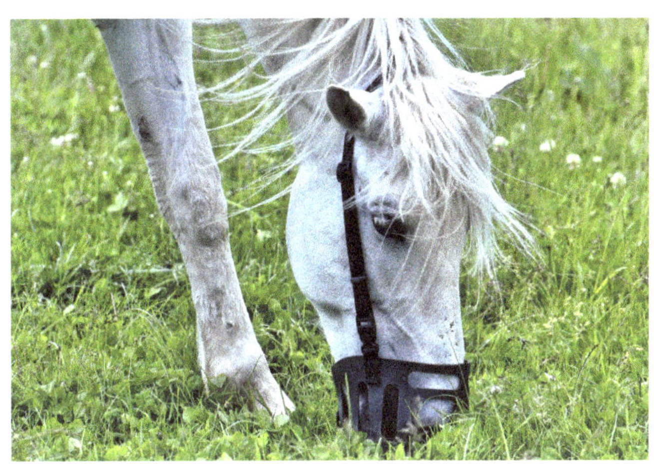

Grazing muzzle
(photo: Alexas fotos)

Make sure the muzzle fits well and has a panic snap. This is important to prevent the horse from being injured if he gets caught on something. Normally the muzzle does not prevent the horse from drinking. Make sure this is the case. Check regularly that the muzzle is still properly attached. When a horse that is used to restricted grazing loses a muzzle he could easily overeat with all the associated risks.

Some horses resent the muzzle and refuse to eat. Others do not understand that they are still able to eat. Reassure them by pushing some grass through the holes. The muzzle can be completely or partially closed off with duct tape. The horse will get his movement, without being able to graze too much.

Wearing a grazing muzzle may cause stress. This especially needs to be avoided in PPID horses. They have too much cortisol in their bodies already and stress will increase the levels further (as described on 95 under 'Stress').

Some horses get so skilful at grazing with a muzzle that more grazing restrictions, as described on the following pages, are needed.

If the grazing muzzle causes problems, realise the horse is better off in a paddock with hay than out on pasture with a grazing muzzle.

> The different types of grass growing in the pasture influence the effectiveness of a grazing muzzle as well. Some grass varieties are tastier than others. For example, horses prefer meadow fescue to English rye grass. Fescue grows more upright and is therefore easier to eat with a grazing muzzle. If this tastier variety grows abundantly in the pasture a grazing muzzle will be noticeably less effective.

Pasture management

Short, overgrazed grass contains high NSC levels. Always prevent pasture from becoming overgrazed. The stronger grass varieties will survive better than the weaker types. Strong grass however contains more NSC than more fragile plants.

Grass flower heads are high in NSC. Try to avoid grass from blooming by proper pasture management like strip grazing, pasture rotation or restricted grazing. Even mowing could be a solution at times when other measures have not been effective.

Strip grazing

With electric fencing a grazing area can be moved daily, or made bigger or smaller as required.

Pasture rotation

- Divide your pasture, depending on the size, into a maximum of six plots.
- Let the horses graze each plot until the grass is about 4 cm (1 1/2") high.
- By mowing the grass, root sprouts and suckers are stimulated to multiply.
- Remove manure and weeds after the horses have been moved. The plot can then be fertilised and left to rest and regrow.
- About three weeks after mowing and fertilising grass is ready to be grazed again.

Limited pasture access

Horses that are prone to laminitis (overweight, EMS, PPID, high risk breeds) should not be given too much pasture time. Preferably they will have no access to pasture at all. Only allow grazing at times when NSC levels are low.
At other times they can be kept in a sand paddock, riding arena or for instance in a yard that is fenced off with electric tape.

You will be amazed at how inventive horses become to reach tufts of grass from underneath a fence. Use electric tape to keep them away, or remove it by spraying or covering with weed mat or plastic.

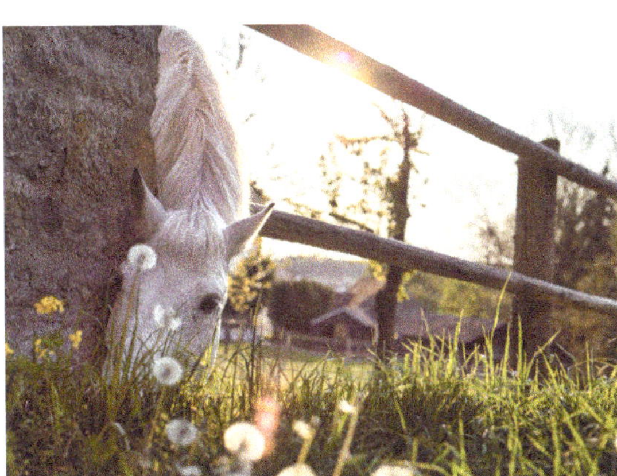

Inventive grazing
(photo: Rainer Maiores)

Removing horses from their herd may cause them to become upset. The stress caused by separation anxiety will have a negative effect on the healing process. Apart from the effect it has on cortisol levels (see page 95 under 'Stress') a separated horse could start moving too much out of insecurity. He will move compulsively, trying to find the herd. Make sure he is able to see his friends or give it the company of one of them, or a sheep or a goat. Only provide close company to horses with severe or acute laminitis if they are still able to move. Otherwise the company may urge them to move more than is good for them. In the section 'Social interaction' there is more on this subject.

- Be extra vigilant once grazing restrictions have been reduced. At the first laminitic signs or deterioration, you will have to limit grazing again.

MOWING

Be careful with mowing. Short grass receives more sunlight which increases sugar production. Plantain, clover and dandelion leaves lay flat on the ground and are not touched by the lawn mower. They do however, contain high fructan levels. Thistles, also high in fructan, grow new shoots after mowing. Obviously grass clippings should not be fed to horses.

THE LEARNING EFFECT OF RESTRICTED GRAZING

In 2011, a study on the uptake of grass and hay quantities by ponies that were restricted in grazing showed some remarkable results. In the first week of the study, the ponies ate a quantity equivalent to about half a percent of their body weight during the 3 hours they were given access to pasture each day. After six week the amount they ate in the same time had doubled to nearly one percent. During the six weeks the animals learned that they should hurry up eating while they were out on the pasture.

In 2012, another study showed that restricted grazing has no negative effect on the acidity of the intestines, as long as the limitation does not exceed 12 hours.

Weather conditions

Clear blue skies after a frosty night? No grazing! Even night temperatures below 5 °C (41 °F) increase the risks considerably.

> ➤ At least three nights with temperatures over 5 °C (41 °F) are required before horses can be safely taken out on pasture early in the morning without feeding them hay.

During a long period of drought, especially combined with bright sunshine, the risk of high NSC increases considerably. Some grass varieties will produce extra simple sugars, others more fructans. Once it starts raining after a period of drought, the new growth will contain high NSC levels as well. Rule of thumb: grazing is only recommended once grass stems have grown at least two leaves.

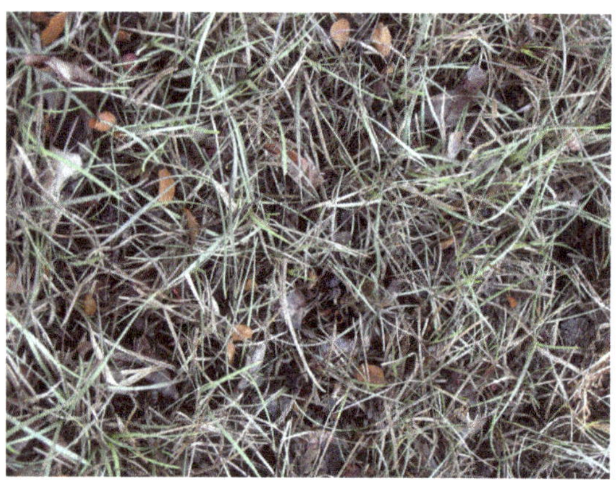

Drought-damaged grass
(photo: Katie Fitzgerald)

On sunny days after warm nights, NSC levels increase steadily during the day. On those days the morning is the most suitable time to put your horse out on pasture. On warm, cloudy days NSC levels decline throughout the day. On days like these, the afternoon and evening are more suitable for grazing.

Shade

Light plays an important role in photosynthesis. Pastures with more shade are therefore often safer. Trees and barns can provide shade, but do note what trees you give your horse access to. The ground beneath oak or beech trees can be scattered with acorns or beechnuts. It is best to fence these areas off.

Plant fast-growing trees like birch, willow, poplar or maple. The honey locust is a very fast growing tree with dense foliage of small leaves that gives plenty of shade. There are varieties without thorns. Having trees in or around pasture provides another advantage. Their roots prevent the fertile top layer of the soil from being washed away.

Forest grazing is a very good alternative as well. Let go of the idea that only pasture is an appropriate environment for horses. An additional advantage is the extra exercise horses get in a forest because it is more challenging than a field. Keep your eyes open for the presence of anything potentially dangerous like toxic plants, rabbit holes and obstacles like stumps or old fences. Protect trees with shallow roots against damage by horse feet by fencing them off with electric tape. Lastly you will want to make sure that you provide enough roughage in the absence of grass.

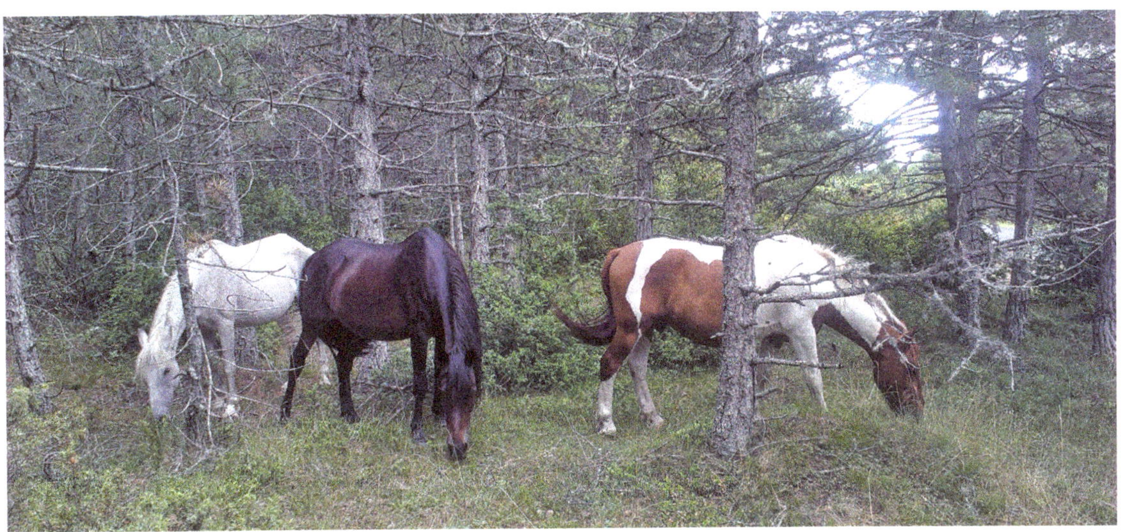

A forest plot as a housing alternative

HAY, GRASS, HERBS AND WEEDS

Hay can be analysed for NSC content at a laboratory for soil and crop research. If this is not possible, try to determine how the horse responds by observation. Horses prone to developing laminitis show signs fairly quickly, for instance by a reduction or enlargement of their neck size (see page 81 under 'Cresty Neck Score'). By soaking hay NSC levels can be decreased (see sidebar 'Soaking hay' on page 117).

> ➤ Oat and barley hay are usually considered safe. The assumption is that the majority of carbohydrates is located in the seeds. However, oat and barley grains are harvested when they are filled with starch. High concentrations of WSC are left behind in the stem.

NSC CONTENT OF DIFFERENT GRASS VARIETIES

Different sources contradict each other on this aspect. Therefore, do not just focus on the variety of the grass, but consider all aspects described in this chapter when making a pasture risk assessment.

Uncultivated grass varieties that originate and naturally grow in certain regions are well adapted to the local conditions and usually lower in NSC.

Agricultural grass varieties are often especially selected to produce high NSC in order to generate a high milk or meat yield. English rye grass is such a variety. Consider resowing pasture with a horse pasture mix (see sidebar 'Reseeding pasture' on page 182).

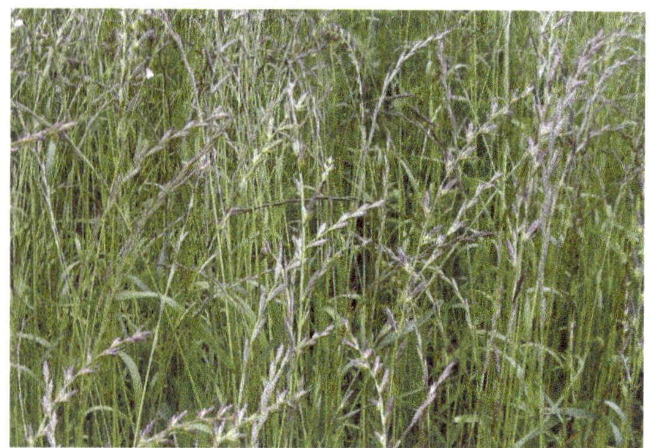

Italian rye grass
(photo: Jirí Kamenícek)

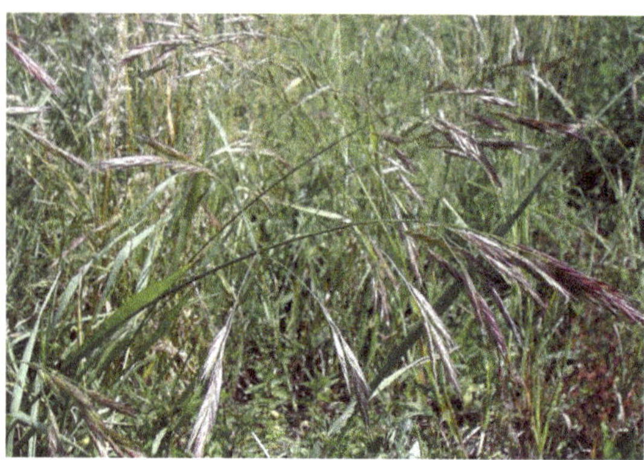

Brome grass
(photo: Radim Paulic)

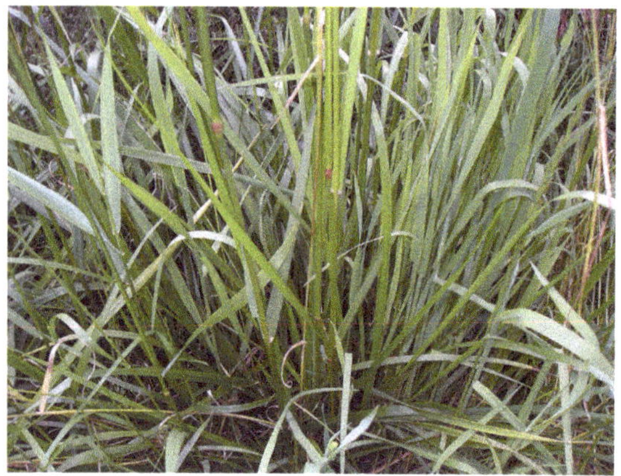

Tall fescue
(photo: Václav Hrdina)

NSC CONTENT PER GRASS VARIETY

HIGH
• English and Italian rye grass • Brome grass • Tall fescue • Meadow fescue
AVERAGE
• Kentucky bluegrass
LOW
• Creeping soft grass • Meadow foxtail • Orchard grass • Phleum (specifically timothy grass) • Red fescue

HERBS AND WEEDS

Herbs and weeds can contain very high concentrations of NSC. Keep pasture free from proliferating weeds. Sheep can be a valuable help for this.

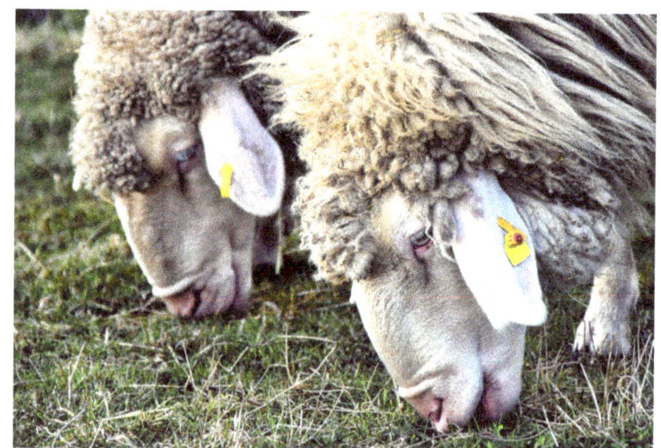

Ecological weed killers
(photo: Ulrich Leone)

FERTILISING

Pasture with only one type of grass on nutrient-poor soil can increase the risk of high NSC levels. A lack of nutrients prevents plants from growing well causing these levels to accumulate. Nitrogen and phosphorus deficiencies play an especially important role in this. Have the soil analysed and ask for fertilisation advice. Clearly indicate that the land is being used for grazing horses. Potassium levels need extra attention when pasture is used for horses prone to laminitis (see sidebar).

> This does not apply to natural, species-rich pastures. The grass and herb species that are characteristic of the present soil, grow well on nutrient-poor soil.

> Fertilising reduces the NSC content per plant, but increases the quantity of grass. Keep in mind that across the turf NSC quantity can actually rise because of the increased grass density. By strip grazing, the use of grazing muzzles and restricting grazing time, grass consumption can be controlled.

Unfortunately different laboratories provide varying test results and opinions. Make sure the minerals calcium, magnesium, sodium and sulphur (and possibly cobalt, copper, iron, and manganese) are included in the analysis, as well as the acidity of the soil. Do not forget to ask for an interpretation of the test results.

POTASSIUM

By over-fertilising for years with both organic and inorganic fertiliser the soil may contain a surplus of potassium. Dried chicken manure especially contains high levels of potassium. Too much potassium in the soil, and therefore in the plant, interferes with the ability of grass to absorb calcium and magnesium. As a result, protein production within the plant is disturbed. This leads to the production of excessive amounts of NSC in the grass.

By ingesting too much potassium horses can develop difficulties absorbing magnesium, on top of the already lower available concentrations in the grass. The beneficial effects of a magnesium supplement can therefore be less than expected.

Consult an agricultural laboratory for fertilisation advice that keeps potassium levels as low as possible, without causing potassium deficiency. Both magnesium levels in the grass and the magnesium absorption capacity of the horse will rise once potassium levels are normalised.

Soil acidity is easy to optimise by applying lime. The pH of horse pasture should be between 6.5 and 7.2 but tends to become too acidic over time. Loam and clay soils are easier to maintain at the right level than sandy or sandy loam soil.

Spreading compost (man-made), or preferably humus (naturally decomposed organic matter), is a relatively safe way of fertilising. The disadvantage is their composition cannot be adjusted to the deficiencies of the soil.

Low NSC grasses (especially timothy grass, fescue and orchard grass) do not thrive on poor or calcium deficient soils.

DROUGHT

Insufficient water means plants are unable to grow properly. Drought can be fought by irrigation or by planting trees, as tree roots will help retain moisture.

Pasture high in salt content suffers similar effects as pasture in periods of drought, and often the two are related. The soil's salt content is determined by all mineral salts combined. Usually, years of fertilising with chemical fertiliser, organic manure, compost and humus have added these salts to the soil.

In times of drought, when water evaporates from the soil, its salt concentration increases. Roots get damaged because water is being extracted from their cells by the saline soil. Plants are then unable to absorb enough water. By irrigating, drying out of the plants can be prevented to some extent.

Agricultural laboratories can test soil samples for salt content. Knowing your land has been fertilised intensively for many years might already provide a clue.

EXTERNAL FACTORS

Grass can get damaged by unexpected frost, hail, trampling, insect damage and so on. When flowering is adversely affected by external factors the seed cannot develop and NSC will then remain behind in the stem.

HOUSING

Earlier in this chapter, keeping horses on pasture was discussed from the perspective of the horse's diet. Now we look at pasture as a way of keeping or housing horses. Obviously, the environment horses live in needs to be safe, without dangerous objects or fences they can injure themselves on. We will focus on ways to keep your horse that will have a positive impact on laminitis.

STABLING

Box rest is not a solution for laminitis but can be part of the cause. Stabling limits the horse in his movement, restricting adequate blood flow to the hooves. In addition, stabling causes stress with all its negative effects.

When NSC risks are manageable, horses can be offered continuous grazing with a natural shelter or walk-in stable. In case you do not have pasture at your disposal, turn your horse out in a paddock or arena as much as possible. In the absence of a paddock you might be able to create an acceptable temporary solution by fencing off part of the yard with an electric fence. If this is all impossible, you might be able to join several stables to create a bigger space.

If you don't have any other option than to offer your horse solitary confinement in a stable, consider carefully whether it might be possible for someone else, somewhere else, to take care of the horse temporarily.

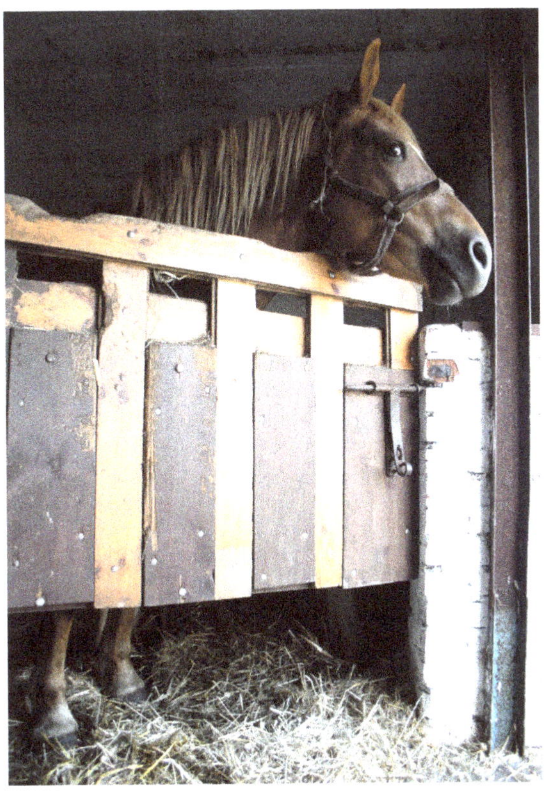

Box rest can be part of the cause
(photo: Justyna Furmanczyk)

Bedding

In both normal stables as walk-in stables it is recommended to provide bedding only that is covering half of the surface, or just one corner. That way horses can decide for themselves whether they use it or not. Often, they prefer hard ground over standing on soft bedding. Horses that can barely stand because of the pain will choose to lie down on the soft bedding. Make sure it remains clean.

Sawdust strongly absorbs moisture and dries out hooves. Leave mud on the hooves and don't pick them when bringing the horse in. The sawdust then draws moisture from the mud instead of the hooves.

> Design recommendations for paddock paradises used to include watering holes to prevent hooves from drying out. However, recent studies have shown that water has hardly any influence on the moisture level of the hoof wall.

Surface

If your boarding facility has a varied and partly paved surface, make sure the laminitic horse has no need to walk across gravel and stony areas. The sole will be too thin and sensitive.

Slow feeders, drinking water and salt lick should be placed as far apart as possible.

The ground should certainly not be too wet. The grass will be trampled and destroyed in the mud. Install efficient drainage.

Paddock paradise

A great way of housing horses is the paddock paradise, a concept developed by Jaime Jackson. A wide track is created around the property, at some points giving access to some bigger areas or paddocks. The track system stimulates the natural urge to move. The concept is based on the observation of wild horses following the same fixed routes to grazing areas, watering holes, minerals and other places of interest.

In a paddock paradise, it is possible to create all kinds of natural elements and challenges to stimulate movement. More movement means increased circulation, better wear patterns and faster growing hooves. Besides, it creates better physical and mental health in general.

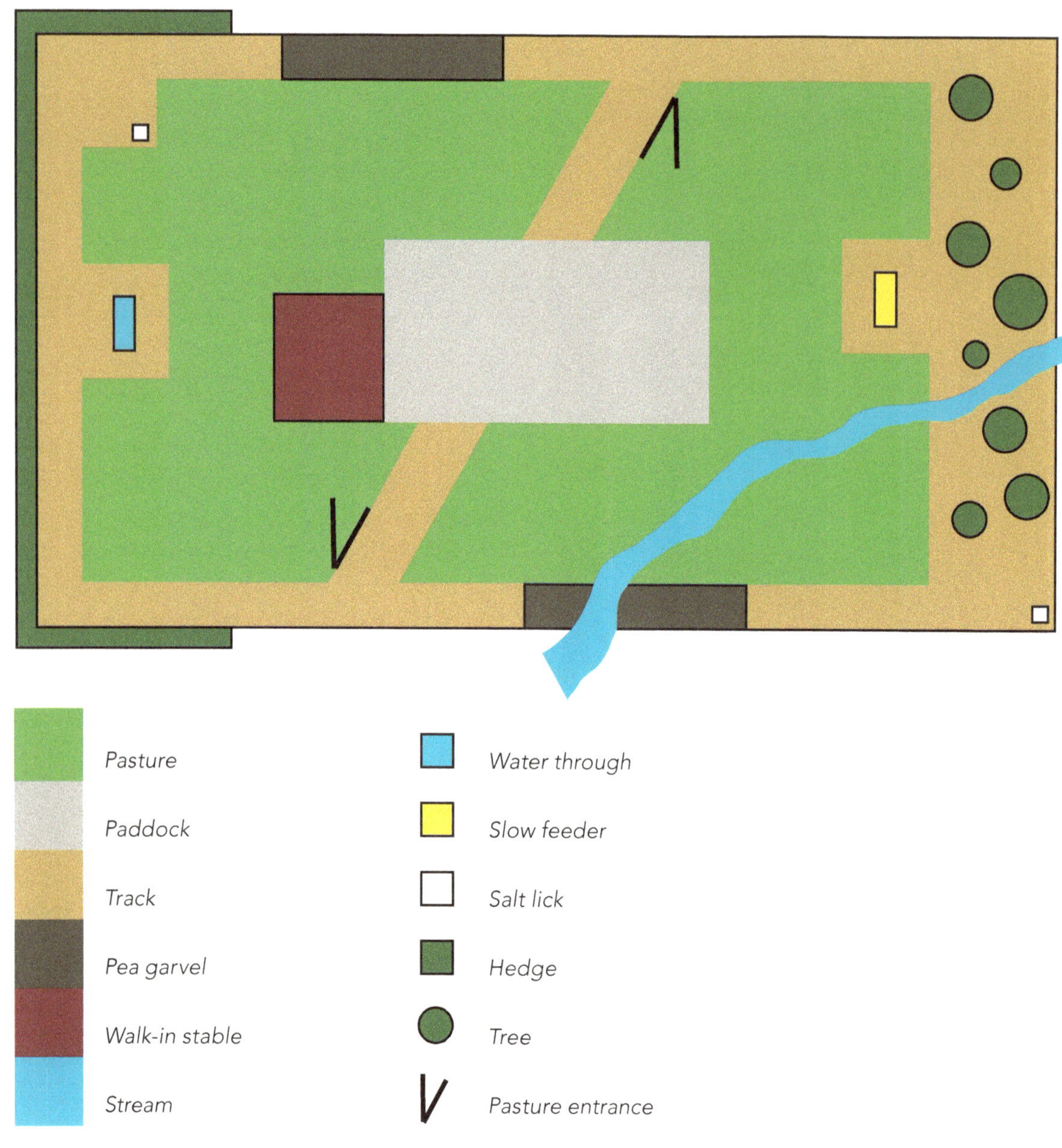

Example of a paddock paradise

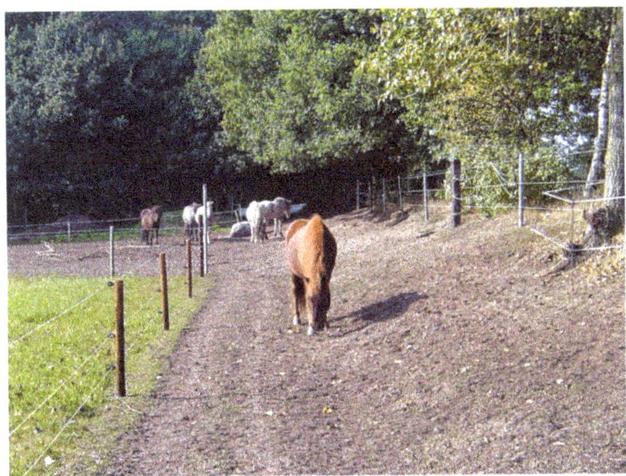

Taking a stroll in a paddock paradise
(photo: Marja van Run)

Some possibilities:

- Place several hay feeders, water troughs and salt licks, as far from each other as possible
- Provide walk-in stables or natural shelters
- Integrate hedgerows or tree lines
- Create height differences
- Provide different kind of footing with pavers, concrete slabs, pea gravel and rocks.

Pea gravel

Laminitic horses often benefit significantly from a surface covered with pea gravel. It distributes the force optimally over the painful underside of the hoof. You will be able to see that your horse benefits from this solution if it stands in it when given the choice and spends more time there than elsewhere. Often we also notice improvement in posture, movement and behaviour. A good gravel layer is at least 10 centimetres (4") deep and is made of pea gravel with a diameter of approximately 5 to 10 millimetres (0.2 - 0.4"). Gravel grains that are too small can get stuck in the collateral grooves and penetrate the stretched white line or lamellar wedge. Gravel grains that are too large can bruise the sole. It is best to deposit the gravel on a layer of white sand covered with anti-root cloth (weed mat).

SOCIAL INTERACTION

As soon as the laminitic horse is able to move again, it is good to give it company. Choose a quiet horse as a companion, preferably a horse the patient is already bonded with. If possible, reintroduce the horse back into the herd. Make sure the herd is not too large. Each horse needs at least half a hectare (one acre).

If the above is not possible, consider providing the company of a sheep or goat. Horses also get along well with donkeys. However, the company of donkeys does pose an increased risk of lung worm infection in horses. By worming with ivermectin or moxidectin, this risk can be controlled.

> Do not rely on faecal egg count when it comes to lung worms in horses. The eggs of this worm cannot be found in manure.

For a laminitic horse social interaction is of great importance. It not only provides a more natural environment and stimulates the horse to move more, but it also makes the horse feel better. Who feels better, heals faster.

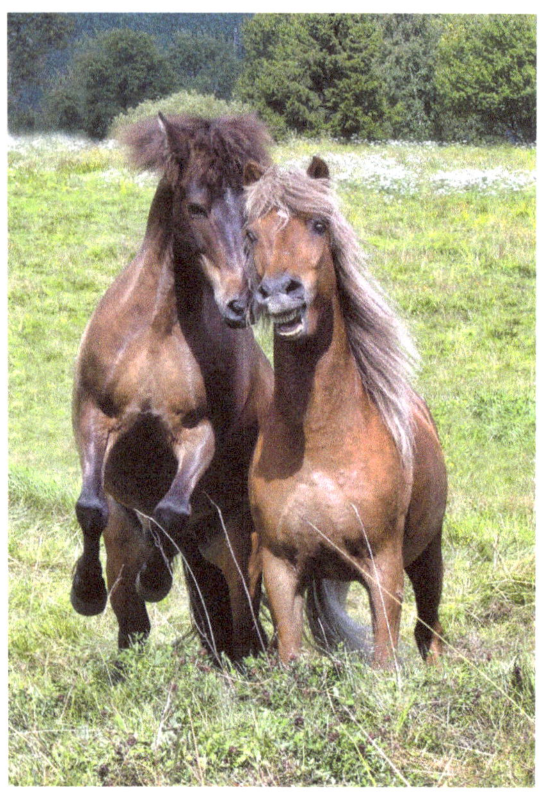

Who feels better, heals faster
(photo: Hanna Dalberg)

Social interaction between the horse and its caretaker are equally important. Do not leave your laminitic horse to face its trouble on its own. Providing the necessary treatments and measures are of course of vital importance, but the horse will heal faster if it gets your loving attention as well. Let it feel that you are both in the battle against laminitis together. If you do not think this will make a difference, at least observe how your own motivation and perseverance increase by it.

Horses are strongly attached to their existing social relationships, whether it is with another horse or a donkey, goat or sheep. Separation can be stressful. Should your horse need to go to a clinic, consider allowing the whinnying, braying or bleating friend to come along.

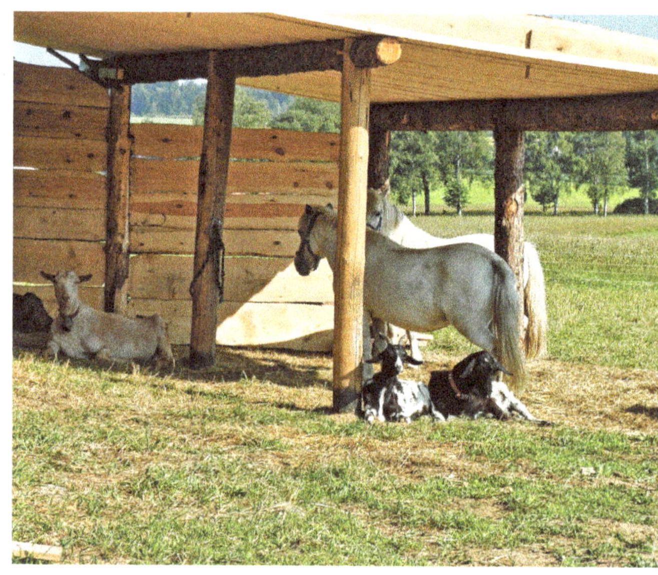

Social relationships are very important to horses

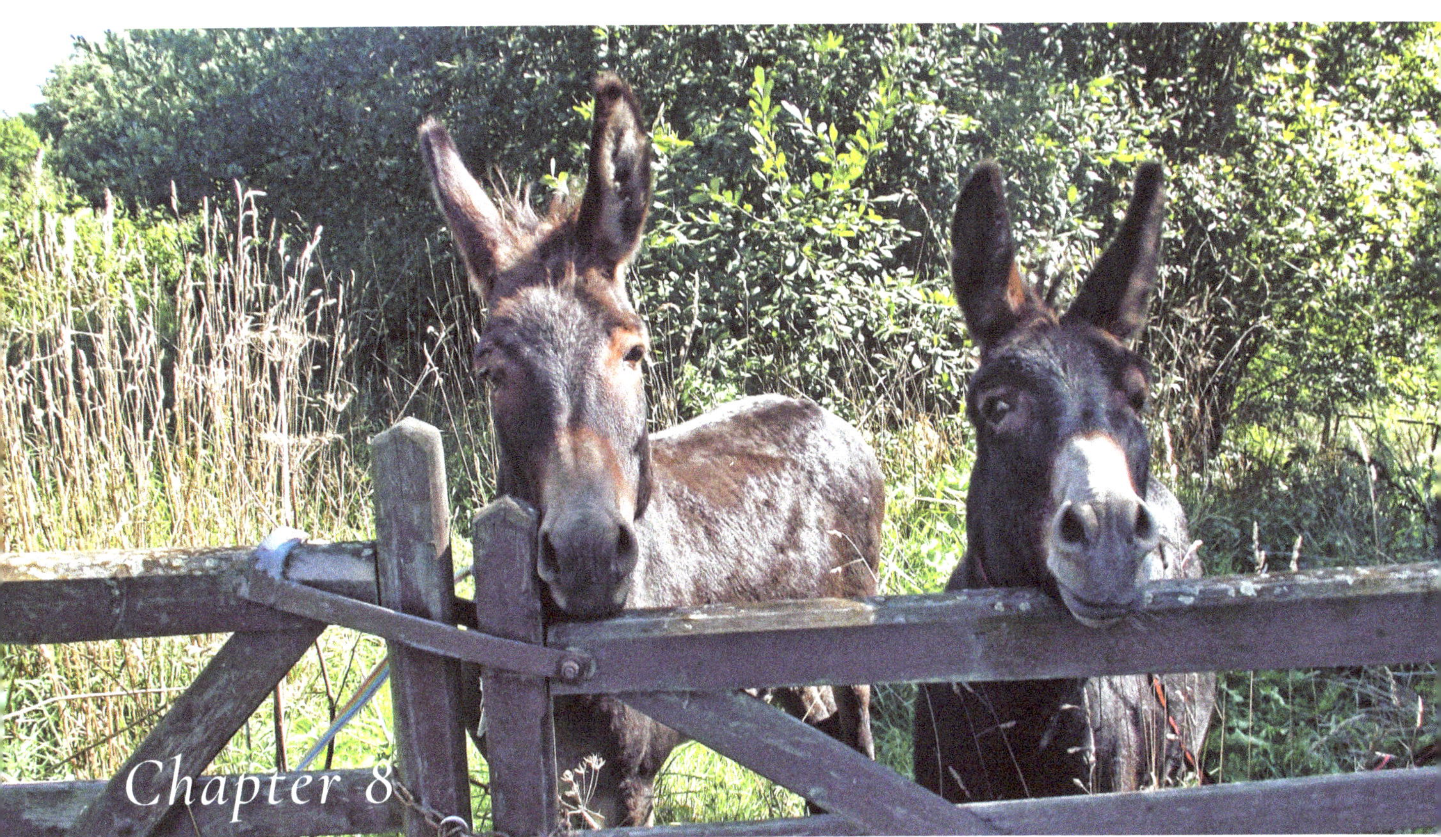

Chapter 8

DONKEYS

Despite the many differences between donkeys and horses, donkeys are all too often regarded as difficult and noisy, small horses with long ears. Both veterinarians, hoof care providers and donkey owners are guilty of this prejudice which is not only unjustified, but can be detrimental to donkeys as well.

Donkeys are, just like horses, susceptible to laminitis. This final chapter focuses on the key differences between donkeys and horses with respect to the diagnosis, treatment and prevention of laminitis.

As said, we will now have a look at the donkey. For mules and hinnies some aspects differ slightly. Hinnies (horse stallion x donkey mare) tend to have more donkey like characteristics, while mules (donkey stallion x horse mare) tend to look more like horses. Onagers and other varieties of wild ass species are not covered in this book for reasons of convenience.

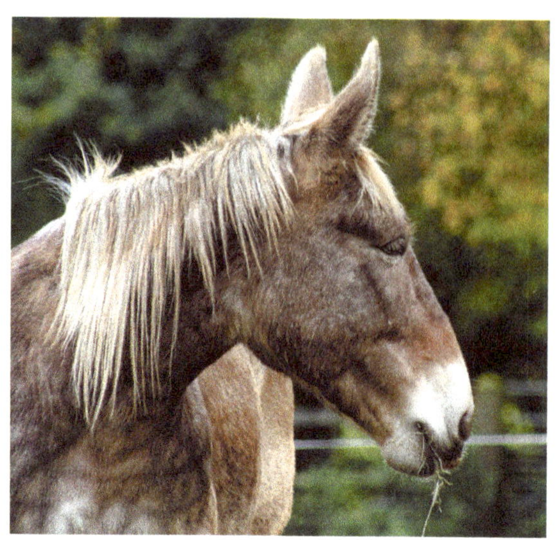

Mule
(photo: Mulography)

PHYSIOLOGICAL DIFFERENCES

The most notable physiological differences between horses and donkeys in the context of laminitis include:

- Body temperature
- Pulse
- Respiratory rate
- Body condition score

Body temperature

Donkeys have a lower body temperature than horses. For an adult donkey the average temperature is 36.8 °C (98 °F). The average horse temperature is almost a whole degree Celsius (2 °F) higher at 37.7 °C (100 °F). A raised temperature or fever could be a clinical sign of acute laminitis. In donkeys increased temperature starts at lower levels.

Pulse

Another clinical sign of acute laminitis is a strong pulse with a higher frequency than usual. The normal heart rate of a donkey is between 36 and 48 beats per minute. A heart rate of 48 beats per minute could be alarming for a horse. The horse's heart beats between 28 and 40 times per minute.

Respiratory rate

Donkeys also have a higher respiratory rate, ranging between 12 and 28 breaths per minute versus 8 to 14 in horses.

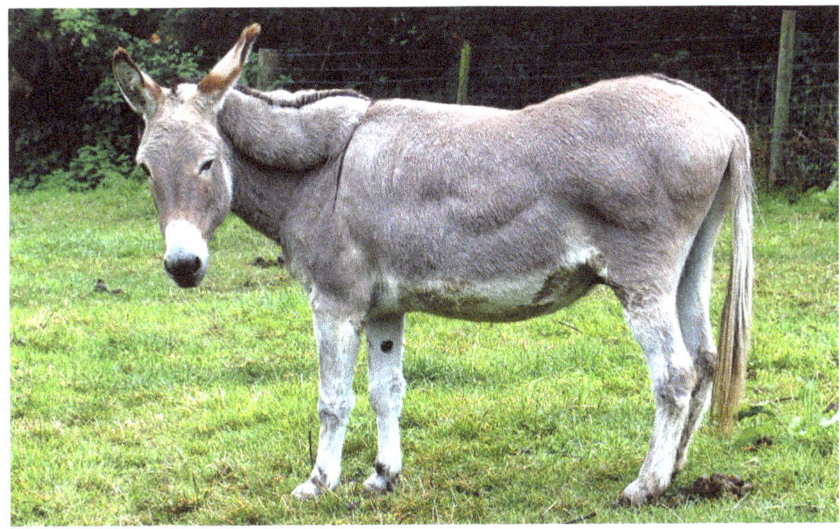

Donkey with a body condition score of 5
(photo: The Donkey sanctuary)

Body condition score

The body condition score (BCS) is a rating system that can be used to determine the body condition of horses. A too high BCS is an indication of an increased risk of laminitis.

The BCS as used for horses is not suitable for donkeys. The same bcs that would rate a horse as 'ideal' would mean 'fat' for a donkey. Many donkeys are overweight without the owner realising this. On the following page is a BCS chart adapted to donkeys.

PATHOPHYSIOLOGICAL DIFFERENCES

With regard to pathophysiology (the physiology of disordered function) differences can be found in relation to:

- Fluid balance
- Pain threshold
- EMS
- PPID
- Hyperlipidemia
- Traumatic laminitis

Fluid balance

Donkeys are desert-adapted and their fluid balance differs to that of horses. They will not show signs of dehydration quickly. Therefore, water intake and loss of fluids from urine and manure must be monitored extra carefully when donkeys are ill.

BODY CONDITION SCORE (BCS) - DONKEYS

	NECK	WITHERS	BACK AND LOIN	RIBS	HIND QUARTERS
1. POOR	Neck thin, all bones easily felt. Neck meets shoulder abruptly, shoulder bones felt easily, angular.	Dorsal spine of withers prominent and easily felt	Backbone prominent, can feel dorsal and transverse processes easily	Ribs can be seen from a distance and felt with ease. Belly tucked up.	Hip bones visible and felt easily.
2. MODERATE	Some muscle development overlying bones. Slight step where neck meets shoulders.	Some cover over dorsal withers, spinous processes felt but not prominent	Dorsal and transverse processes felt with light pressure	Ribs not visible but can be felt with ease	Poor muscle cover on hindquarters, hipbones felt with ease. Poor muscle development.
3. GOOD	Good muscle development, bones felt under light cover of muscle/fat. Neck flows smoothly into shoulder.	Good cover of muscle/fat over dorsal spinous processes. Withers flow smoothly into back.	Cannot feel individual spinous or transverse processes. Muscle development either side of midline is good.	Ribs just covered by light layer of fat/muscle, ribs can be felt with light pressure. Belly firm with good muscle tone.	Good muscle cover in hindquarters, hipbones can be felt with light pressure
4. FAT	Neck thick, crest hard, shoulder covered in even fat layer	Withers broad, bones felt with firm pressure	Can only feel dorsal and transverse processes with firm pressure. Slight crease along midline.	Ribs dorsally only felt with firm pressure, ventral ribs may be felt more easily. Belly overdeveloped.	Hindquarters rounded, bones felt only with firm pressure. Fat deposits evenly placed.
5. VERY FAT	Neck thick, crest bulging with fat and may fall to one side. Shoulder rounded and bulging with fat.	Withers broad, unable to feel bones	Back broad, unable to feel spinous or transverse processes. Deep crease along midline bulging fat on either side.	Large, often uneven fat deposits covering dorsal and possibly ventral aspect of ribs. Ribs not palpable. Belly pendulous.	Cannot feel hipbones, fat may overhang either side of tail head. Fat often uneven and bulging.

Pain threshold

Donkeys have a higher pain threshold than horses. They hardly show pain because of their stoic nature, even when their limits have been reached. Maybe people just do not recognise their expressions of pain very well. Anyway, it can complicate the physical examination by a veterinarian or hoof care provider.

It may take some time before a donkey owner notices something serious is going on. Sole perforation for example, when the coffin bone penetrates the sole, is seen more often in laminitic donkeys than in horses. Also primary causes like colic or infection are often overlooked because of the silent suffering of the donkey.

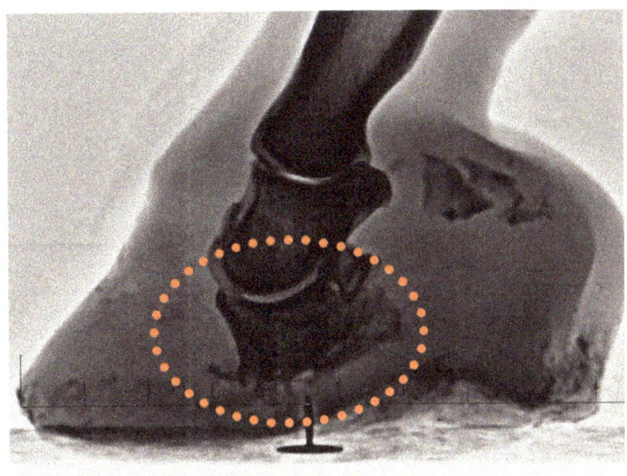

Advanced case of coffin bone deformation in a donkey's hoof *(photo: Alfons Geerts)*

EMS

During evolution the donkey's metabolic system has perfectly adapted to the harsh North African conditions. Its digestive system is still most suitable to process foods that contain little NSC and consist mainly of slow digesting crude fibres.

Unfortunately, nowadays many donkeys are condemned to a lazy life as ecological lawn mower which causes many of them to suffer from equine metabolic syndrome (EMS). This disease, extensively described on page 80, makes donkeys prone to developing laminitis. We have to realise that there is not much of a difference between the way donkeys and horses should be housed and fed and their need for movement.

PPID

As mentioned before in this book ACTH is a hormone secreted by the pituitary gland that controls the production of cortisol. Increased cortisol levels enhance the risk of laminitis. When donkeys are handled by veterinarians often a twitch is used on their upper lip. The use of the twitch instantly causes a sharp rise in ACTH levels in the blood of the donkey. This influences the test results for determining PPID (see page 72 under 'ACTH test').

Especially in the early stages, the clinical signs of PPID in donkeys are less evident. Laminitis can be a consequence of PPID without the owner being aware that the donkey suffers from this condition.

Hyperlipidemia

Vasoconstriction caused by hyperlipidemia can cause or aggravate laminitis. Donkeys are more prone to hyperlipidemia than horses, partly because they lose their appetite (anorexia) in response to pain. A drastically reduced food intake causes hyperlipidemia which in donkeys can lead to organ failure and death. Donkeys are prone to suffer from hyperlipidemia during or after a period of stress.

Traumatic laminitis

In traumatic laminitis hoof tissue is damaged because of overloading. One or more feet can be loaded excessively in order to unload another part of the body that is hurting, for example as a result of nerve damage, bone fractures or joint infections. This specific cause of laminitis is often encountered in donkeys. Their high pain threshold combined with sensitivity to hoof problems such as white line disease and thrush makes traumatic laminitis easy to be overlooked.

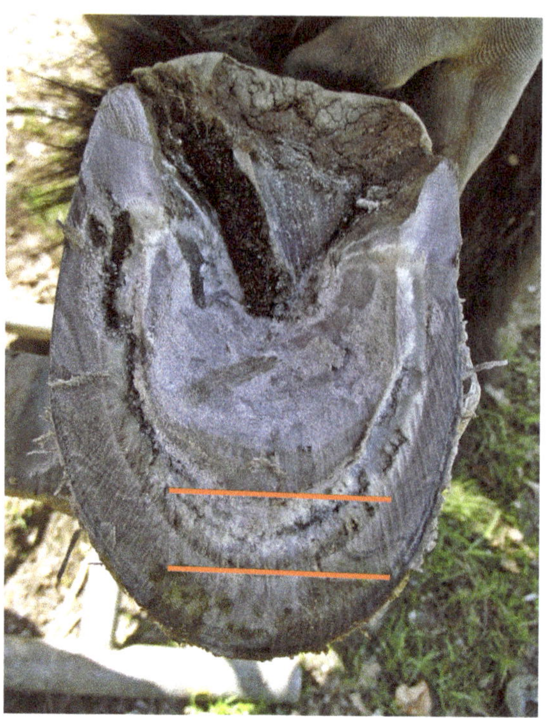

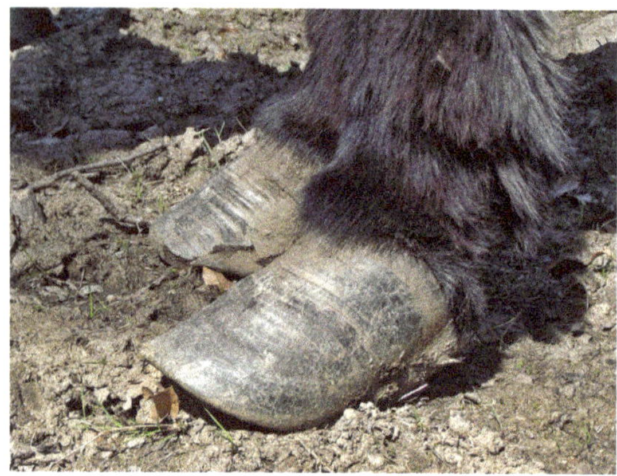

Traumatic laminitis

The long hoof wall pulls on the lamellar connection like a lever

BEHAVIOUR

As many people have experienced, donkeys can be difficult. However, a lot of their difficult behaviour can be explained. Let's have a look at the following four aspects of donkey behaviour:

- Picking up feet
- Defence mechanism
- Social behaviour
- Performance

Picking up feet

Handling donkeys can be difficult, especially when in pain, because they are often less well trained or not used to being handled. Donkeys are extremely attached to standing on all four legs. When picking up feet, allow them some time to find their balance, especially when their feet are hurting. It is important to keep the lifted leg underneath their body because of their narrow build. When a leg is pulled sideways, donkeys will lose their balance quickly and react in the manner described below.

Defence mechanism

Where as horses are flight animals, donkeys are more likely to respond to threatening situations by freezing than fleeing. Therefore, to force a donkey into doing something often has the opposite effect. Chances are that he then moves on to the attack. Donkeys will give out less warning signals in advance than we are accustomed to in horses. A laminitic donkey in pain experiences a great deal of stress. From its frozen state he can kick out with a hind leg very unexpectedly to chase away the hoof care provider he experiences as an assailant. A donkey is able to forcefully kick sideways and can even hit you in the head with a hind leg when you are holding a front foot. Being kicked in the forehead is another risk, even when you are holding the hind leg as bent as possible.

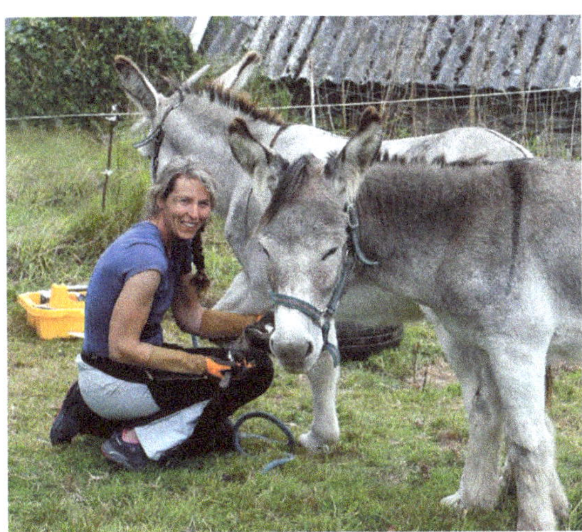

Help a donkey find its balance

Instead of putting up a fight, the donkey might choose to run off. Once that decision is made it will be difficult to stop the donkey from doing so. Trimming a laminitic donkey in the open field is a particularly bad idea. It is better to choose a safe enclosed area. Donkeys accept being tied up on a short rope better than horses. A twitch is less effective in donkeys. You can hold a donkey securely by gripping the head tightly under your arm and clasping the ear at the base.

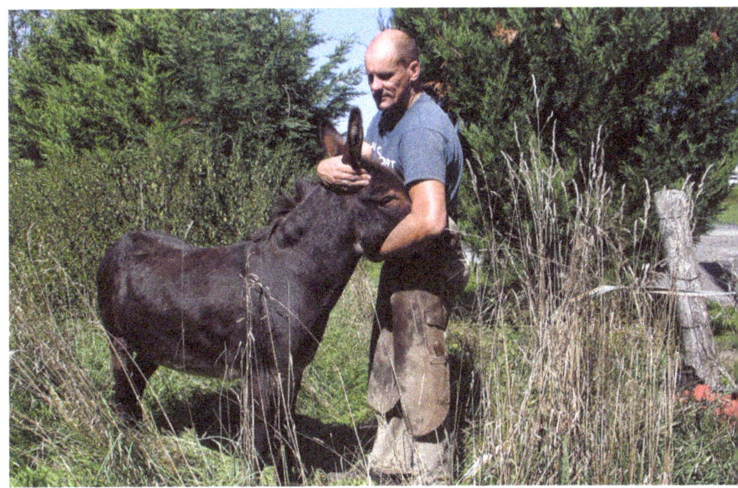

Fixation of a donkey

Social behaviour

Donkeys are very social animals, even more so than horses. They develop intense relationships with other donkeys, horses or even-toed ungulates such as goats or sheep. Yet often donkeys are kept in isolation. This results in chronic stress that causes hormonal, blood sugar and blood circulation problems. These three types of problems, as you have read in this book, are strongly related to the development of laminitis.

Performance

Usually, donkey are not handled as much as horses. After all, they are rarely used for sports or recreation. Subtle changes in performance due to a reduced health or condition often remain unnoticed in donkeys that are kept in the pasture compared to horses that are handled and used daily. However, these subtle changes are often the first and most important signs that the animal is developing or suffering from laminitis.

HOOVES

Even though laminitis is not a hoof disease, its worst and most obvious characteristics are found in the hooves. To be able to correctly interpret signs of laminitis in donkeys it is necessary to know the following.

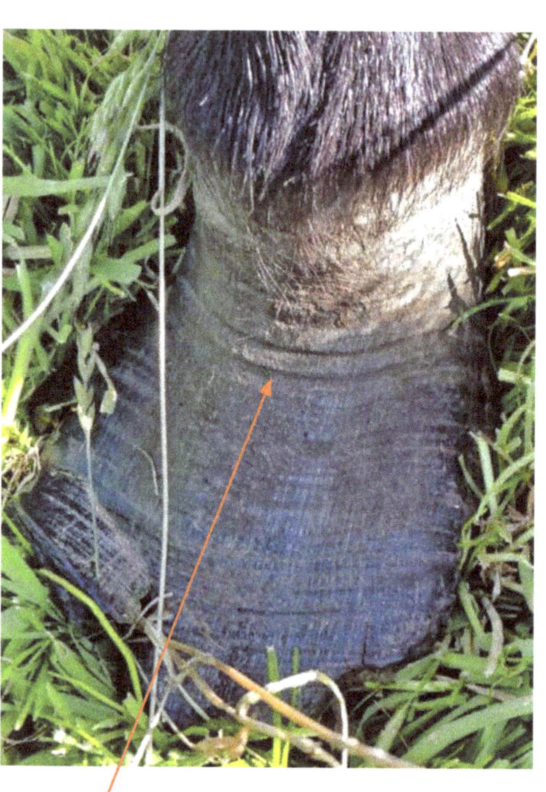

Laminitic rings

Laminitic rings

The horizontal ridges (laminitic rings) in the hoof wall caused by laminitis are less evident in donkey hooves than in horse hooves.

Coffin bone

A donkey coffin bone has a slightly different shape than that of a horse. It is important to keep this in mind when evaluating radiographs.

Lamellar connection

The lamellar connection of a donkey hoof consists of fewer lamellae than can be counted in a horse hoof. This is the reason why donkeys are more prone to white line separation, the partial detachment of the connection between hoof wall and coffin bone.

White line disease

Donkeys are also more susceptible to white line disease, the deterioration of the white line by a combination of bacteria and fungi. The sole of a donkey hoof grows almost at the same rate as the hoof wall. Find a hoof care provider that has experience with the maintenance of donkey feet.

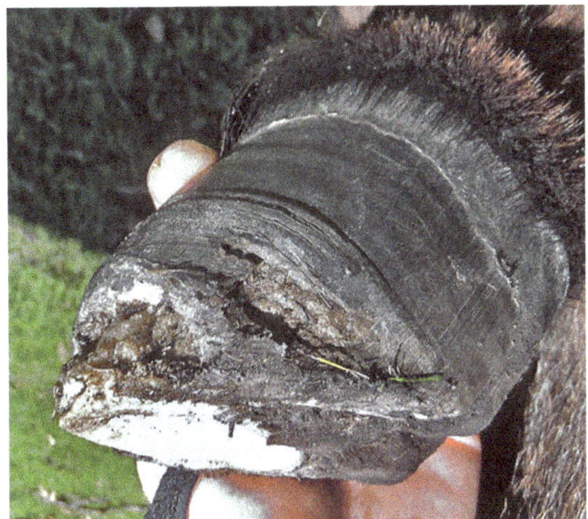

White line disease
(photo: Marika Haase)

Trim

The toe angle of donkey hooves is often trimmed too acute. As a result the rotated coffin bone will then press harder onto the sole and cause more pain. Also in donkey hooves the goal is to trim the coffin bone parallel to the ground.

Many donkeys do not get enough hoof maintenance because of the following three reasons. Firstly, because the sole grows considerably the hoof wall looks like it is only sticking out a little. In reality, both hoof wall and sole can be centimetres (inches) too long. Secondly, many hoof care providers find donkeys difficult or annoying to deal with. It can be difficult to find someone who is willing to trim your donkey. Finally, there is the value of the donkey. When the donkey is just the pasture buddy of the riding horse it may be lower down on the list of priorities. The owner might not want to spend a lot of money on the donkey. If the hoof care provider says that donkeys only need two trims per year, chances are slim the donkey will get sufficient hoof care. A donkey should be trimmed just as often as a horse.

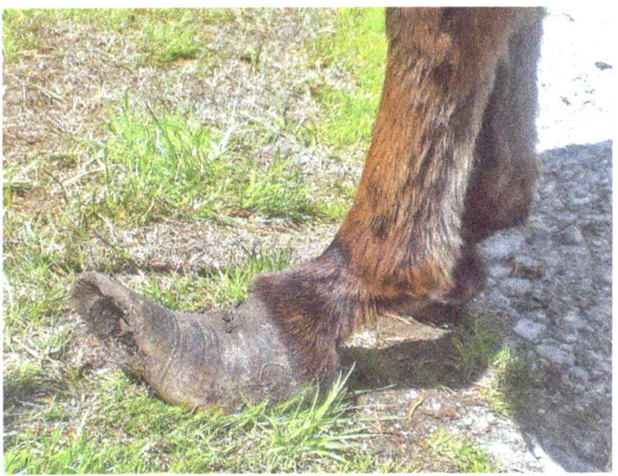

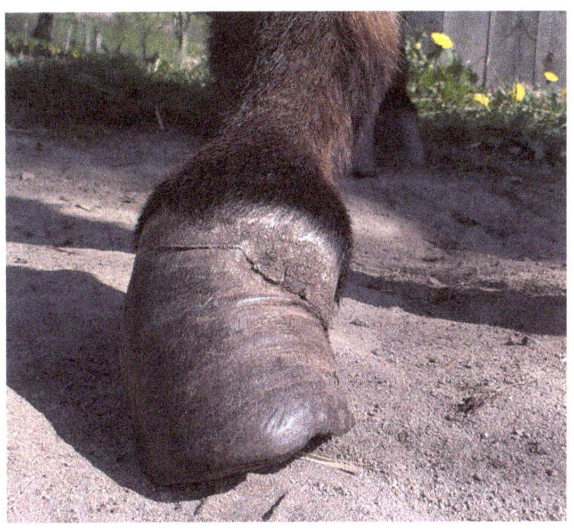

Two cases of lack of hoof maintenance

NUTRITION

FOOD CHOICE

Donkeys search for a greater variety of food and are more selective in their choice of food than horses. They look for food with lots of crude fibre that is low in NSC. They are able to digest this food better than horses. Because of their digestive efficiency domestic donkeys are at greater risk of developing obesity in our lavish pastures. Obesity is a notorious cause of laminitis. Grazing limitation by pasture rotation, strip grazing, restricted grazing or grazing muzzles is needed for donkeys sooner than for horses.

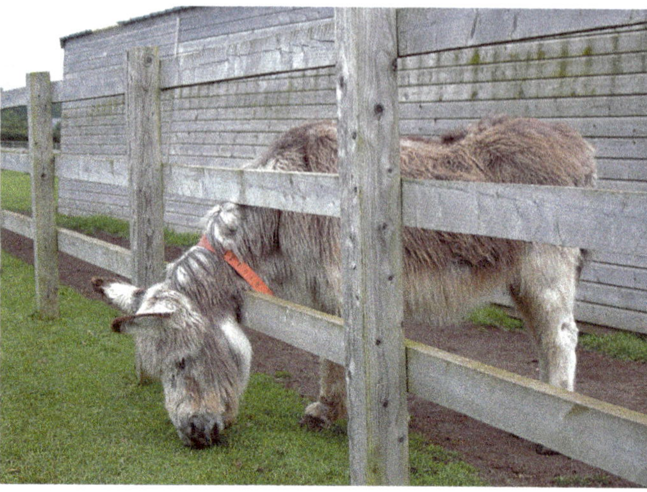

Creative grazing

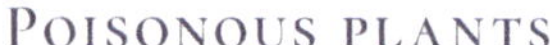

POISONOUS PLANTS

By browsing for a varied diet the risk of ingestion of poisonous plants increases slightly. Toxins in plants may harm the body or cause a disorder that subsequently facilitates laminitis.

Never underestimate the ingenuity of a donkey. If he can escape, he will escape. Then you will not have control over what (and how much) he eats.

DRUGS

Drugs are not always administered to donkeys at an adjusted dosage. Unfortunately, the donkey's body responds differently to certain types of drugs. The advantage is that side effects occur less frequently. Some analgesic anti-inflammatory drugs (NSAIDs) are degraded so rapidly that they are useless as a painkiller. Other drugs are broken down so much slower by donkeys than by horses that the risk of overdosing is high.

EPILOGUE

It is possible that after reading all the information in this book you feel quite overwhelmed. Maybe you don't completely agree with some of it. Especially the concept of resolving severe laminitis without horseshoes often encounters resistance. Remember that there might be different solutions for the same problem. For example, the fact described in this book that anticoagulant drugs are not needed does not mean they are bad by definition. For each therapy, each remedy, or each dietary modification that works for one horse another horse can be found that benefits from the opposite. Select from this book what you think will work for your horse. Ask critical questions to anyone that is involved in the recovery of your horse. Ask these questions especially to yourself.

New articles appear regularly on understandinglaminitis.com and fb.me/understandinglaminitis.

www.understandinglaminitis.com

fb.me/understandinglaminitis

ACKNOWLEDGEMENTS

Not many books were ever written without the help from others. For this book, I would like to thank Cynthia Cooper, Gretschen Fathauer, Brian Hampson and Christoph von Horst. Brian and Christoph have provided me with unique material and Cynthia and Gretschen have sent me many beautiful pictures. In addition, Cynthia has actively mediated with other photographers and horse owners. And it was Cynthia who strongly encouraged me to have my book translated. A very big thank you to translator Heleen Davies for the splendid work she has done.

I have been touched by the enthusiasm so many people around the world have shown in allowing me to use their photographic material. Every effort has been made to identify and contact the copyright holders of the images. All photographers (and their web sites) are listed on page 221. Please contact me via www.understandinglaminitis.com in case of any omissions.

Frans Veldman, Koen Theys and Heleen Davies have contributed to the actuality, completeness and accuracy of the information in this book by giving their critical input. Philip Johnson has explained the difficult matter of PPID to me very patiently. Polly-Anne and Howard Lloyd proved to be very secure proofreaders.

I have been influenced by many people in writing this book. The privilege of working with my clients and, of course, their horses, ponies and donkeys has been the reason why I am always happy to go to work. For this I am most grateful of all.

Clermont-Ferrand (France), november 2020

Remco Sikkel

RESOURCES

BOOKS

- Adams and Stashak's lameness in horses / Gary Baxter (ed.). - 2011, ISBN : 978-0-813-81549-7
- Clinical anatomy of the horse / Hillary Clayton (et al.). - 2005, ISBN: 0-7234-3302-X
- Color atlas of the horse's foot / Christopher Pollitt. - 2000, ISBN: 0-7234-1765-2
- Consumer's guide to alternative therapies in the horse / David Ramey. - 1999, ISBN: 1-58245-062-5
- Current therapy in equine medicine / Edward Robinson. - 2008, ISBN: 1-4160-5475-8
- Diagnosis and management of lameness in the horse / Michael Ross (et al.). - 2003, ISBN: 978-0-7216-8342-3
- Diagnostic techniques in equine medicine / Frank taylor (et al.). - 2009, ISBN: 978-0-7020-2792-5
- Diseases and disorders of the horse / Derek Knottenbelt, Reginald Pascoe. - 2003, ISBN: 0-7020-2743-X
- Equine behavior: a guide for veterinarians and equine scientists / Paul McGreevy. - 2004, ISBN: 0-7020-2634-4
- Equine clinical nutrition: feeding and care / Lon Lewis. - 1995, ISBN: 0-8121-1636-4
- The equine distal limb: an atlas of clinical anatomy and comparative imaging / Jean-Marie Denoix. - 2000, ISBN: 1-84076001-X
- Equine exercise physiology: the science of exercise in the athletic horse / Kenneth Hinchcliff (et al.). - 2008, ISBN: 978-0-7020-2857-1
- Equine laminitis: current concepts / Christopher Pollitt. - 2008, ISBN: 1-74151-651-X
- Equine laminitis: managing pasture to reduce the risk / Kathryn Watts. - 2010, ISBN: 1-74254-036-8
- Equine nutrition and feeding / David Frape. - 2010, ISBN: 1-4051-9546-0
- Equine pathology / James Rooney. - 1999, ISBN: 0-8138-2334-X
- Equine podiatry / Andrea Floyd. - 2007, ISBN: 0-7216-0383-1
- Equine science / Rick Parker. - 2007, ISBN: 1-4180-3254-9
- Essential fatty acid supplementation as a preventative for carbohydrate overload-induced laminitis / K. Neely, D. Herthel
- Explaining laminitis and its prevention / Robert Eustace. - 1996, ISBN: 0-9518974-0-3
- Feed your horse like a horse: optimize your horse's nutrition for a lifetime of vibrant health / Juliet Getty. - 2009, ISBN: 1-60844-214-4

- Forages: an introduction to grassland agriculture / Robert Barnes (ed.). - 2003, ISBN: 0-8138-0421-3
- Founder: prevention and cure the natural way / Jaime Jackson. - 2001, ISBN: 0-9658007-3-3
- Horse journal: guide to equine supplements and nutraceuticals / Eleanor Kellon. - 2008, ISBN: 1-59921-178-5
- The horse nutrition handbook / Melyni Worth. - 2010, ISBN: 1-60342-541-1
- Horse owner's veterinary handbook / Tom Gore, Paula Gore, James Giffin. - 2008, ISBN: 0-470-12679-5
- Horse owners guide to natural hoof care / Jaime Jackson. - 2002, ISBN: 0-9658007-6-8
- Improving the foot health of the domestic horse: the relevance of the feral horse foot model / Brian Hampson and Christopher Pollitt. - 2011, ISBN: 978-1-74254-319-2
- Insulin-induced laminitis: an investigation of the disease mechanism in horses / Melody de Laat (et al.). - 2011, ISBN: 978-1-74254-295-9
- Keeping a horse the natural way: a natural approach to horse management for optimum health and performance / Jo Bird. - 2002, ISBN: 0-7641-5411-7
- Knottenbelt and Pascoe's color atlas of diseases and disorders of the horse / Derek Knottenbelt (et al.). - 2014, ISBN: 978-0-7234-3660-7
- The lame horse / James Rooney. - 1998, ISBN: 0-929346-55-6
- Laminitis explained / David Ramey. - 2006, ISBN: 1-872119-55-7
- Making natural hoof care work for you / Pete Ramey. - 2003, ISBN: 0-9658007-7-6
- Manual of equine lameness / Gary Baxter. - 2011, ISBN: 978-1-118-30137-1
- More insights into: laminitis in the Arabian horse / Tobias Reuben Menis. - 2012, ISBN: 1-4461-5693-1
- Natural methods for equine health and performance / Mary Bromiley. - 2009, ISBN: 1-4051-7929-5
- Paard natuurlijk: gezondere paarden en betere prestaties in sport en recreatie / Frans Veldman, Ilona Kooistra. - 2007, ISBN: 90-809285-3-4
- Practical guide to lameness in horses / Ted Stashak, Cherry Hill. - 1996, ISBN: 0-683-07985-9
- Preventing laminitis in horses: a practical guide to decreasing the risk of laminitis (founder) in your horse / Christine King, Richard Mansmann. - 2000, ISBN: 0-9674926-1-0
- Understanding equine medications: your guide to horse health care and management / Barbara Forney. - 2007, ISBN: 1-58150-151-X
- Understanding laminitis / Fran Jurga (et al.). - 1998, ISBN: 0-9390499-8-8
- Understanding the equine foot / Fran Jurga. - 1998, ISBN: 0-939049-96-1
- Veterinary advice on laminitis in horses / Rebecca Hamilton-Fletcher. - 2004, ISBN: 1-86054-247-6
- Who's afraid of founder?: laminitis demystified: causes, prevention, and holistic rehabilitation / Hiltrud Strasser. - 2003, ISBN: 978-0-9685988-4-9

ARTICLES

- Adiponectin and leptin are related to fat mass in horses / C. Kearns (et al.), *Vet. J.* 172.3 (2006): 460-465
- Adipokine, chemokine, and cytokine expression profiles in adipose tissue depots of lean and overweight ponies / P. Weber (et al.) *J. Equine Vet. Sci.* 33.10 (2013): 846
- The anatomy and physiology of the suspensory apparatus of the distal phalanx / C. Pollitt, *Vet. Clin. North Am. Equine Pract.* 26.1 (2010): 29-49
- Black walnut extract: an inflammatory model / J. Belknap, *Vet. Clin. North Am. Equine Pract.* 26.1 (2010): 95-101
- Carbohydrate alimentary overload laminitis / C. Pollitt, *Vet. Clin. North Am. Equine Pract.* 26.1 (2010): 65-71
- Changes in proportions of dry matter intakes by ponies with access to pasture and haylage for 3 and 20 hours per day respectively, for six weeks / J. Ince (et al.), *J. Equine Vet. Sci.* 31.5 (2011): 283
- Chronic laminitis: managing the foundered horse / D. Walsh, *homesteadvet.net*
- Clinical anatomy and physiology of the normal equine foot / C. Pollitt, *Equine Vet. Educ.* 4.5 (1992): 219-224
- Clinical and genetic investigation of Connemara hoof wall separation syndrome / C. Finnp (et al.), *J. Equine Vet. Sci.* 33.10 (2013): 857
- Clinical outcome of 14 obesity-associated laminitis cases managed with the same rehabilitation protocol / D. Taylor (et al.), *J. Equine Vet. Sci.* 33.10 (2013): 870
- Clinical presentation, diagnosis, and prognosis of chronic laminitis in Europe / R. Eustace, *Vet. Clin. North Am. Equine Pract.* 26.2 (2010): 391-405
- Clinical updates I: Laminitis / J. Orsini, *J. Equine Vet. Sci.* 30.9 (2010): 455-459
- Comparison of hair follicle histology between horses with pituitary pars intermedia dysfunction and excessive hair growth and normal aged horses / M. Innera (et al.), *Vet. Dermatol.* 24.1 (2013): 212-217
- Comparison of insulin sensitivity of horses adapted to different exercise intensities / S. turner (et al.), *J. Equine Vet. Sci.* 31.11 (2011): 645-649
- Continuous digital hypothermia initiated after the onset of lameness prevents lamellar failure in the oligofructose laminitis model / A. van Eps (et al.), *Equine Vet. J.* 46.5 (2014): 625-630
- A comparison of weight estimation methods in adult horses / E. Wagner (et al.), *J. Equine Vet. Sci.* 31.12 (2011): 706-710
- Comparison of weight loss, with or without dietary restriction and exercise, in standardbreds, Andalusians and mixed breed ponies / S. Potter (et al.), *J. Equine Vet. Sci.* 33.5 (2013): 339
- Contrasting structural morphologies of 'good' and 'bad' footed horses / R. Bowker, *Proc. Am. Assoc. Equine Pract.* 49 (2003): 186–209
- Corticosteroid-associated laminitis / S. Bailey, *Vet. Clin. North Am. Equine Pract.* 26.2 (2010): 277-285
- Cresty neck scoring: how to? / T. Cubitt, *www.poulingrain.com*

- Current concepts on the pathophysiology of pasture-associated laminitis / R. Geor, *Vet. Clin. North Am. Equine Pract.* 26.2 (2010): 265-276
- Current understanding of the equine metabolic syndrome phenotype / R. Geor (et al.), *J. Equine Vet. Sci.* 33.10 (2013): 841-844
- Decreased expression of p63, a regulator of epidermal stem cells, in the chronic laminitic equine hoof / R. Carter (et al.), *Equine Vet. J.* 43.5 (2011): 543-551
- Deep digital flexor tendon force and digital mechanics in normal ponies and ponies with rotation of the distal phalanx as a sequel to laminitis / M. McGuigan (et al.), *Equine Vet. J.* 37.2 (2005): 161-165
- Diabetes, insulin resistance, and metabolic syndrome in horses / P. Johnson (et al.), *J. Diabetes Sci. Technol.* 6.3 (2012): 534-540
- Diagnosis and treatment of foot infections / B. Agne, *J. Equine Vet. Sci.* 30.9 (2010): 510-512
- Dietary fructan carbohydrate increases amine production in the equine large intestine: implications for pasture-associated laminitis / C. Crawford (et al.), *J. Anim. Sci.* 85.11 (2007): 2949-2958
- Dietary management of obesity and insulin resistance: countering risk for laminitis / R. Geor, *Vet. Clin. North Am. Equine Pract.* 25.1 (2009): 51-65
- Digital hypothermia inhibits early lamellar inflammatory signalling in the oligofructose laminitis model / A. van Eps (et al.), *Equine Vet. J.* 44.2 (2012): 230-237
- Documentation of the clinical outcome of four laminitis cases managed with the same hoof care and dietary management protocol / D. Taylor (et al.), *J. Equine Vet. Sci.* 30.2 (2010): 114-115
- The effect of airflow on thermographically determined temperature of the distal forelimb of the horse / S. Westermann (et al.), *Equine Vet. J.* 45.5 (2013): 637-641
- Effects of a supplement containing chromium and magnesium on morphometric measurements, resting glucose, insulin concentrations and insulin sensitivity in laminitic obese horses / K. Chameroy (et al.), *Equine. Vet. J.* 43.3 (2011): 494-499
- Effects of barefoot trimming and shoeing on the joints of the lower forelimb and hoof morphology of mature horses / D. Proske (et al.), *The Prof. Anim. Scientist* 33.4 (2017): 483-489
- Effects of clopidogrel and aspirin on platelet aggregation, thromboxane production, and serotonin secretion in horses / B. Brainard (et al.), *J. Vet. Intern. Med.* 25.1 (2011): 116-122
- Effect of environmental conditions on degree of hoof wall hydration in horses / B. Hampson (et al.), *Am. J. Vet. Res.* 73.3 (2012): 435-438
- The effect of hoof angle variations on dorsal lamellar load in the equine hoof / G. Ramsey (et al.), *Equine Vet. J.* 43.5 (2011): 536-542
- The effect of oral metformin on insulin sensitivity in insulin-resistant ponies / K. Tinworth (et al.), *Vet. J.* 191.1 (2012): 79-84
- The effect of soaking on carbohydrate removal and dry matter loss in orchardgrass and alfalfa hays / K. Martinson (et al.), *J. Equine Vet. Sci.* 32.6 (2012): 332-338
- The effect of soaking on protein and mineral loss in orchardgrass and alfalfa hay / K. Martinson (et al.), *J. Equine Vet. Sci.* 32.12 (2012): 776-782

- Effects of a "two-hit" model of organ damage on the systemic inflammatory response and development of laminitis in horses / E. Tadros (et al.), *Vet. Immunol. Immunopathol.* 150.1-2 (2012): 90-100
- Effects of incretin hormones on beta-cell mass and function, body weight, and hepatic and myocardial functions / S. Mudaliar (et al.), *Am. J. Med.* 123.3 (2010): S19-27
- Effects of industrial polystyrene foam insulation pads on the center of pressure and load distribution in the forefeet of clinically normal horses / J. Schleining (et al.), *Am. J. Vet. Res.* 72.5 (2011): 628-633
- Effects of intracecal buffer solution treatment in apoptosis of epidermal lamellar cells in horses with experimental laminitis / A. Souza (et al.), *J. Equine Vet. Sci.* 30.2 (2010): 113
- Effects of Ω-3 (n-3) fatty acid supplementation on insulin sensitivity in horses / T. Hess (et al.), *J. Equine Vet. Sci.* 33.6 (2013): 446-453
- Effects of oral administration of levothyroxine sodium on serum concentrations of thyroid gland hormones and responses to injections of thyrotropin-releasing hormone in healthy adult mares / C. Sommardahl (et al.), *Am. J. Vet. Res.* 66.6 (2005): 1025-1031
- Effect of orally administered sodium bicarbonate on caecal pH / E. Taylor (et al.), *Equine Vet. J.* 46.2 (2013): 223-226
- Effect of restricted grazing on hindgut pH and fluid balance / P. Sicilliano, *J. Equine Vet. Sci.* 32.9 (2012): 558-561
- Effects of the insulin-sensitizing drug pioglitazone and lipopolysaccharide administration on insulin sensitivity in horses / J. Suagee (et al.), *J. Vet. Intern. Med.* 25 (2011): 356-364
- Endocrine disorders and laminitis / E. Tadros (et al.), *Equine Vet. Educ.* 25.3 (2013): 152-162
- Endocrinopathic laminitis / C. McGowan, *Vet. Clin. North Am. Equine Pract.* 26.2 (2011): 233-237
- Endocrinopathic laminitis in the horse / P. Johnson (et al.), *Clin. Tech. Equine Pract.* 3.1 (2004): 45-56
- Endocrinopathic laminitis, obesity-associated laminitis, and pasture-associated laminitis / N. Frank, *Proc. Am. Assoc. Equine Pract.* 54 (2008): 341-346
- Endocrinopathic laminitis: reducing the risk through diet and exercise / N. Menzies-Gow, *Vet. Clin. North Am. Equine Pract.* 26.2 (2010): 371-378
- Epidemiological study of pasture-associated laminitis and concurrent risk factors in the South of England / N. Menzies-Gow (et al.), *Vet. Rec.* 167.18 (2010): 690-694
- Equine hyperlipaemia: a review / K. Hughes (et al), *Aus. Vet. J.* 82.3 (2004): 136-142
- Equine laminitis: a revised pathophysiology / C. Pollitt, *Proc. Am. Assoc. Equine Pract.* 45 (1999): 189-192
- Equine metabolic syndrome / N. Frank, *Vet. Clin. North Am. Equine Pract.* 27.1 (2011): 73-92
- Equine metabolic syndrome: more unknowns than knowns / Kentucky Equine Research, *J. Equine Vet. Sci.* 26 (2006): 543-545
- Equine pituitary pars intermedia dysfunction / D. McFarlane, *Vet. Clin. North Am. Equine Pract.* 27.1 (2011): 93-113
- Estimation of the body weight of Icelandic horses / G. Hoffmann (et al.), *J. Equine Vet. Sci.* 33.11 (2013): 893-895

- Evaluation of systemic immunological hyperreactivity after intradermal testing in horses with chronic laminitis / I. Wagner (et al.), *Am. J. Vet. Res.* 64 (2003): 279-283
- De ezel, net even anders / Ellen Graaf-Roelfsema (et al.), *Diergeneeskundig Memorandum* 56.3 (2009): 1-76
- Factors affecting the glucose response to insulin injection in mares: epinephrine, short- and long-term prior feed intake, cinnamon extract, and omega-3 fatty acid supplementation / L. Earl (et al.), *J. Equine Vet. Sci.* 32.1 (2012): 15-21
- Fecal pH and microbial populations in thoroughbred horses during transition from pasture to concentrate feeding / M. van den Berg (et al.), *J. Equine Vet. Sci.* 33.4 (2013): 215-222
- Feeding naturally / L. Ross-Williams, *www.naturalhorsetalk.com*
- Fructose-induced leptin resistance exacerbates weight gain in response to subsequent high-fat feeding / A. Shapiro (et al.), *Am. J. Physiol. Regul. Integr. Comp. Physiol.* 295.5 (2008): 1370-1375
- Functional anatomy of the cartilage of the distal phalanx and digital cushion in the equine foot and a hemodynamic flow hypothesis of energy dissipation / R. Bowker (et al.), *Am. J. Vet. Res.* 59.8 (1998): 961-968
- Gastrointestinal derived factors are potential triggers for the development of acute equine laminitis / J. Elliott (et al.), *J Nutr.* 136.7 suppl. (2006): 2103S-2107S
- Glucose transport in the equine hoof / K. Asplin (et al.), *Equine Vet. J.* 43.2 (2011): 196-201
- The growth and adaptive capabilities of the hoof wall and sole: functional changes in response to stress / R. Bowker, *Proc. Am. Assoc. Equine Pract.* 49 (2003): 146-168
- Histological and morphometric lesions in the pre-clinical, developmental phase of insulin-induced laminitis in Standardbred horses / M. de Laat (et al.), *Vet. J.* 195.3 (2013): 305-312
- Histopathological examination of chronic laminitis in Kaimanawa feral horses of New Zealand / B. Hampson (et al.), *N. Z. Vet. J.* 60.5 (2012): 285-289
- Histopathology of equine hoof wall, skin and chestnut in acute spontaneous laminitis / O. Wattle (et al.), *J. Equine Vet. Sci.* 30.2 (2010): 116
- Home care for horses with chronic laminitis / J. Orsini (et al.), *Vet. Clin. North Am. Equine Pract.* 26.1 (2010): 215-223
- Home care nursing for the laminitic horse / J. Wrigley, *J. Vet. Sci.* 31.10 (2011): 605-609
- Hoof mass, motion and the mythos of P3 rotation / J. Jackson, *SRP Bulletin* 113 (2006)
- Hyperinsulinemic laminitis / M. de Laat (et al.), *Vet. Clin. North Am. Equine Pract.* 26.2 (2010): 257-264
- Hyperlipaemia in a donkey / J. Tarrant (et al.), *Aus. Vet. J.* 76.7 (1998): 466-469
- Insulin dysregulation / N. Frank (et al.), *Equine Vet. J.* 46.1 (2014): 103-112
- The interaction of grazing muzzle use and grass species on forage intake of horses - a preliminary study / E. Glunk (et al.), *J. Equine Vet. Sci.* 33.5 (2013): 357
- Lamellar metabolism / O. Wattle, C. Pollitt, *Clin. Tech. Equine Pract.* 3.1 (2004): 22-33
- Laminar leukocyte accumulation in horses with carbohydrate overload-induced laminitis / R. Faleiros (et al.), *J. Vet. Intern. Med.* 25.1 (2011): 107-115
- Laminitis and the equine metabolic syndrome / P. Johnson (et al.), *Vet. Clin. North Am. Equine Pract.* 26.2 (2010): 239-255

- Laminitis attack: the first line of defense / D. Walsh (et al.), *www.safergrass.org*
- Laminitis in feral horses: where, when, and why? / B. Hampson, *J. Equine Vet. Sci.* 31.10 (2011): 594-595
- Laminitis in przewalski horses kept in a semireserve / K. Budras, *J. Vet. Sci.* 2.1 (2001): 1-7
- Laminitis: recognition of at-risk individuals, and methods of prevention / B. Ange, *J. Equine Vet. Sci.* 30.9 (2010): 471-474
- Laminitis theory: shots around the target / C. Pollitt, *www.laminitisreserach.org*
- Laminitis treatment: a natural medicine perspective / J. Harman, *Hoofcare & Lameness: J. Equine Foot* 73 (s.a.)
- Leidingwater, water uit de put of een stromend beekje: wat is de beste keuze voor jouw paard / H. Boon, *CAP* 5 (2010): 56-60
- Magnesium disorders in horses / A. Stewart, *Vet. Clin. North Am. Equine Pract.* 27.1 (2011): 149-163
- Managing hoof abscesses: options for treating this frequent and frustrating cause of lameness / S. O'Grady, *www.equipodiatry.com*
- Managing obesity in pasture-based horses / I. Becvarova (et al.), *Compend. Contin. Educ. Vet.* 34.4 (2012): 1-4
- Maggot debridement therapy for laminitis / S. Morrison, *Vet. Clin. North Am. Equine Pract.* 26.2 (2010): 447-450
- Medical acupuncture for equine laminitis / L. Lancaster, *J. Equine Vet. Sci.* 31.10 (2011): 604
- Metabolic predispositions to laminitis in horses and ponies: obesity, insulin resistance and metabolic syndromes / R. Geor, *J. Equine Vet. Sci.* 28.12 (2008): 753-759
- Microbial events in the hindgut during carbohydrate-induced equine laminitis / G. Milinovich (et al.), *Vet. Clin. North Am. Equine Pract.* 26.1 (2010): 79-94
- Morphometry and abnormalities of the feet of Kaimanawa feral horses in New Zealand / B. Hampson (et al.), *Aust. Vet. J.* 88.4 (2010): 124-131
- A multicenter, matched case-control study of risk factors for equine laminitis / P. Alford (et al.), *Prev. Vet. Med.* 49.3-4 (2001): 209-222
- Neuropathic pain management in chronic laminitis / B. Driessen (et al.), *Vet. Clin. North Am. Equine Pract.* 26.2 (2010): 315-337
- Nutrition and exercise in the management of horses and ponies at high risk for laminitis / R. Geor, *J. Equine Vet. Sci.* 30.9 (2010): 463-470
- Overview of current laminitis research / S. Eades, *Vet. Clin. North Am. Equine Pract.* 26.1 (2010): 51-63
- Pasture-associated laminitis / R. Geor, *Vet. Clin. North Am. Equine Pract.* 25.1 (2009): 39-50
- Pasture management to minimize the risk of equine laminitis / K. Watts, *Vet. Clin. North Am. Equine Pract.* 26.2 (2010): 361-369
- Pasture nonstructural carbohydrates and equine laminitis / A. Longland (et al.), *J. Nutr.* 136.7 (2006): 2099-2100
- Pathophysiology and clinical features of pituitary pars intermedia dysfunction / D. McFarlane, *Equine Vet. Educ.* 26.11 (2014): 592-598

- Pathology of the distal phalanx in equine laminitis: more than just skin deep / J. Engiles, *Vet. Clin. North Am. Equine Pract.* 26.1 (2010): 155-165
- The perils of excess potassium / B. Lee, *albrechtsanimals.typepad.com*
- Pregnancy-associated laminitis in mares / P. Johnson (et al.), *J. Equine Vet. Sci.* 29.1 (2009): 42-46
- A preliminary study into the use of manual lymphatic drainage to support recovery from laminitis / H. Powell, *J. Equine Vet. Sci.* 33.10 (2013): 872
- Preventing laminitis in the contralateral limb of horses with non-weight-bearing lameness / R. Redden, *Clin. Tech. Equine Pract.* 3.1 (2004): 57-63
- Primer on dietary carbohydrates and utility of the glycemic index in equine nutrition / P. harris (et al.), *Vet. Clin. North Am. Equine Pract.* 25.1 (2009): 23-37
- Probiotic use in horses - what is the evidence for their clinical efficacy? / A. Schoster (et al.), *J. Vet. Intern. Med.* 28 (2014): 1640-1652
- Prognostic indicators of poor outcome in horses with laminitis at a tertiary care hospital / J. Orsini (et al.), *Can Vet J* 51.6 (2010): 623-628
- Prosthetics: science, not science fiction / S. Wenholz, *The Horse* juli 01(2005)
- Psyllium lowers blood glucose and insulin concentrations in horses / S. Moreaux (et al.), *J. Equine Vet. Sci.* 31.1 (2011): 160-165
- Recent research into laminitis / P. Huntington (et al.), *www.ker.com*
- Regional intravenous limb perfusion compared to systemic intravenous administration for marimastat delivery to equine lamellar tissue / C. Underwoord (et al.), *J. Vet. Pharmacol. Therap.* 38 (2015): 392-399 A reproducible model for long-term rehabilitation of the foundered equine metabolic syndrome horse / D. Bicking, *J. Equine Vet. Sci.* 33.10 (2013): 870-871
- Review of equine piroplasmosis / L. Wise (et al), *J. Vet. Intern. Med.* 27 (2013): 1334-1346
- A review of factors affecting carbohydrate levels in forage / K. Watts (et al.), *J. Equine Vet. Sci.* 24.2 (2004): 84-86
- A review of unlikely sources of excess carbohydrate in equine diets / K. Watts, *J. Equine Vet. Sci.* 25.8 (2005): 338-344
- Risk factors for development of acute laminitis in horses during hospitalization: 73 cases (1997-2004) / C. Parsons (et al.), *J. Am. Vet. Med. Assoc.* 230.6 (2007): 885-889
- Risk factors for equine laminitis: a systematic review with quality appraisal of published evidence / C. Wylie (et al.), *Vet. J.* 193.1 (2012): 58-66
- Ruwvoer: vaak onderschat, maar van onschatbare waarde / N. Rietman, *In de strengen* 67.21 (2005): 16-21
- Short-term incubation of equine laminar veins with cortisol and insulin alters contractility in vitro: possible implications for the pathogenesis of equine laminitis / J. Keen (et al.), *J. Vet. Pharmacol. Ther.* 3 (2012)
- Some laminitis problems in horses may be caused by excessive iron intake / D. Pitzen, *www.naturalhorsetrim.com*
- Stress bij paarden / A. ten Napel, *www.holistischdierenarts.nl*
- The structure, innervation and location of arteriovenous anastomoses in the equine foot / C. Pollitt (et al.), *Equine. Vet. J.* 26.4 (1994): 305-312

- Supporting limb laminitis / A. van Eps (et al.), *Vet. Clin. North Am. Equine Pract.* 26.2 (2010): 287-302
- Treating laminitis: beyond the mechanics of trimming and shoeing / W. Baker, *Vet. Clin. North Am. Equine Pract.* 28.2 (2012): 441-455
- Venograms for use in laminitis treatment / S. Eastman (et al.), *J. Equine Vet. Sci.* 32.11 (2012): 757-759
- What's new in laminitis research I - pathophysiology and prevention / J. Orsini (et al.), *J. Equine Vet. Sci.* 32.10 (2012): 641-647
- What's new in laminitis research II - advances in laminitis treatment / N. Grenager (et al.), *J. Equine Vet. Sci.* 32.10 (2012): 647-653
- Winter care of the insulin resistant horse / E. Kellon, *www.naturalhorsejourney*

WEB SITES

- www.animalhealthfoundation.com
- www.deepdyve.com
- www.hoofrehab.com
- www.j-evs.com
- jn.nutrition.org
- journalofanimalscience.org
- www.ker.com/library/
- www.laminitisresearch.org
- www.naturalhorsetrim.com
- www.naturalhorseworld.com
- www.ncbi.nlm.nih.gov/pubmed
- www.paardnatuurlijk.nl
- www.paddockparadijs.nl
- www.safergrass.org
- www.thehorse.com
- www.thelaminitissite.org

PHOTOGRAPHERS

- Advanced equine therapies
- Albert Uderzo
- Alexas fotos
- Alfaromeogirl
- Alfons Geerts
- Andrew Grimm
- Brian Hampson
- Carlton veterinary hospital
- Caroline Wang-Andresen
- Cathy Dee
- Christoph von Horst
- Cheryl Henderson
- Chris Pollitt
- Cindy Altorf
- Claudia Beutel
- Claudia Garner
- Cynthia Cooper
- David Stephens
- Deanna Fenwick
- Dominic Morel

- The Donkey sanctuary
- Elizabeth Fish
- Esther Bosch
- František Brabec
- František Pleva
- Gretschen Fathauer
- Haiku farm
- Hanna Dalberg
- Hasan Jerbi
- Heidi Billing
- Helen Morrell
- Heleen Davies
- Ilona Kooistra
- Ilse Bartholomeeusen
- Inka Piegsa-Quischotte
- Ivan Procházka
- Jamie Berning
- The Japanese society of equine science
- John Baird
- James H. Miller
- Jan Ševcík
- Janice Hutchinson
- Jirí Kamenícek
- Jirí Novák
- Justyna Furmanczyk
- Karan Rawlins
- Karin Schouwenburg
- Kate Light
- Kathmann Vital
- Katie Fitzgerald
- Kelly Wilson
- Kim Hillegas
- Kim Starr
- Klaas Feuth
- Lacelynn Seibel
- Laura Vos
- Leslie Potter
- The Liphook equine hospital
- Linda Lebesque
- Lisa Lancaster
- Liz Jaynes
- Lubomír Klátil
- Lucy Priory
- Maria Alexandra
- Marika Haase
- Marion Ryan
- Marja van Run
- Mark DePaolo
- Marlou van Blitterswijk
- Mary Bayard Fitzpatrick
- Matthias Zomer
- Michael Kesl
- Michael Porter
- Mike Harris
- Mike van Dijk
- Milan Korínek
- Miran Rijavec
- Mulography
- Museum für Naturkunde, Berlin
- Myhre equine clinic
- N. Irlbeck
- Novus
- Patrick Brunner
- Pavel Buršík
- Pavel Šinkyrík
- Peter Kocna
- Petr Voboril
- Polyplas
- Rainer Maiores
- Radim Paulic
- Rebekah Wallace
- Robert Vidéki
- Rood & Riddle stem cell laboratory
- Rose Kingery-Potter
- Ruth Steele
- Sabine Baron
- Sarah Bernier
- Scott Morrison
- Sherilyn Allen
- Simon Constable
- Soft-ride
- Sophie Gent

- Stanislav Krejcík
- Tamara Horová
- Tanja Boeve
- Theodore Webster
- Tomas Figura
- Tomas Leibelt
- Tomáš Machácek
- Tracy Dunn
- Triton barns
- Ulrich Leone
- University of Veterinary Medicine Hanover
- Václav Hrdina
- Vladimír Motycka
- Vladimír Nejeschleba
- Vojtech Herman
- W. Ellenberger
- Wesley De Candt
- Wide open pets

BOTANICAL NOMENCLATURE

Botanical nomenclature is the formal, scientific naming of plants. Below you will find the botanical names of the plants and trees mentioned in this book.

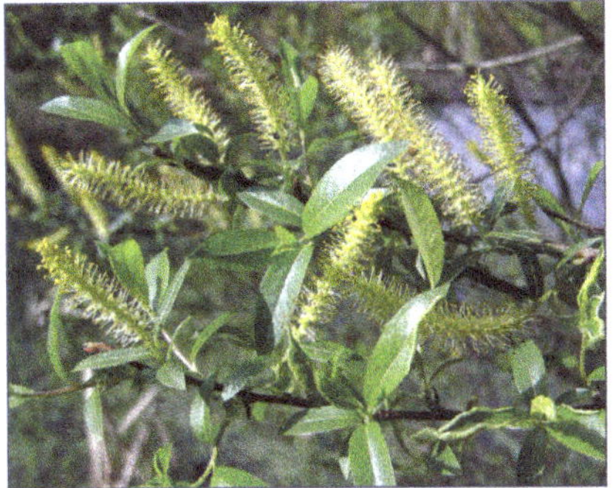

(photo: František Brabec)

ALMOND WILLOW

Family: Salicaceae
Genus: Salix
Species: Salix Triandra

Also known as: Almond-leaved willow.

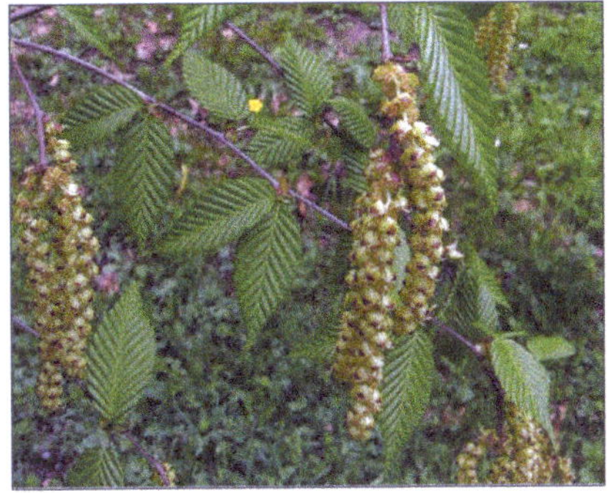

Yellow birch
(photo: Radim Paulic)

BIRCH

Family: Betulaceae
Genus: Betula

The genus Betula contains 60 species amongst which the yellow birch (Betula Alleghaniensis).

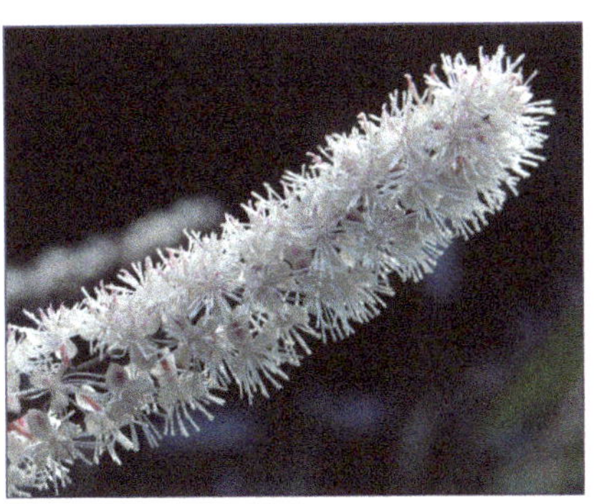

(photo: Tamara Horová)

BLACK COHOSH

Family: Ranunculaceae
Genus: Actaea
Species: Actaea Racemosa

Also known as: Black bugbane, black snakeroot, black baneberry, fairy candle.

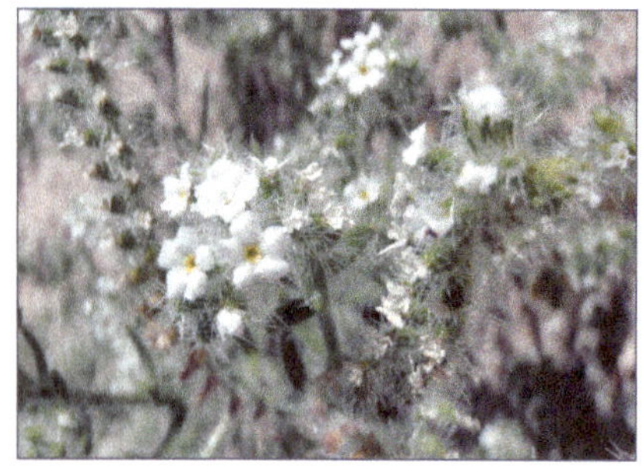

(photo: Stacy Manson)

BLOND PSYLLIUM

Family: Plantaginaceae
Genus: Plantago
Species: Plantago Ovata

Also known as: Flea seed, blond plantain, che qian zi, englishman's foot, spogel.

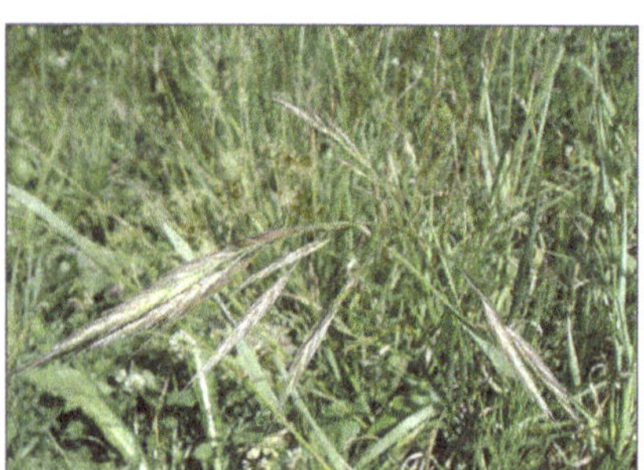

(photo: Radim Paulic)

BROME GRASS

Family: Poaceae
Genus: Bromus

The genus Bromus contains 170 species.
Also known as: Brome grass, cheat grass, chess grass.

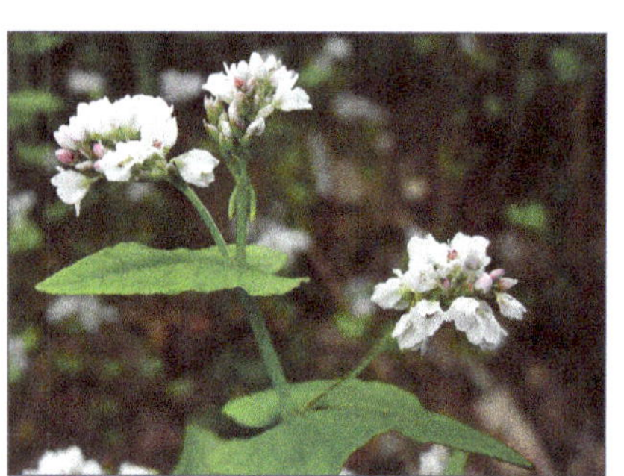

(photo: Stanislav Krejcík)

BUCKWHEAT

Family: Polygonaceae
Genus: Fagopyrum
Species: Fagopyrum Esculentum

Also known as: Japanese buckwheat, silverhull buckwheat.

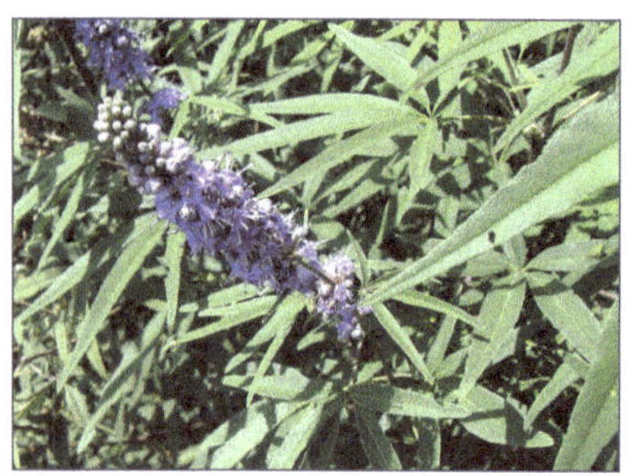

(photo: František Pleva)

CHASTETREE BERRY

Family: Lamiaceae
Genus: Vitex
Species: Vitex Agnus-Castus

Also known as: Chasteberry, Abraham's balm, lilac chastetree, monk's pepper.

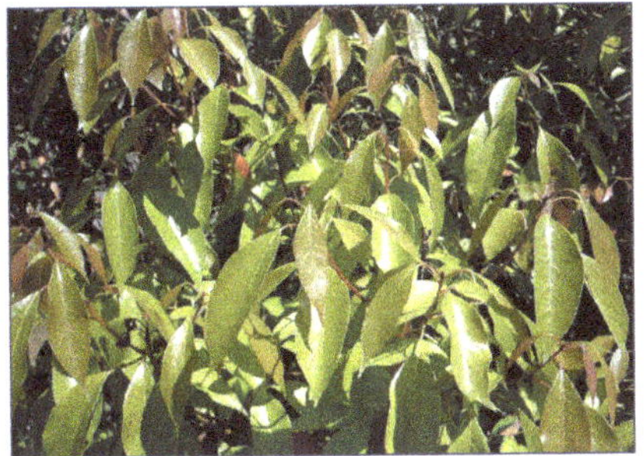
Camphor laurel
(photo: Tamara Horová)

CINNAMON

Family: Lauraceae
Genus: Cinnamomum

The genus Cinnamomum contains over 300 species amongst which Camphor laurel (Cinnamomum Camphora).

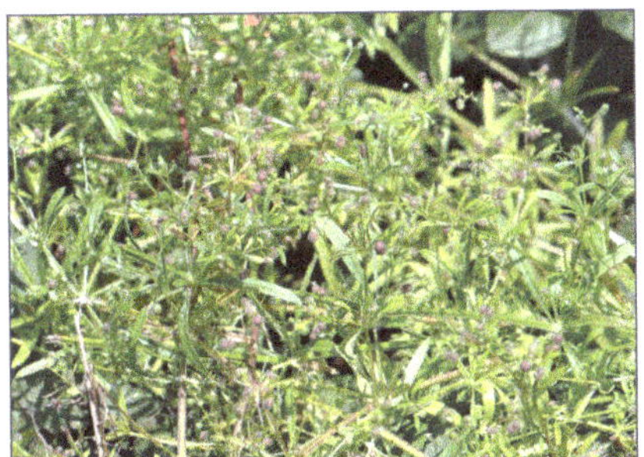
(photo: Lubomír Klátil)

CLEAVERS

Family: Rubiaceae
Genus: Galium
Species: Galium Aparine

Also known as: Clivers, goose grass, catchweed, sticky weed, robin-run-the-hedge, sticky willy, sticky willow, velcro weed, grip grass.

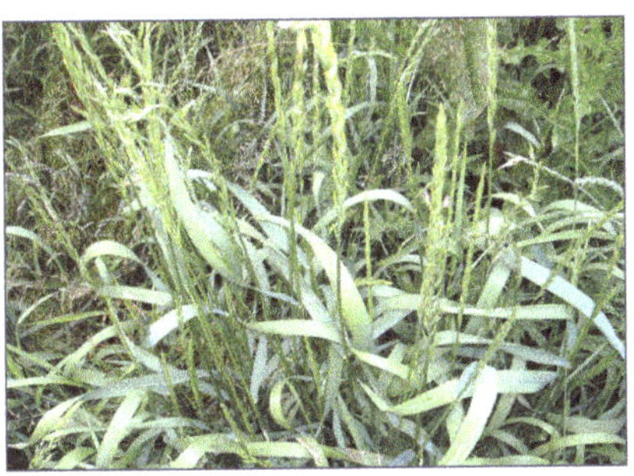
(photo: Radim Paulic)

COUCH GRASS

Family: Poaceae
Genus: Elymus
Species: Elymus Repens

Also known as: Common couch, twitch, quick grass, quitch (grass), dog grass, quack grass, scutch grass, witch grass.

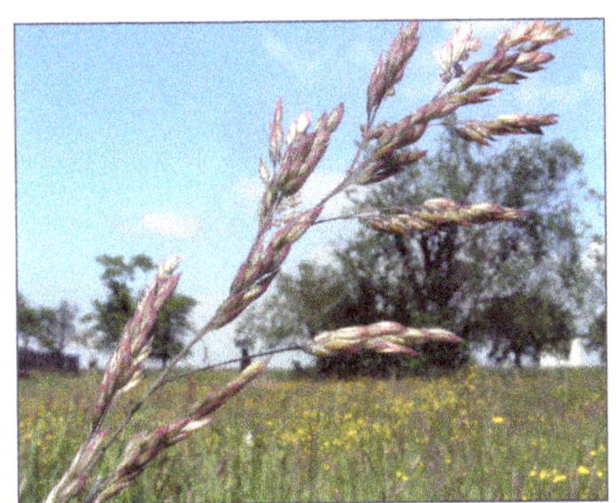
(photo: Jirí Kamenícek)

CREEPING SOFT GRASS

Family: Poaceae
Genus: Holcus
Species: Holcus Lanatus

Also known as: Common velvet grass, creeping velvet grass, fog grass, meadow soft grass, mesquite grass, tufted soft grass, woolly soft grass, Yorkshire fog.

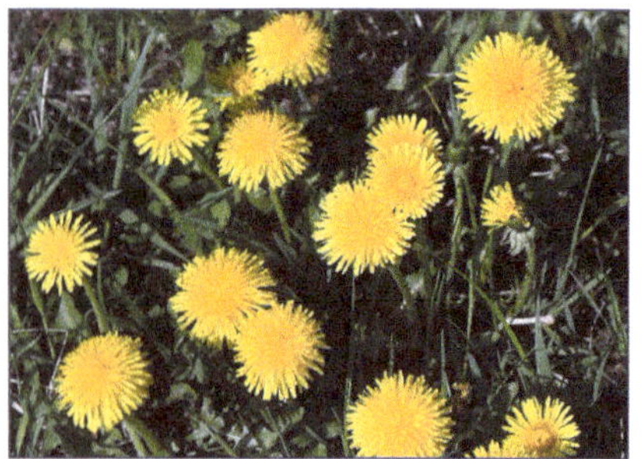

(photo: Stanislav Krejcík)

DANDELION

Family: Asteraceae
Genus: Taraxacum

The genus Taraxacum contains 34 species amongst which the common dandelion (Taraxacum Officinale) and the red seeded dandelion (Taraxacum Erythrospermum).

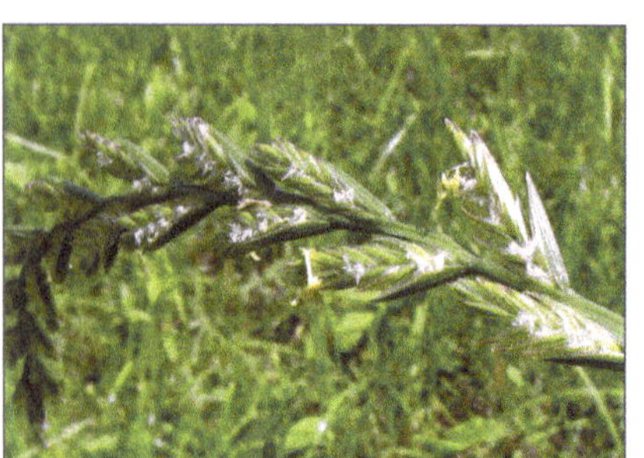

(photo: Jirí Kamenícek)

ENGLISH RYE GRASS

Family: Poaceae
Genus: Lolium
Species: Lolium Perenne

Also known as: Perennial rye grass, winter rye grass.

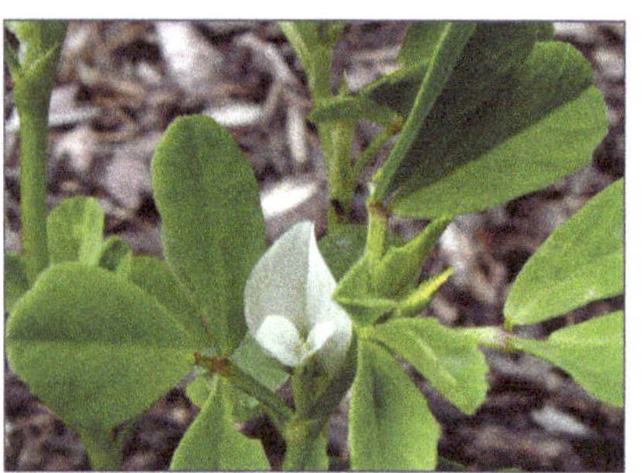

(photo: Michael Kesl)

FENUGREEK

Family: Fabaceae
Genus: Trigonella
Species: Trigonella Foenum-Graecum

Also known as: Sicklefruit fenugreek.

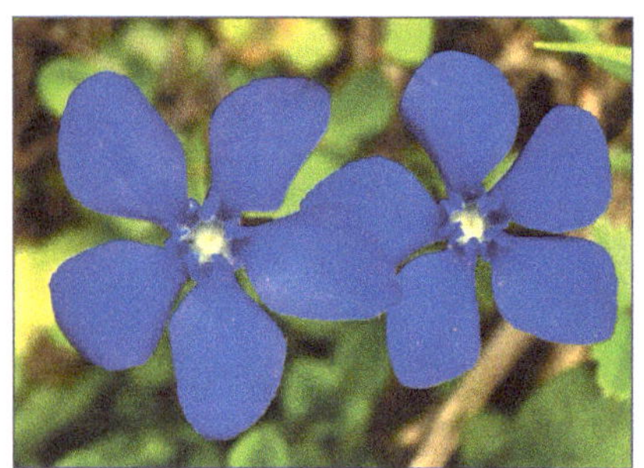

Spring gentian
(photo: Vladimír Nejeschleba)

GENTIAN

Family: Gentianaceae
Genus: Gentiana
Species: Gentiana

The genus Gentiana contains 400 species amongst which the spring gentian (Gentiana Verna).

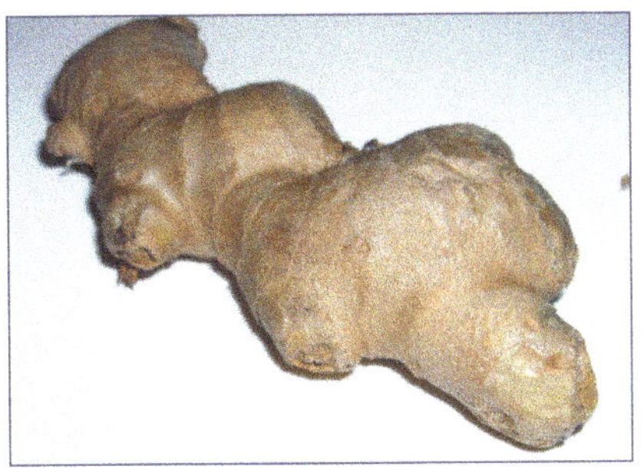

(photo: Miran Rijavec)

GINGER

Family: Zingiberaceae
Genus: Zingiber
Species: Zingiber Officinale

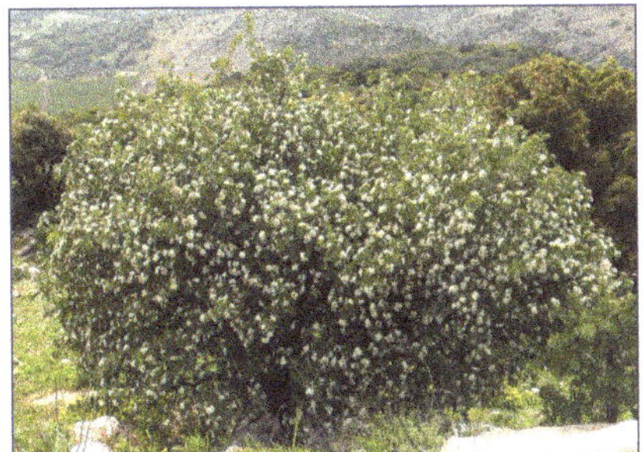

(photo: Pavel Buršík)

HAWTHORN

Family: Rosaceae
Genus: Crataegus

The genus Crataegus contains approximately 200 species amongst which the Azarole (Crataegus Azarolus).

Also known as: Thornapple, may-tree, white thorn, hawberry.

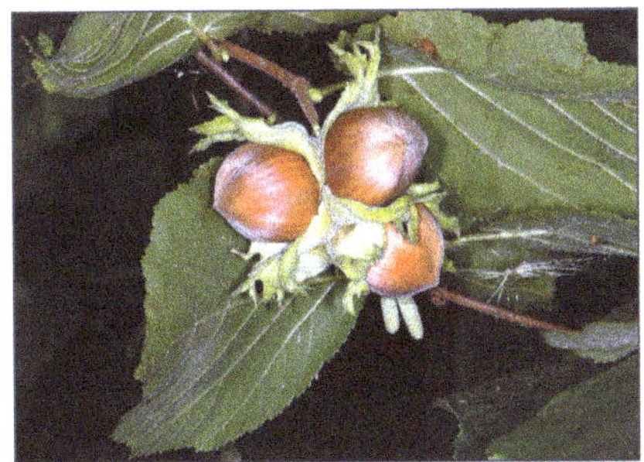

(photo: Vladimír Motyka)

HAZEL

Family: Betulaceae

Genus: Corylus

The genus Corylus contains 18 species amongst which the common hazel (Corylus Avellana).

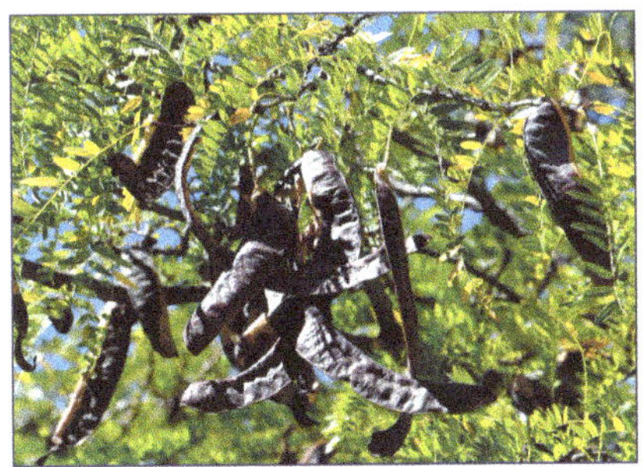

(photo: Tomáš Machácek)

HONEY LOCUST

Family: Fabaceae
Genus: Gleditsia
Species: Gleditsia Triacanthos

Also known as: False locust, thorny locust.

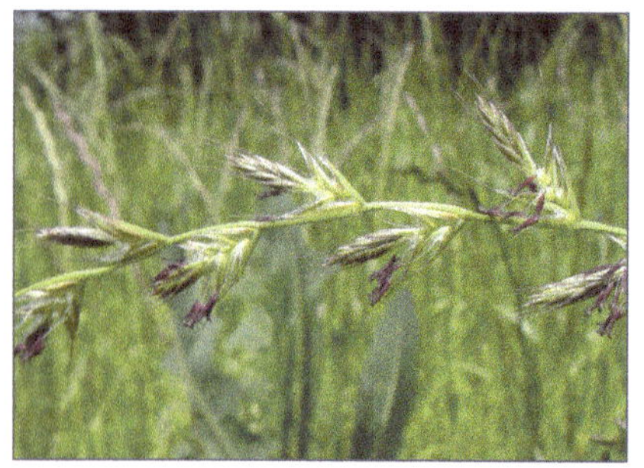
(photo: Jirí Kamenícek)

ITALIAN RYE GRASS

Family: Poaceae
Genus: Lolium
Species: Lolium Multiflorum

Also known as: Annual rye grass.

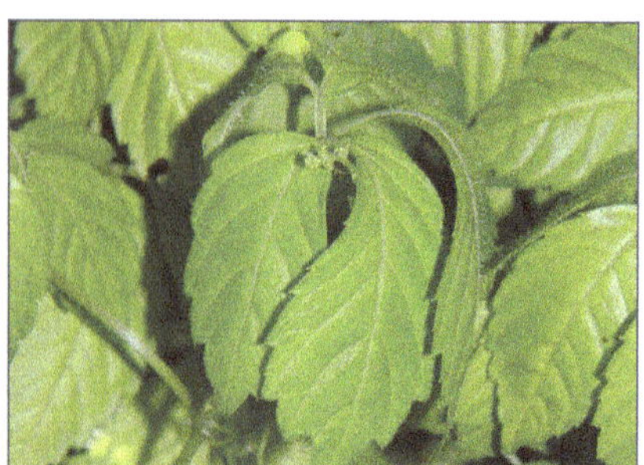
(photo: Petr Voboril)

JIAOGULAN

Family: Cucurbitaceae
Genus: Gynostemma
Species: Gynostemma Pentaphyllum

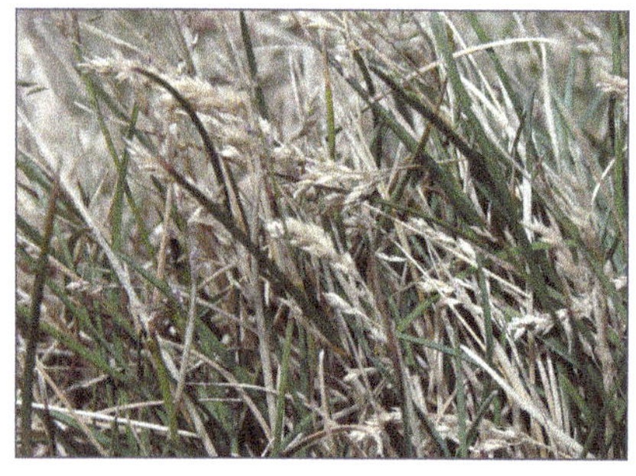
(photo: Kim Starr)

KENTUCKY BLUE GRASS

Family: Poaceae
Genus: Poa
Species: Poa Pratensis

Also known as: Smooth meadow grass, common meadow grass.

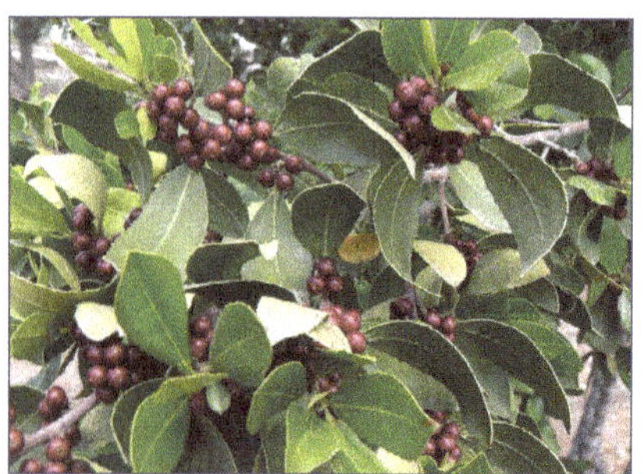
Bay laurel
(photo: Pavel Buršík)

LAUREL

Family: Lauraceae
The family Lauraceae contains more than 50 genera and more than 3000 plants amongst which the bay laurel (Laurus Nobilis).

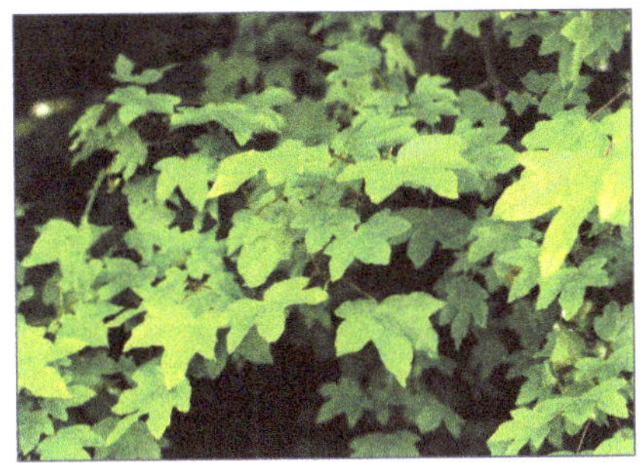

(photo: Tomas Figura)

MAPLE

Family: Aceraceae or Sapindaceae
Genus: Acer

The genus Acer contains 128 species amongst which the field maple (Acer Campestre).

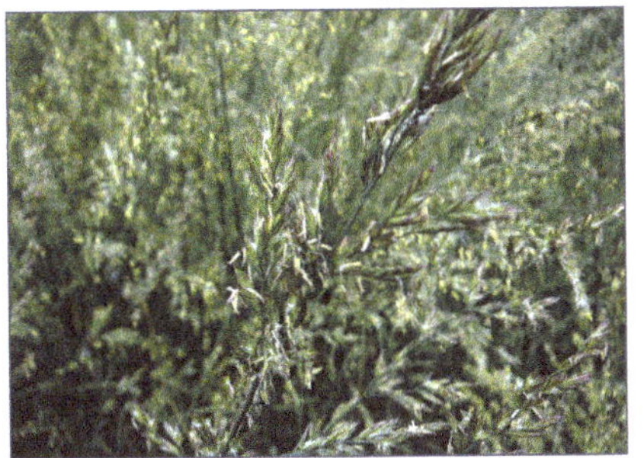

(photo: Ivan Procházka)

MEADOW FESCUE

Family: Poaceae
Genus: Festuca
Species: Festuca Pratensis

Also known as: English blue grass.

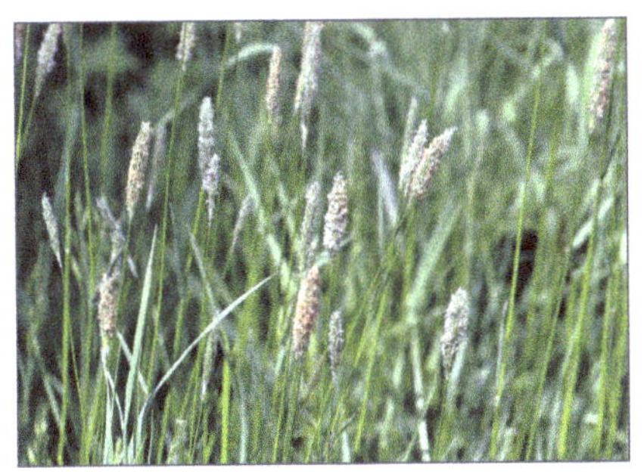

(photo: Lubomír Klátil)

MEADOW FOXTAIL

Family: Poaceae
Genus: Alopecurus
Species: Alopecurus Pratensis

Also known as: Field meadow foxtail.

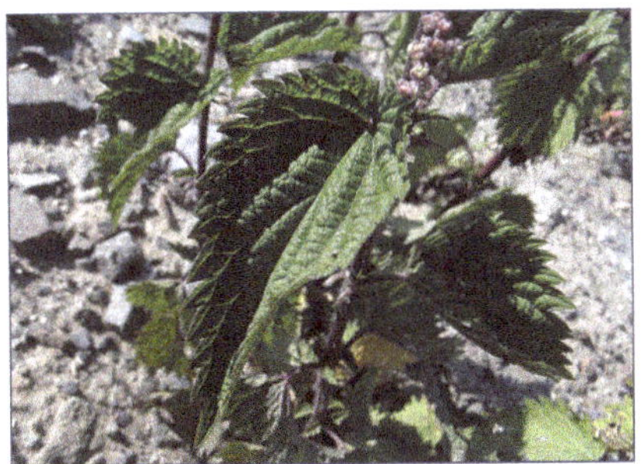

Stinging nettle
(photo: Jirí Kamenícek)

NETTLE

Family: Urticaceae
Genus: Urtica

The genus Urtica contains 45 species amongst which the stinging nettle (Urtica Dioica) and burning nettle (Urtica Urens).

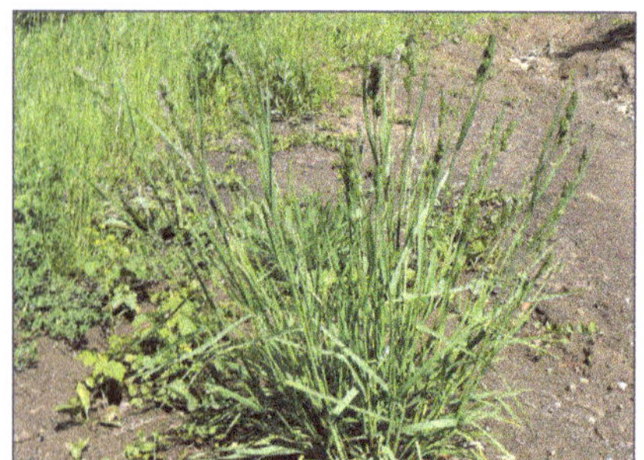

(photo: Vojtech Herman)

ORCHARD GRASS

Family: Poaceae
Genus: Dactylis
Species: Dactylis Glomerata

Also known as: Cock's foot grass.

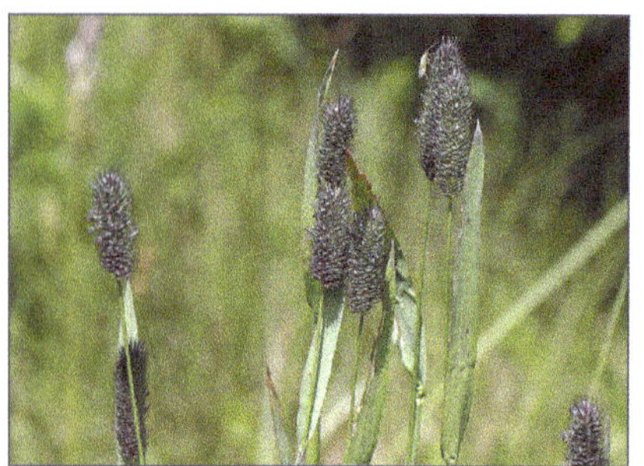

Alpine cat's tail
(photo: Jan Ševcík)

PHLEUM

Family: Poaceae
Genus: Phleum

The genus Phleum contains 18 species amongst which timothy grass (Phleum Pratense) and alpine cat's tail (Phleum Alpinum).

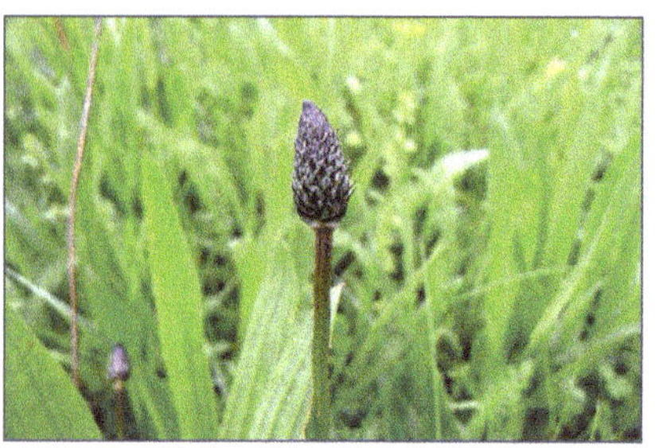

Narrowleaf plantain
(photo: Pavel Šinkyrík)

PLANTAIN

Family: Plantaginaceae
Genus: Plantago

The genus Plantago contains 18 species amongst which narrowleaf plantain (Plantago Lanceolata) and broadleaf plantain (Plantago Major).

Also known as: Fleawort.

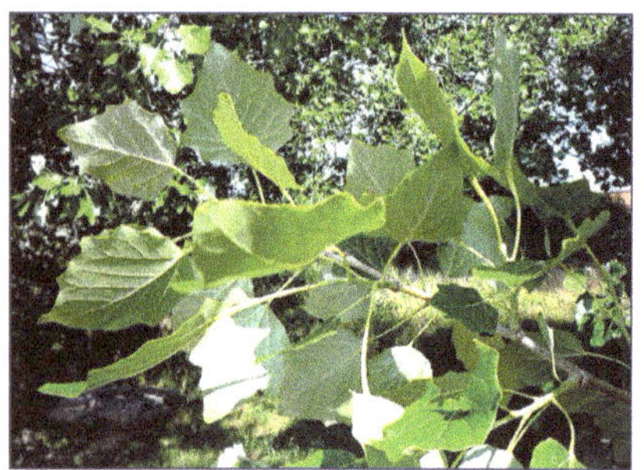

White poplar
(photo: Jirí Kamenícek)

POPLAR

Family: Salicaceae
Genus: Populus

The genus Populus contains 35 species amongst which the white poplar (Populus Alba).

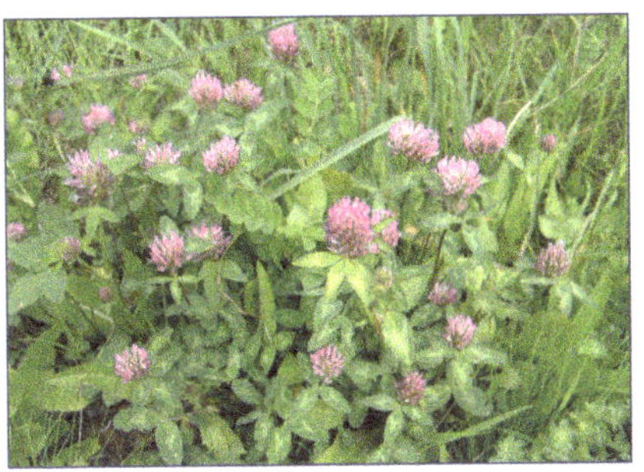
(photo: Lubomír Klátil)

RED CLOVER

Family: Fabaceae
Genus: Trifolium
Species: Trifolium Pratense

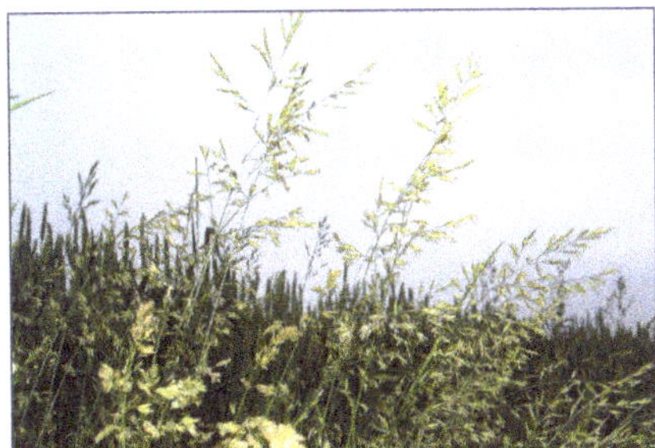
(photo: Václav Hrdina)

RED FESCUE

Family: Poaceae
Genus: Festuca
Species: Festuca Rubra

Also known as: Creeping red fescue.

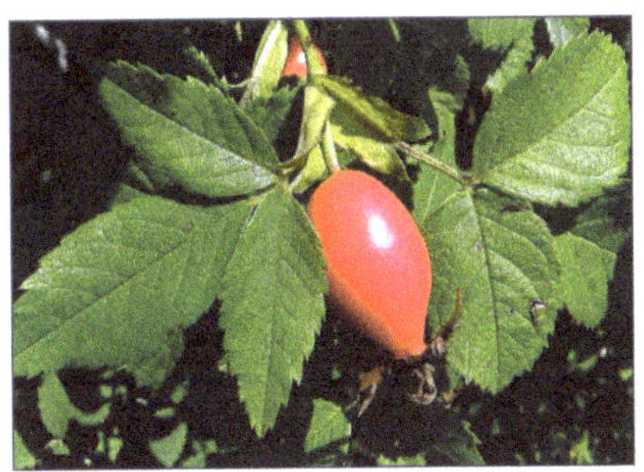
(photo: Peter Kocna)

ROSEHIP

Family: Rosaceae
Genus: Rosa
Species: Rosa Canina

Also known as: Rose haw, dog rose.

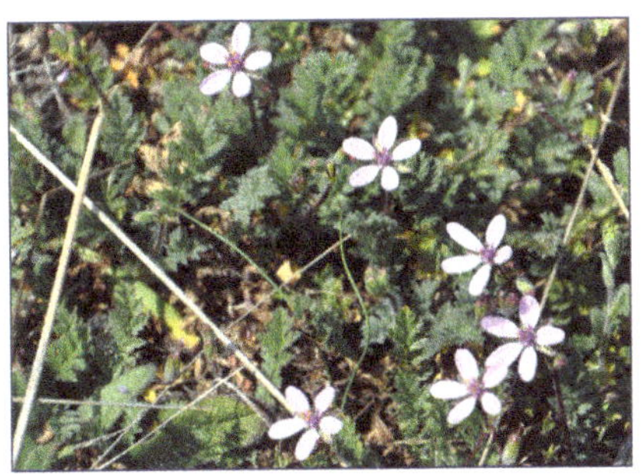
(photo: Lubomír Klátil)

STORK'S BILL

Family: Geraniaceae
Genus: Erodium
Species: Erodium Cicutarium

Also known as: Redstem filaree, pinweed.

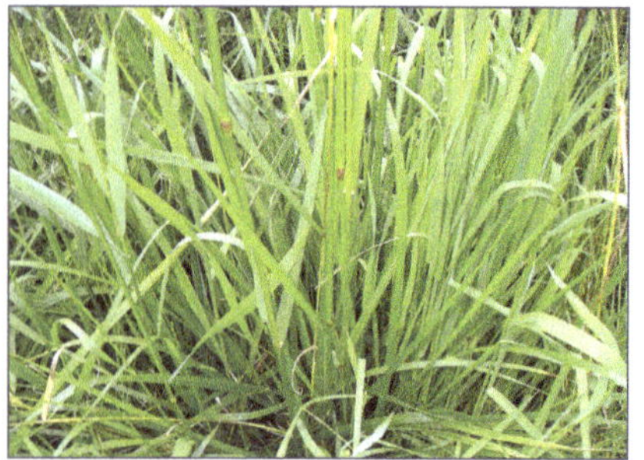
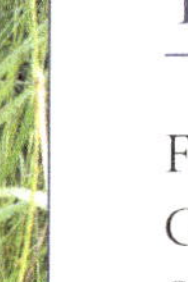

(photo: Václav Hrdina)

TALL FESCUE

Family: Poaceae
Genus: Festuca
Species: Festuca Arundinacea

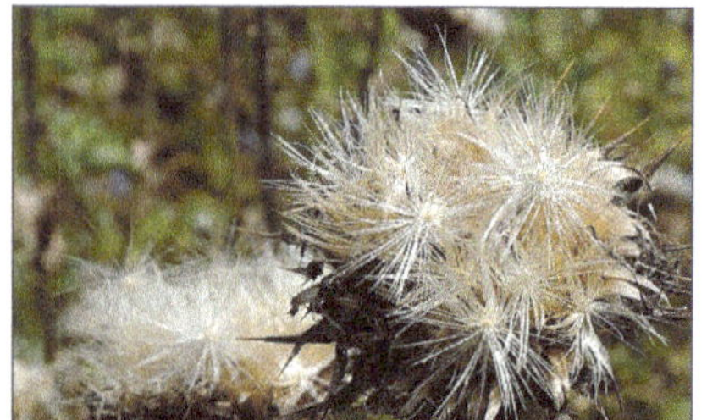

Milk thistle
(photo: Milan Korínek)

THISTLE

Family: Asteraceae
The family Asteraceae contains 14 genera amongst which the milk thistle (Silybum Marianum) and the musk thistle (Carduus Nutans).

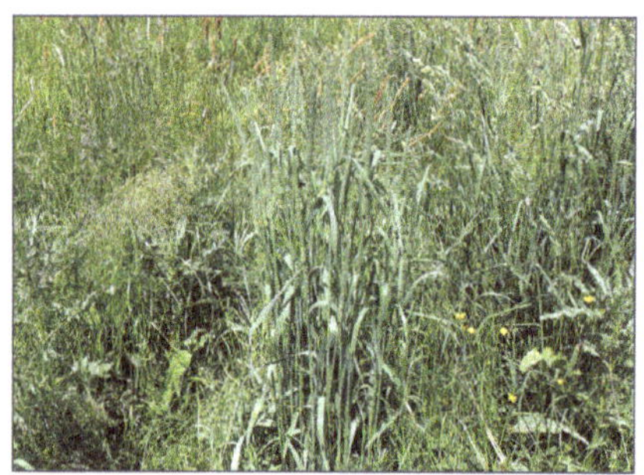

(photo: Vojtech Herman)

TIMOTHY GRASS

Family: Poaceae
Genus: Phleum
Species: Phleum Pratense

Also known as: Meadow cat's tail.

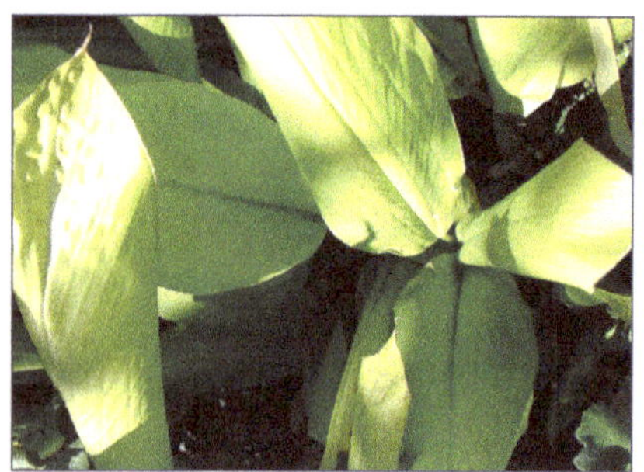

(photo: Kim Starr)

TURMERIC

Family: Zingiberaceae
Genus: Curcuma
Species: Curcuma Longa

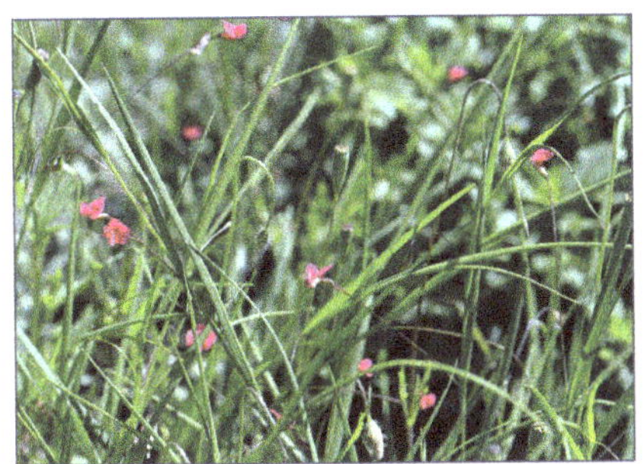
Grass vetchling
(photo: Jan Ševcík)

VETCH

Family: Fabaceae
Genus: Vicia

The genus Vicia contains 140 species amongst which the grass vetchling (Lathyrus Nissolia).

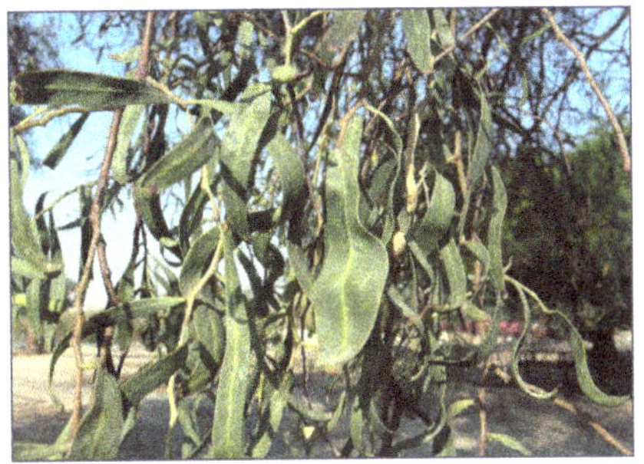
Willow acacia
(photo: Pavel Buršík)

WILLOW

Family: Salicaceae
Genus: Salix

The genus Salix contains 400 species amongst which the almond willow (Salix Triandra) and the willow acacia (Acacia Salicina).

Also known as: Sallow.

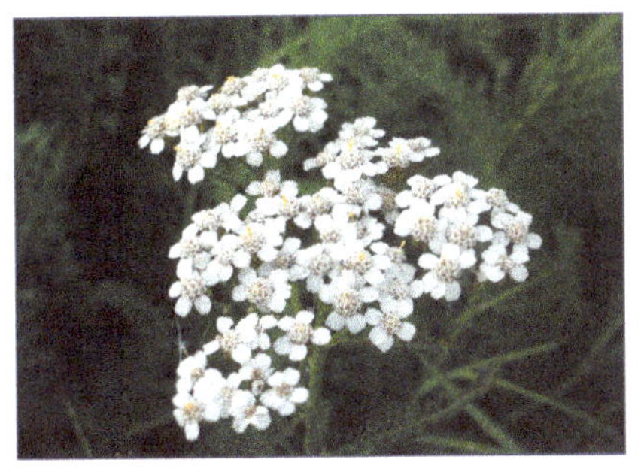
(photo: Tomas Leibelt)

YARROW

Family: Asteraceae
Genus: Achillea
Species: Achillea Millefolium

CHECKLIST

Owner

Name: ______________________________

Address: ____________________ Postal code: __________

City: ____________________

Phone: ____________________ Mobile phone: ____________________

E-mail: ____________________

Veterinarian

Name: ______________________________

Practice: ______________________________

Address: ____________________ Postal code: __________

City: ____________________

Phone: ____________________ Mobile phone: ____________________

E-mail: ____________________

Horse

Name: ____________________

Sex: ☐ mare ☐ gelding ☐ stallion

Age: __________

Breed: ____________________

Laminitis since: __________

First time laminitis, or a new episode of laminitis after the horse was sound without pain relief for at least 14 days: yes/no

Diagnosed by: ☐ veterinarian ☐ hoof care provider ☐ last/other hoof care provider
☐ owner ☐ other: ____________________

State of the hooves:

Stance *(for example laminitic stance, all four feet close together)*:

Movement:

Obel: ☐ 1 ☐ 2 ☐ 3 ☐ 4
Neck size: ___________
Weight: ___________
Method: ☐ weigh bridge ☐ Carrol & Huntington ☐ weight tape
Overweight: yes/no
CNS: ☐ 0 ☐ 1 ☐ 2 ☐ 3 ☐ 4
BCS: ☐ 1 ☐ 2 ☐ 3 ☐ 4 ☐ 5 ☐ 6

Underlying diseases:
☐ PPID
☐ EMS
☐ reduced renal and/or liver function
☐ vitamin- and/or mineral deficiency
☐ Lyme disease/piroplasmosis
☐ hyperlipidemia
☐ other: ______________________________

History of the horse

With owner since: ___________
Has had laminitis before: yes/no
If yes, when: ___________
Cured: yes/no
Hereditary (*for example breed, bloodline*): yes/no
Stress factors:

Diagnosis

Add pictures, veterinary reports and research results if possible.

Cause:

Diagnosed by: ☐ veterinarian ☐ hoof care provider ☐ last/other hoof care provider
☐ owner ☐ other: ____________________

Description physical examination (*knocking on the hoof wall, hoof testers, walking on a circle or lunging*):

Medical imaging:
☐ thermography
☐ radiography
☐ venography
Short description of the outcome:

Blood tests:
☐ insulin
☐ leptin
☐ glucose (tolerance)
☐ ACTH
☐ cortisol
Has PPID and/or EMS/insulin resistance been determined: yes/no

Differential diagnosis:
☐ sole bruise(s)
☐ arthritis
☐ trimming and/or shoeing errors
☐ other: ____________________

COMPLICATIONS

Abscesses: ☐ LF ☐ RF ☐ LH ☐ RH
Specify (*for example RF coronary band medial*):

Hospitalization necessary: yes/no
Receives treatment: yes/no
Short description treatment: ______________________________

Sole perforation: ☐ LF ☐ RF ☐ LH ☐ RH
Hospitalization necessary: yes/no
Receives treatment: yes/no
Short description treatment: ______________________________

Coronary band prolapse: ☐ LF ☐ RF ☐ LH ☐ RH
Hospitalization necessary: yes/no
Receives treatment: yes/no
Short description treatment: ______________________________

White line disease: ☐ LF ☐ RF ☐ LH ☐ RH
Receives treatment: yes/no
Short description treatment: ______________________________

Frog infection: ☐ LF ☐ RF ☐ LH ☐ RH
Receives treatment: yes/no
Short description treatment: ______________________________

Sepsis: yes/no
Hospitalization necessary: yes/no
Receives treatment: yes/no
Short description treatment: ______________________________

Treatment, prevention

Description treatment:

Medication:
☐ antibiotic drugs
☐ analgesic and anti-inflammatory drugs *(NSAIDs: fenylbutazon, flunixine, ketoprofen, suxibuzone, firocoxib, fentanyl)*
☐ nerve blocking drugs
☐ antihypertensive drugs
☐ anticoagulant drugs *(heparin, aspirin)*
☐ vasodilator drugs *(pentoxifylline, acepromazine)*
☐ antidiabetic drugs *(metformin, pioglitazon)*
☐ antihistamine drugs
☐ enzyme inhibiting drugs *(marimastat, batimastat)*
☐ anti-oxidants *(DMSO, DMG, MSM)*
☐ botox
☐ other: ______________________

Preventive remedies:
☐ paraffin or vegetable oils
☐ intestinal cleansing *(activated carbon, Fuller's earth, Hippo-ex-laminitis)*
☐ probiotics
☐ buffer solution *(sodium bicarbonate, Equishure)*
☐ other: ______________________

Supplements:
- minerals and vitamins
  ☐ magnesium, chromium, vanadium
  ☐ manganese
  ☐ selenium
  ☐ vitamin E

- fatty acids
  - ☐ omega-3
  - ☐ arginine
- hoof growth promoters
  - ☐ methionine
  - ☐ sulphur
  - ☐ zinc
  - ☐ biotin

Phytotherapeutic remedies:
☐ IR related *(cinnamon, fenugreek, blond psyllium, turmeric)*
☐ analgesic, anti-inflammatory *(for example No-Bute)*
☐ other: ______________________

Hormones:
☐ thyroid hormones *(for example levothyroxine)*
☐ dopamine-agonists, serotonin-antagonists *(pergolide, permax, periactin, celance, bromocriptine)*

(Complementary) therapies:
☐ cold therapy
☐ acupuncture, acupressure, shiatsu
☐ massage
☐ essential oils: ______________________

Surgery:
☐ tenotomy, desmotomy
☐ hoof wall-/coronary band resection
☐ other: ______________________

Hoof protection:
☐ none (barefoot)
☐ shoes pulled
when: __________
short description transition:

☐ emergency insoles
☐ hoof boots
brand/type: ______________________
since: __________

how often, what effect:

☐ fixation
(since) when: ____________
☐ sole protection applied

Trimming *(short description of trimming method)*:

Soil, grass and forage analysis *(outcome and advice)*:

Nutrition management *(for example only (soaked) hay and salt lick)*:

Changes in living circumstances:
☐ horse has a companion *(for example other horse, goat, sheep)*
☐ grazing restrictions
☐ horse removed from pasture
☐ grazing muzzle
☐ strip grazing, pasture rotation, limited pasture access
☐ other: ____________
☐ paddock paradise
☐ other: ____________

Communication agreements

When, how and by whom progress will be evaluated

(for example every two weeks, by e-mail, veterinarian in CC):

Who is allowed to publish pictures and/or information on social media:

Other remarks

This checklist can be downloaded from www.understandinglaminitis.com/checklist.pdf

GLOSSARY

Words that occur frequently in this book, or that are not further specified in the text, are listed in this glossary including a short definition. The definitions are within the context of the subject of this book. The italicised words in the descriptions refer to explanations elsewhere in the glossary. Also the index on page 255 can be used to find specific subjects.

A

ACTH
: Adrenocorticotropic hormone. A *hormone* secreted by the *pituitary gland*.

ADAMTS-4
: A disintegrin like and metalloproteinase with thrombospondin type 1 motif 4. A cartilage degrading *enzyme*.

ADIPOKINE
: Cell signalling protein secreted by fat tissue that acts on the immune system.

ADIPOSITY
: A type of *obesity* that is characterised by abnormal fat deposits.

AMINO ACIDS
: The building blocks of proteins.

ANTIOXIDANT
: A substance that inhibits the oxidation by *free radicals* of other molecules.

APOPTOSIS
: The process of controlled death of abnormal cells.

ARTERIOVENOUS ANASTOMOSIS
: see: Shunt

B

BASEMENT MEMBRANE
: Connective tissue that attaches the (secondary) dermal lamellae to the (secondary) epidermal lamellae.

BCS
: Body condition score. A numerical scale used to evaluate the amount of fat on a horse's body.

BLOOD SERUM
: Bright yellow liquid component of blood that remains after coagulation factors have been removed.

BODY CONDITION SCORE
see: BCS

BONE DEMINERALISATION
A process that reduces the mineral content in bones.

C

CATABOLISM
A type of metabolism that breaks down endogenous tissue.

CATECHOLAMINES
Hormones produced by the adrenal glands: *epinephrine*, *norepinephrine* and *dopamine*.

CELLULOSE
Raw fibre. Cellulose, *hemicellulose* and *lignin* form the group of *structural carbohydrates*.

CNS
Cresty Neck Score. A numerical scale used to evaluate the amount of fat on a horse's neck and therefore its obesity.

COLLAGEN
A major component of connective tissue, cartilage and bones.

CORTICOSTEROID
Chemical variation of the endogenous adrenal *hormone cortisol*.

CORTISOL
Adrenal *hormone* that (under stress) is secreted to quickly convert proteins and fats into *glucose*.

CORONARY BAND RESECTION
The removal of part of the hoof wall just below the coronary band by grinding, rasping or cutting.

CRESTY NECK SCORE
see: CNS

CYTOKINE
A protein involved in the immune system, able to enhance the activity of *MMPs*.

CUSHING'S DISEASE, CUSHING'S SYNDROME
see: PPID

D

DESMOTOMY
The surgical cutting of the check ligament in an attempt to remove the forces that cause rotation of the coffin bone.

DEXAMETHASONE SUPPRESSION TEST
see: DST

DOPAMINE
A *hormone* related to *epinephrine* which has a vasoconstrictive effect.

DOPAMINE-AGONIST
A drug that activates dopamine receptors and therefore stimulates the body's response to *dopamine*.

DOPAMINE-ANTAGONIST
A drug that inhibits dopamine receptors and therefore decreases the body's response to *dopamine*.

DST
Dexamethasone suppression test. This test is used to diagnose *PPID*.

E

EMS
Equine metabolic syndrome. A hormonal problem similar to type 2 diabetes in humans.

Endorphin
An endogenous morphine produced by the body as a natural painkiller.

Endothelin-1
see: ET-1

Endothelium
The thin layer of cells that lines the interior surface of blood vessels and lymphatic vessels.

Endotoxin
Toxic component found in the outer membrane of *gram-negative bacteria*, that is released after the death of these bacteria.

Endotoxin microthrombosis
Small blood clot as a result of *endotoxins*.

Enteroviruses
A group of very small viruses that live in the gastrointestinal tract and faeces.

Enzyme
A type of protein that causes, enables or accelerates a chemical reaction.

Enzyme inhibitor
A compound that binds to an *enzyme* and decreases its activity.

Epinephrine
A *hormone* that is among others responsible for the conversion of *glycogen* into *glucose*. It is released in response to excitement, stress, pain, heat, cold and physical exertion. It causes vasoconstriction.

Equine metabolic syndrome
see: EMS

ESC
see: Ethanol soluble carbohydrates

ET-1
Endothelin-1. *Hormone* produced by the *endothelium* which has a vasoconstrictive effect.

Ethanol soluble carbohydrates
Monosaccharides (among others *glucose* and *fructose*) and disaccharides (among others *sucrose*) together form the group of ethanol soluble carbohydrates.

Exotoxin
A toxin secreted by *gram-positve bacteria*.

F

Fibrocartilage
Very elastic type of cartilage that is able to withstand heavy pressure. The digital cushion partly consists of fibrocartilage.

FIBROSIS
The thickening and scarring of connective tissue, usually as a result of injury.

FOUNDER
The failure of the lamellar connection (rotation and sinking) as a result of laminitis. Synonym for the chronic phase.

FREE RADICAL
Harmful molecular by-product of normal metabolism, inflammation, medication, residual pesticides in foods, strenuous exercise, stress, *obesity* and *adiposity*.

FRUCTANS
A group of certain types of *water soluble non-structural carbohydrates.* This group contains, amongst others, inulin and oligofructose.

FRUCTOSE
Fruit sugar, a simple monosaccharide. Belongs to the group of *ethanol soluble non-structural carbohydrates.*

G

GLUCAGON
A *hormone* produced by the *pancreas* that determines the *glucose* production of the liver.

GLUCOCORTICOIDS
Hormones produced by the adrenal glands that are involved in *glucose* metabolism, suppression of allergic and inflammatory responses. *Cortisol* is the most important glucocorticoid. The production of glucocorticoids is influenced by *ACTH.*

GLUCOSE
A monosaccharide also known as dextrose or grape sugar. Belongs to the group of *ethanol soluble non-structural carbohydrates.*

GLUCOSE TOLERANCE TEST
A medical test to determine how quickly *glucose* is cleared from the blood to determine if hormonal problems occur during this process.

GLUT-1
Glucose transporter 1. An *enzyme* that facilitates the transport of *glucose* to cells with a large demand for glucose, independent of *insulin.*

GLYCOGEN
Glucose that has been transformed by the cells of the liver and the muscles.

GRAM-NEGATIVE BACTERIUM
Bacterium that has an extra outer membrane around the cell wall. When this bacterium dies, *endotoxins* are released.

GRAM-POSITIVE BACTERIUM
Bacterium that possess a thick cell wall that differs in composition from the endogenous cells in the horse's body. This bacterium releases *exotoxins.*

H

HEMICELLULOSE
Raw fibre. Hemicellulose, *cellulose* and *lignin* form the group of *structural carbohydrates.*

HEMIDESMOSOME
A protein structure in the cell membrane that enables horn cells to attach to the *basement membrane.*

HIRSUTISM
see: Hypertrichosis

HISTAMINE
Histamine is involved in the inflammatory response and has a strong vasodilatory effect. It stimulates the production of *ACTH.*

HOOF MECHANISM
The alternate widening and narrowing of the hoof which contributes to blood circulation and shock absorption.

HOOF SLOUGHING
Loss of the hoof capsule caused by the failure of the entire connection between dermis and epidermis of the hoof.

HOOF WALL RESECTION
The complete or partial removal of the hoof wall. In case of laminitis only the toe area of the wall is resectioned.

HORMONE
Substance produced by endocrine glands that selectively alters functional activity of certain organs and tissues.

HYPERGLYCEMIA
A condition in which an excessive amount of glucose circulates in the blood.

HYPERINSULINEMIA
Chronically raised *insulin* levels in the blood as a result of overproduction of this *hormone.*

HYPERLIPIDEMIA
The presence of elevated fat concentrations in the blood, associated with periods of negative energy balance and physiologic stress.

HYPERTRICHOSIS
A long, thick, wavy coat as a result of *PPID.*

HYPOPHYSIS
see: Pituitary gland

I

IGF-1
Insulin-like growth factor 1 is a *hormone* similar in molecular structure to *insulin,* that is among others, responsible for growth of cells and tissues.

INFECTION
Disease caused by a germ such as a bacteria, fungus, virus or parasite.

INFILTRATION
Phase of an inflammation process when white blood cells move from within the blood out to infiltrate into the diseased or inflamed tissues.

INFLAMMATION
A response of the body to tissue damage.

INSULIN
A *hormone* produced by the *pancreas*, responsible for the metabolism of *glucose*.

INSULIN-LIKE GROWTH FACTOR 1
see: IGF-1

INSULIN RESISTANCE
A physiological condition in which cells fail to respond to the normal actions of the *hormone insulin*. *Glucose* in the blood is no longer absorbed efficiently, leading to high blood sugar levels.

K

KERATIN
A fibrous protein that is the key structural material of horn cells.

L

LACTIC ACID BACILLUS
Gram-positive bacterium that can cause fermentation in the horse's hind gut.

LAMELLAR WEDGE
A mass of proliferating horn cells, old blood, dead hoof tissue, and wound fluid which is wedged in the space between the separated hoof wall and coffin bone.

LAMELLAR CONNECTION
The connection between dermal and epidermal lamellae, including the intermediate basement membrane. It ensures the connection between the hoof wall and the coffin bone/hoof cartilage.

LAMINITIC RING
Deep growth ring in the hoof wall as a result of laminitis.

LEPTIN
A *hormone* made by adipose cells that helps to regulate energy balance by inhibiting appetite.

LIGNIN
Raw fibre. Lignin, *cellulose* and *hemicellulose* form the group of *structural carbohydrates*.

M

MATRIX METALLOPROTE(ÏN)ASE
see: MMP

MELANOCORTINS
A group of *hormones* which are produced by the *pituitary gland*, including *ACTH*.

METABOLISM
The complex of physical and chemical processes that take place in living cells for the maintenance, breakdown and construction of tissue and the production of energy.

MICROTHROMBOSIS
Small blood clot.

MMP
Matrix metalloprote(ïn)ase. A *(pro-)enzyme* responsible for breaking down proteins.

MMP-TRIGGER
An *enzyme* that can cause the overproduction of *MMPs*.

MYCOTOXINS
Toxic by-products of moulds, fungi and yeasts.

N

NEUROTRANSMITTER
Endogenous chemical that transmits nerve impulses.

NON-STEROIDAL ANTI-INFLAMMATORY DRUGS
see: NSAIDs

NON-STRUCTURAL CARBOHYDRATES
Non-structural carbohydrates. *Starch*, *fructans* (among others inulin and oligofructose) and sugars (among others *glucose*, *fructose* and *sucrose*) together form the group of non-structural carbohydrates.

NOREPINEPHRINE
A *hormone* related to *epinephrine* that is released in times of stress, pain, heat, cold and physical strain. It causes vasoconstriction.

NSC
see: Non-structural carbohydrates

NSAIDs
Non-steroidal anti-inflammatory drugs. Certain group of drugs that have an analgesic (pain-killing) and anti-inflammatory effect.

O

OBEL GRADING SYSTEM
Evaluation method to classify the progression of laminitis in horses.

OBESITY
Excess body fat that is more or less evenly distributed throughout the entire body.

OEDEMA
A condition characterized by an excess of watery fluid collecting in the cavities or tissues of the body.

OESTROGEN
Primary female sex *hormone*.

OMEGA FATTY ACIDS
Certain types of polyunsaturated fatty acids. Fatty acids are the smallest compounds of fat.

OSTEITIS
Inflammation of bone.

OSTEOLYSIS
Decalcification or dissolution of bone tissue caused by calcium deficiency.

OSTEOMYELITIS
Inflammation of bone or bone marrow, usually due to infection.

Osteopenia
A medical condition in which the protein and mineral content of bone tissue is reduced, but less severely than in *osteoporosis*.

Osteoporosis
A medical condition in which the bones gradually lose their density and strength.

Oxidative stress
Cell damage caused by excess reactive oxygen compounds.

P

Pancreas
A glandular organ, located in the first section of the small intestine (duodenum) that secretes enzymes such as *insulin*, to stimulate the breakdown of easily digestible components like *starch*, fat and protein.

Phytoestrogen
Plant-derived substances that have the ability to cause oestrogenic effects because of their structural similarity with *oestrogen*.

Phytotherapy
The use of plants as medicines or health-promoting agents.

Pituitary gland
An endocrine gland, located at the base of the brain responsible for the excretion of among others *ACTH*.

Pituitary pars intermedia dysfunction
see: PPID

PPID
Pituitary pars intermedia dysfunction. A disease caused by elevated levels of *melanocortins* in the blood.

Pro-enzyme
An inactive *enzyme* precursor.

R

Reperfusion injury
Tissue damage caused when blood supply returns to the tissue after a period of lack of oxygen and nutrients. The restoration of circulation results in inflammation through the induction of *oxidative stress*.

S

Saccharose
see: Sucrose

Serotonin
A neurotransmitter (a compound that carries signals along and between nerves) that is involved in pain suppression and vasoconstriction.

SEROTONIN-ANTAGONIST
A drug that inhibits the action of *serotonin* receptors and therefore decreases the body's response to this neurotransmitter.

SHUNT
A direct connection between a vein and an artery.

SIRS
Systemic inflammatory response syndrome. An inflammatory state affecting the whole body.

STARCH
Insoluble, *non-structural carbohydrate*.

STREPTOCOCCUS LUTETIENSIS
A certain type of *gram-positive bacterium* that lives in the gastrointestinal tract.

STRUCTURAL CARBOHYDRATES
Cellulose, *hemicellulose* and *lignin* are the three types of structural carbohydrates (raw fibre).

SUCROSE
A disaccharide often extracted from either cane or beet sugar. Belongs to the group of *ethanol soluble non-structural carbohydrates*.

SUPEROXIDE DISMUTASE
An *enzyme* that is capable of breaking down the *free radical* superoxide. It is one of the most important antioxidants in the body.

T

TENOTOMY
The surgical transection of the deep digital flexor tendon in an attempt to remove the forces that cause rotation of the coffin bone.

TIMP
Tissue inhibitor of metalloprotease. A protein that regulates the production and activity of *MMPs*.

V

VASCULAR INSULIN RESISTANCE
Insulin resistance as a result of defects in the vasodilatory response to *insulin*.

W

WATER SOLUBLE CARBOHYDRATES
Fructans (among others inulin en oligofructose) and sugars (among others *glucose*, *fructose* and *sucrose*) together form the group of water soluble carbohydrates.

WSC
see: Water soluble carbohydrates

INDEX

A

B

C

D

E

F

G

H

I

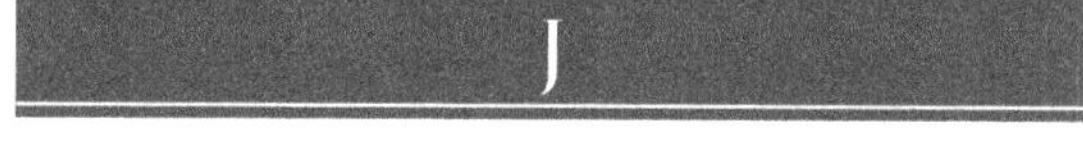

J

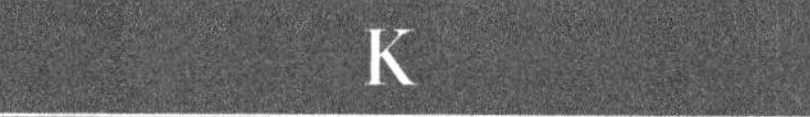

K

L

M

N

O

P

R

S

T

U

V

W

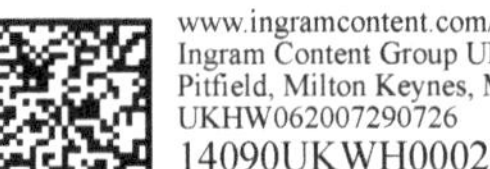

www.ingramcontent.com/pod-product-compliance
Ingram Content Group UK Ltd.
Pitfield, Milton Keynes, MK11 3LW, UK
UKHW062007290726
14090UKWH00022B/1429

9 789493 034099